Transplantation Dermatology

Current Problems in Dermatology

Vol. 43

Series Editors

Peter Itin Basel

Gregor Jemec Roskilde

Transplantation Dermatology

Volume Editors

Peter Häusermann Basel
Jürg Steiger Basel
Jakob Passweg Basel

41 figures, 39 in color, and 16 tables, 2012

KARGER

Basel · Freiburg · Paris · London · New York · New Delhi · Bangkok · Beijing · Tokyo · Kuala Lumpur · Singapore · Sydney

Current Problems in Dermatology

Dr. Peter Häusermann
Leitender Arzt Dermatologie
Universitätsspital Basel
Petersgraben 4
CH-4031 Basel
Switzerland

Prof. Jürg Steiger
Chefarzt Klinik für Transplantationsimmunologie und Nephrologie
Universitätsspital Basel
Petersgraben 4
CH-4031 Basel
Switzerland

Prof. Jakob Passweg
Chefarzt Hämatologie
Universitätsspital Basel
Petersgraben 4
CH-4031 Basel
Switzerland

Library of Congress Cataloging-in-Publication Data

Transplantation dermatology / volume editors, Peter Häusermann, Jürg Steiger, Jakob Passweg.
p. ; cm. -- (Current problems in dermatology, ISSN 1421-5721 ; v.43)
Includes bibliographical references and index.
ISBN 978-3-8055-9855-2 (hard cover : alk. paper) -- ISBN 978-3-8055-9856-9 (e-ISBN)
I. Häusermann, Peter. II. Steiger, Jürg. III. Passweg, Jakob. IV. Series: Current problems in dermatology ; v. 43. 1421-5721
[DNLM: 1. Skin Diseases--etiology. 2. Hematopoietic Stem Cell Transplantation--adverse effects. 3. Immunocompromised Host. 4. Immunosuppressive Agents--adverse effects. 5. Organ Transplantation--adverse effects. 6. Skin Diseases--pathology. 7. Sunscreening Agents--therapeutic use. W1 CU804L v.43 2012 / WR 140]
617.4'7701--dc23

2011053286

Bibliographic Indices. This publication is listed in bibliographic services, including MEDLINE/Pubmed.

www.karger.com
Printed in Germany on acid-free and non-aging paper (ISO 9706) by Kraft Druck GmbH, Ettlingen
ISSN 1421–5721
e-ISSN 1662–2944
ISBN 978–3–8055–9855–2
e-ISBN 978–3–8055–9856–9

Contents

Preface

Transplantation Dermatology provides dermatologists and physicians of other specialities with a comprehensive overview of the most important skin-related issues in the field of solid organ and hematopoietic stem cell transplantation.

The first section summarizes all the important knowledge on solid organ transplantation and skin. The chapters first cover the main principles and concepts of solid organ recipients and end with the most important health-related expectations and future trends of treatment. In between, the related epidemiological, clinical and histological skin problems are discussed. Pre- and posttransplant management and follow-up programs focus on international as well as European and Swiss guidelines. Finally, important knowledge is summarized related to standard, new and upcoming immunosuppressive drugs.

The second section provides the dermatologist with all the relevant information on what is to be expected in recipients of hematopoietic stem cell transplantation. Hallmark historical aspects are summarized and most important information is given in the setting of early, late and very late periods after transplantation. Skin manifestations of graft-versus-host disease and their respective therapeutic options are explained, and the new consensus classification and treatment aspects of chronic graft-versus-host disease are highlighted.

In the final section, the authors give a comprehensive and easy to read review and practical guidance on all the relevant aspects of photoprotection.

We sincerely hope that this book will be of help and interest to all physicians involved in the diagnosis, management and overall care of patients after solid organ and hematopoietic stem cell transplantation. The importance of updated information in that field is underlined by the fact that the number of solid organ and hematopoietic stem cell transplantations is rising worldwide.

The editors would like to thank all the participating authors for their time and effort put into finalizing this project. Many thanks also go to Karger Publishers for their support and to the sponsors of this book.

Finally, I would like to dedicate this book to my dearest Katharina, Maxine, Renée and Niggi.

Peter Häusermann, Basel

Häusermann P, Steiger J, Passweg J (eds): Transplantation Dermatology.
Curr Probl Dermatol. Basel, Karger, 2012, vol 43, pp 1–8

Organ Transplantation and Skin – Principles and Concepts

Günther F.L. Hofbauer · Sandra N. Freiberger · Guergana Iotzova-Weiss · Bahar Shafaeddin · Piotr J. Dziunycz

Dermatologische Klinik, Universitätsspital Zürich, Zürich, Switzerland

Abstract

Solid organ transplantation influences the biology of the skin profoundly. In the wake of transplantation, inflammatory, infectious and neoplastic disorders arise, often with atypical clinical presentation. Inflammatory disorders mainly relate to pathogen-driven conditions such as seborrheic dermatitis and pityrosporum folliculitis and to drug reactions. Infectious disorders are dominated by viral infections of human papilloma virus and by infections and reactivations of herpes family members. Neoplastic disorders are greatly increased with squamous cell carcinoma of the skin as most relevant clinical problem which is increased 65- to 100-fold following transplantation. This dramatic increase in cutaneous carcinogenesis results from the isolated effect of ultraviolet light on the skin with immunosuppression and DNA damage and of immunosuppressants which drive skin cancer formation by properties unrelated to immunosuppression and from the combined effect of UV light and immunosuppressive drugs on immunomodulation which results in impaired antitumor response as well as chronic tumorigenic inflammation.

The primary function of our immune system is the distinction between self and non-self. The realm of self contains the functioning cells of the organism which are to be protected. The immune system thus learns tolerance by central and peripheral mechanisms to protect normal cells from attack. Any deviation towards self-antigen reactivity results in autoimmunity. The realm of non-self is the outside world with infectious agents such as bacteria, virus, fungi, and parasites as well as abnormal cells such as cancer cells. Here, the immune system needs to act quickly and efficiently against foreign, non-self antigen to protect the body from harm. Any deviation from foreign antigen recognition results in anergy or tolerance with potentially fatal outcome (cf. fig. 1a).

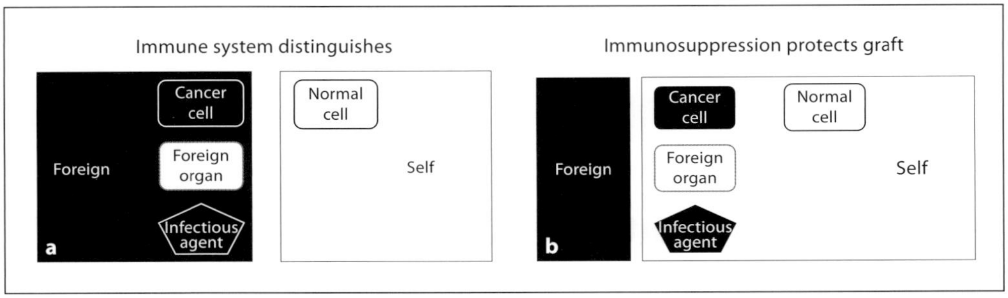

Fig. 1. **a** The main function of the immune system is the distinction between self-antigen and non-self, foreign antigen. While this protects the organism from infection and cancer, it triggers graft rejection of a foreign transplanted organ, an allograft. **b** Immunosuppressive drugs have proved very efficient at suppressing this graft rejection by expanding the realm of the tolerated antigens. These drugs, however, affect the immune system's capacity against other targets. The price for achieving graft preservation is an increase in infection and cancer.

While organ transplantation has provided many recipients of solid organs such as a heart, a liver or a lung with a new life or with a greatly improved quality of life such as in kidney or pancreas transplantation, the basic problem of introducing foreign antigen into another organism remains. The recipient's immune system will mount a multi-pronged immune response resulting in rejection of the transplanted organ. The breakthrough of solid organ transplantation relies in large part on the development of immunosuppressive drugs which suppress this rejection response by the immune system and thus achieve graft tolerance. The realm of tolerated antigen is thus expanded [1]. This expansion, however, comes at a price: The use of immunosuppressive drugs entails an increase in infection and cancer (fig. 1b) [2].

Inflammation, Infection and Cancer

Next to the increase in infection and cancer, recipients of solid organs suffer from a number of inflammatory skin conditions that occur more frequently than in the general population. We will briefly refer to inflammation and infection first, as these are discussed in more detail later in this volume. Thereon, we will discuss skin cancer in more detail.

Inflammatory Skin Disorders

The colonization of the skin with usually innocuous fungi increases with medical immunosuppression. As a consequence, skin conditions such as seborrheic dermatitis and pityrosporum folliculitis that are driven by skin colonization with *Pityrosporum ovale* occur more frequently, are often widespread and tend to be harder to treat than in the general population [3]. Other inflammatory disorders may occur such as steroid-induced acne or more atypical inflammatory disorders [4].

Inflammatory reactions also comprise drug reactions. Solid organ transplantation typically needs a conditioning treatment as well as immunosuppression based on two or three immunosuppressants following transplantation. Many centers use antimicrobial drugs to prevent opportunistic infections. In addition, further drugs are frequently needed to counteract hypertension, diabetes, renal failure, all common findings in organ transplant recipients (OTR). In spite of their impaired immune system, drug reactions develop in many OTR [5, 6] and may render decision-making difficult in the management of such patients. Bircher and Scherer Hofmeier [this vol., pp. 150–164] address drug reactions in the setting of hemopoietic stem cell transplantation.

Infections

Viral infections in particular occur more frequently and persist more than in the immunocompetent patients. Prime examples are human papilloma viruses (HPV) whose prevalence is greatly increased in OTR [7] and to whom the chapter by Arnold and Hofbauer [this vol., pp. 49–56] is dedicated in particular with a view on HPV and their contribution to skin cancer. Next to HPV, other virus types reappear: molluscum contagiosum is frequently seen in children, but as the immune system evolves, typically ends as a self-limited disease. While the immunocompetent patients show molluscum contagiosum as a limited sexually transmitted infection at times, immunosuppression changes this natural course greatly. AIDS patients show a clear inverse correlation between number of molluscum contagiosum lesions and their CD4+ counts in peripheral blood [8, 9]. Similarly, molluscum contagiosum can occur in OTR, where atypical presentations are commonly seen (fig. 2) [10].

Cutaneous Carcinogenesis

One of the major consequences of solid organ transplantation for the skin is increased skin cancer formation. This cutaneous carcinogenesis reaches impressive numbers with a 65- to 100-fold increase for squamous cell carcinoma (SCC) as compared to the general population [2]. The two main driving forces behind this increase are photodamage by ultraviolet light and the use of immunosuppressants. The effects of either photodamage or immunosuppressant or both combine into different mechanisms that all contribute to the greatly increased incidence of SCC of the skin (cf. fig. 3).

Photodamage is a well-known risk factor for non-melanoma skin cancer in general and SCC in particular [11, 12]. Mainly, it is the cumulative sun damage at low daily

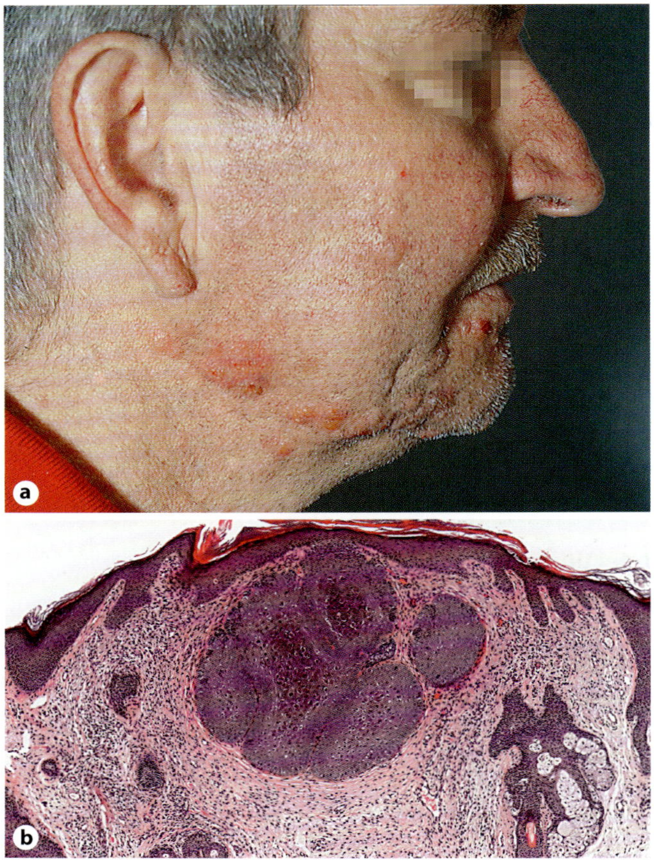

Fig. 2. Folliculitis barbae in a lung transplant recipient (**a**) with an uncommon clinical presentation of molluscum contagiosum, clearly identified on histology (**b**).

exposure over long periods of time that induces so-called field cancerization [13], i.e. a widespread induction of atypical cells harboring mutations in p53 and other genes typical for in situ and invasive SCC [14, 15]. Such photodamage is favored in the OTR population by the long-term intake of photosensitizing drugs. These photosensitizers may be part of immunosuppressive regimens like azathioprine [16, 17] or of further medication regimes commonly used in the OTR population before and after transplantation, in particular antibiotics such as ciprofloxacin [5], antifungals such as voriconazole [18] and thiazide diuretics [19]. The issue of photoprotection is therefore of high importance and impact in the primary and secondary prevention of SCC [20, 21] and is addressed in depth in the chapter by Surber et al. [this vol., pp. 171–196].

Immunomodulation is the joint result of ultraviolet light and immunosuppressive drugs acting on the skin [2]. Ultraviolet light on its own is known to induce cutaneous and systemic immunosuppression, thus also impairing the cutaneous immune reaction against evolving skin cancer cells [22]. In conjunction with immunosuppressive medication, the local inflammatory infiltrate in SCC is reduced in quantity in OTR

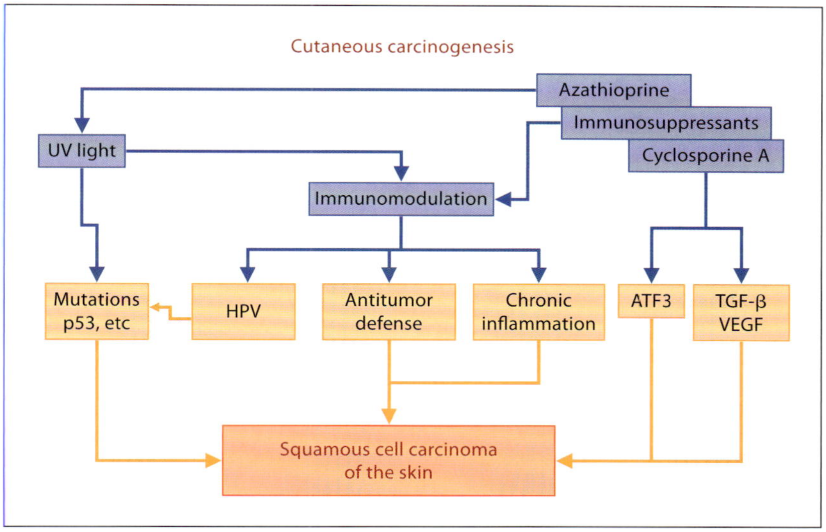

Fig. 3. Cutaneous carcinogenesis in OTR is a multifactorial process. Ultraviolet light and immunosuppressive drugs represent the two main drivers of cancer formation. UV light induces DNA mutations as a first step towards cancer. Immunosuppressants have properties separate from immunosuppression such as photosensitization by azathioprine and increase in transcription factor ATF3 and cytokines TGF-β and VEGF by cyclosporine A. Both ultraviolet light and immunosuppressive drugs combine to allow an increased colonization of the skin by HPV, qualitative and quantitative changes of the immune reaction against SCC including chronic inflammation. All these pathways contribute in parallel to the greatly increased cutaneous carcinogenesis in OTR.

[23] and changes its qualitative composition resulting in a reduction of the immune response against tumor cells [24–26].

Still, while OTR are on a regime of immunosuppressive drugs effectively suppressing rejection of the grafted organ, inflammation is not abolished altogether. Thus, even though inflammation is impaired in and around SCC of OTR, some amount of inflammation can still be observed [23]. It is thus not without interest that low-level smoldering inflammation has been related to carcinogenesis in several organs [27]. Such chronic inflammation as a driver of cancer formation has also been suggested for the epidermal compartment, e.g. for the feed-forward loop of S100A8 and S100A9 proteins stimulating SCC development via the RAGE receptor [28]. Ongoing work in human keratinocytes derived from normal skin and SCC in OTR suggests that such chronic inflammation as in the feed-forward loop of S100A8A9-RAGE may be of relevance in the formation of SCC in OTR [29].

Lastly, immunosuppressants have pharmacological properties of their own independent of their immunosuppressive action [30]. From clinical use, a single drug class cannot be easily identified as a sole culprit for increased SCC formation. Rather, the total amount of immunosuppression seems to rule the induction of SCC formation [14]. Research over the past decades has allowed the delineation of several mechanisms by which immunosuppressants contribute to cutaneous carcinogenesis.

Calcineurin inhibition is the cornerstone of most immunosuppressive regimes. The most commonly used inhibitor of calcineurin, cyclosporine A, as well as tacrolimus as second most used compound in this class can directly induce tumor growth in murine models and increase the secretion of TGF-β and VEGF, conducive to SCC formation [31, 32]. Recently, calcineurin inhibition was recognized to selectively induce the expression of activating transcription factor 3 (ATF3). ATF3 downregulates p53 expression by direct negative regulation of p53 mRNA expression and thus increases SCC formation in vitro, in mouse models and in human SCC [33].

The capacity of azathioprine to sensitize the skin to ultraviolet A light has been mentioned above. Azathioprine is a purine analog resulting in the incorporation of 6-thioguanine in the DNA of replicating cells. The use of azathioprine in the past has been connected to increased incidence of SCC as well as of other malignant tumors such as non-Hodgkin's lymphoma, liver cancer, bile duct cancer, gallbladder cancer, and others. Animal models have provided evidence of increased microsatellite instability and cancer [34, 35]. There is little compelling evidence for direct carcinogenicity of prednisone besides its immunosuppressive effect [35, 36]. Mycophenolate mofetil (MMF) and mTOR inhibitors such as rapamycin are newer drugs reportedly associated with impaired angiogenesis and outgrowth of tumor implants [35] and in particular with beneficial effects in murine models of UV carcinogenesis [37]. mTOR inhibitors and MMF thus seem useful in improving cutaneous carcinogenesis in OTR. The chapter by Stucker et al. [this vol., pp. 36–48] discusses the rationale for the critical selection of immunosuppressants in further detail.

Conclusions

Solid organ transplantation influences the biology of the skin profoundly. The spectrum encompasses inflammatory, infectious and neoplastic disorders. The most relevant clinical problem is SCC of the skin which is increased 65- to 100-fold following transplantation. The underlying factors for this pronounced cutaneous carcinogenesis reside in the isolated and combined effects of ultraviolet light and immunosuppressive drugs on the skin.

References

1 Keller MR, Burlingham WJ: Loss of tolerance to self after transplant. Semin Immunopathol 2011;33: 105–110.
2 Hofbauer GF, Bavinck JN, Euvrard S: Organ transplantation and skin cancer: basic problems and new perspectives. Exp Dermatol 2010;19:473–482.
3 Lally A, Casabonne D, Newton R, Wojnarowska F: Seborrheic dermatitis among Oxford renal transplant recipients. J Eur Acad Dermatol Venereol 2010;24:561–564.
4 Hofbauer GF, Boehler A, Speich R, Burg G, Nestle FO: Painless erythema of the hands associated with non-Hodgkin's lymphoma in a lung transplant recipient. J Am Acad Dermatol 2002;46:S159–S160.
5 Sailer E, Kamarachev J, Boehler A, Speich R, Hofer M, Benden C, et al: Persistent photodamage following drug photosensitization in a lung-transplant recipient. Photodermatol Photoimmunol Photomed 2011;27:213–215.
6 Marcollo Pini A, Kerl K, Kamarachev J, French LE, Hofbauer GF: Interstitial granulomatous drug reaction following intravenous ganciclovir. Br J Dermatol 2008;158:1391–1393.
7 Proby CM, Harwood CA, Neale RE, Green AC, Euvrard S, Naldi L, et al: A case-control study of betapapillomavirus infection and cutaneous squamous cell carcinoma in organ transplant recipients. Am J Transplant 2011;11:1498–1508.
8 Schwartz JJ, Myskowski PL: Molluscum contagiosum in patients with human immunodeficiency virus infection. A review of twenty-seven patients. J Am Acad Dermatol 1992;27:583–588.
9 Theiler M, Kempf W, Kerl K, French LE, Hofbauer GF: Disseminated molluscum contagiosum in a HIV-positive child. Improvement after therapy with 5% imiquimod. J Dermatol Case Rep 2011;5:19–23.
10 Feldmeyer L, Kamarashev J, Boehler A, Irani S, Speich R, French LE, et al: Molluscum contagiosum folliculitis mimicking tinea barbae in a lung transplant recipient. J Am Acad Dermatol 2010;63:169–171.
11 Zwald FO, Brown M: Skin cancer in solid organ transplant recipients: advances in therapy and management. II. Management of skin cancer in solid organ transplant recipients. J Am Acad Dermatol 2011;65:263–279, quiz 80.
12 Zwald FO, Brown M: Skin cancer in solid organ transplant recipients: advances in therapy and management. I. Epidemiology of skin cancer in solid organ transplant recipients. J Am Acad Dermatol 2011;65:253–261, quiz 62.
13 Slaughter DP, Southwick HW, Smejkal W: Field cancerization in oral stratified squamous epithelium; clinical implications of multicentric origin. Cancer 1953;6:963–968.
14 Euvrard S, Kanitakis J, Claudy A: Skin cancers after organ transplantation. N Engl J Med 2003;348: 1681–1691.
15 Geusau A, Dunkler D, Messeritsch E, Sandor N, Heidler G, Rodler S, et al: Non-melanoma skin cancer and its risk factors in an Austrian population of heart transplant recipients receiving induction therapy. Int J Dermatol 2008;47:918–925.
16 Hofbauer GFL, Attard NR, Harwood CA, McGregor JM, Dziunycz P, Iotzova-Weiss G, et al: Reversal of UVA skin photosensitivity and DNA damage in kidney transplant recipients by replacing azathioprine. Am J Transplant 2012;12:218–225.
17 O'Donovan P, Perrett CM, Zhang X, Montaner B, Xu YZ, Harwood CA, et al: Azathioprine and UVA light generate mutagenic oxidative DNA damage. Science 2005;309:1871–1874.
18 Cowen EW, Nguyen JC, Miller DD, McShane D, Arron ST, Prose NS, et al: Chronic phototoxicity and aggressive squamous cell carcinoma of the skin in children and adults during treatment with voriconazole. J Am Acad Dermatol 2010;62:31–37.
19 Jensen AO, Thomsen HF, Engebjerg MC, Olesen AB, Sorensen HT, Karagas MR: Use of photosensitising diuretics and risk of skin cancer: a population-based case-control study. Br J Cancer 2008;99: 1522–1528.
20 Green A, Williams G, Neale R, Hart V, Leslie D, Parsons P, et al: Daily sunscreen application and betacarotene supplementation in prevention of basal-cell and squamous-cell carcinomas of the skin: a randomised controlled trial. Lancet 1999; 354:723–729.
21 Ulrich C, Jurgensen JS, Degen A, Hackethal M, Ulrich M, Patel MJ, et al: Prevention of non-melanoma skin cancer in organ transplant patients by regular use of a sunscreen: a 24 months, prospective, case-control study. Br J Dermatol 2009;161(suppl 3): 78–84.
22 Beissert S, Schwarz T: Ultraviolet-induced immunosuppression: implications for photocarcinogenesis. Cancer Treat Res 2009;146:109–121.
23 Muehleisen B, Petrov I, Gachter T, Kurrer M, Scharer L, Dummer R, et al: Immunohistochemical characterization of inflammatory infiltrate of intraepidermal and invasive squamous cell carcinoma of the skin in immunocompetent patients and organ transplant recipients. Exp Dermatol 2007;16:200.

24 Kosmidis M, Muhleisen B, Scharer L, Dummer R, Hofbauer GF: Regulatory T cells within the inflammatory infiltrate of squamous cell carcinoma of the skin in immunocompetent patients versus solid organ transplant recipients. Exp Dermatol 2007;16:257.
25 Pettersen JS, Fuentes-Duculan J, Suarez-Farinas M, Pierson KC, Pitts-Kiefer A, Fan L, et al: Tumor-associated macrophages in the cutaneous SCC microenvironment are heterogeneously activated. J Invest Dermatol 2011;131:1322–1330.
26 Bluth MJ, Zaba LC, Moussai D, Suarez-Farinas M, Kaporis H, Fan L, et al: Myeloid dendritic cells from human cutaneous squamous cell carcinoma are poor stimulators of T-cell proliferation. J Invest Dermatol 2009;129:2451–2462.
27 Kamp DW, Shacter E, Weitzman SA: Chronic inflammation and cancer: the role of the mitochondria. Oncology (Williston Park) 2011;25:400–410.
28 Gebhardt C, Riehl A, Durchdewald M, Nemeth J, Furstenberger G, Muller-Decker K, et al: RAGE signaling sustains inflammation and promotes tumor development. J Exp Med 2008;205:275–285.
29 Iotzova-Weiss G, Dziunycz P, Vogl T, Hofbauer G: Inflammation as a driver of squamous cell carcinoma of the skin. J Invest Dermatol 2010;130:S52.
30 Guba M, Graeb C, Jauch KW, Geissler EK: Pro- and anti-cancer effects of immunosuppressive agents used in organ transplantation. Transplantation 2004;77:1777–1782.
31 Hojo M, Morimoto T, Maluccio M, Asano T, Morimoto K, Lagman M, et al: Cyclosporine induces cancer progression by a cell-autonomous mechanism. Nature 1999;397:530–534.
32 Maluccio M, Sharma V, Lagman M, Vyas S, Yang H, Li B, et al: Tacrolimus enhances transforming growth factor-beta1 expression and promotes tumor progression. Transplantation 2003;76:597–602.
33 Wu X, Nguyen BC, Dziunycz P, Chang S, Brooks Y, Lefort K, Hofbauer GF, Dotto GP: Opposing roles for calcineurin and ATF3 in squamous skin cancer. Nature 2010;465:368–372.
34 International Agency for Research on Cancer: Azathioprine. Overall Evaluations of Carcinogenicity IARC Monographs on the Evaluation of Carcinogenic Risk of Chemicals to Humans. Lyon, International Agency for Research on Cancer, 1987, pp 119–120.
35 Watorek E, Boratynska M, Smolska D, Patrzalek D, Klinger M: Malignancy after renal transplantation in the new era of immunosuppression. Ann Transplant 2011;16:14–18.
36 International Agency for Research on Cancer: Prednisone. Overall Evaluations of Carcinogenicity IARC Monographs on the Evaluation of Carcinogenic Risk of Chemicals to Humans. Lyon, International Agency for Research on Cancer, 1987, pp 326–327.
37 de Gruijl FR, Koehl GE, Voskamp P, Strik A, Rebel HG, Gaumann A, et al: Early and late effects of the immunosuppressants rapamycin and mycophenolate mofetil on UV carcinogenesis. Int J Cancer 2010;127:796–804.

PD Dr. Günther Hofbauer
Dermatologische Klinik
Universitätsspital Zürich
Gloriastrasse 31
CH–8091 Zürich (Switzerland)
Tel. +41 44 255 46 20, E-Mail hofbauer@usz.ch

Häusermann P, Steiger J, Passweg J (eds): Transplantation Dermatology.
Curr Probl Dermatol. Basel, Karger, 2012, vol 43, pp 9–17

Skin Problems in Immunodeficient Patients

Peter H. Itin[a] · Manuel Battegay[b]

[a]Dermatology and [b]Hospital Epidemiology, University Hospital Basel, Basel, Switzerland

Abstract

The most important function of the skin besides social communication is active protection against mechanical, chemical and microbial threat. The epidermis has biochemical, physical, immunological and anti-infective properties, and is the most important shield against aggressors. Chronic immunosuppression impairs this cutaneous quality and therefore numerous mucocutaneous complications can occur. The physiological colonization of commensal microbes helps to limit the expansion of pathogenic bacteria, viruses and fungi by a continuous release of antimicrobial peptides from keratinocytes. Genetic or acquired immunodeficiency influences these factors. Malignant neoplastic diseases such as leukemia or lymphomas can also lead to severe immunodeficiency. Drug-induced immunodeficiency is common in organ-transplanted patients with the aim to prevent organ rejection. Such patients with prolonged immunodeficiency often develop atypical presentations of mucocutaneous infections. This is the reason why such patients should be biopsied liberally. In addition to the conventional histology, a part of the biopsy should be used for microbiological cultures. Long-term complications of oncogenic viruses have to be considered leading to epithelial cancers (HPV), Kaposi sarcomas (HHV8), lymphomas (EBV) and Merkel cell tumor (polyomavirus) apart from more known acute infections of the skin. Important mucocutaneous markers of immunosuppression such as oral hairy leukoplakia, oral candidiasis and eczema molluscatum exist. This work reviews the pathophysiology of skin protection and describes typical mucocutaneous problems in immunosuppressed patients.

The global number of drug-induced immunosuppressed patients is increasing continuously. It is estimated that in the USA more than 140,000 patients are living with an allogeneic organ and at the same time are kept under immunosuppressive chemotherapy [1]. Long-term immunosuppression impacts strongly on skin functions. In addition, neoplastic diseases such as leukemia or lymphomas can lead to severe immunodeficiency, and most systemic chemotherapies against malignant tumors result in time-limited immunosuppression.

Table 1. Barriers against microbial agents

Physical barrier	Stratum corneum, corneocytes and keratinocytes, desmosomes
Biochemical barrier	Lipids, organic acids, lysozymes, antimicrobial peptides
Microbial barrier	Normal skin flora (commensal microbes)
Immunologic barrier	Innate, acquired, inflammatory cells

Different Barrier Systems of the Skin

The main function of the skin is protection against aggressors from the environment. These include UV radiation, irritants and microbial pathogens. To limit growth of bacteria, fungi and viruses, different types of epithelial barriers and continuous maintenance of biochemical and structural proteins as well as lipids are necessary (table 1) [2]. Physical epithelial barrier is mainly composed by the stratum corneum and its corneocytes. In addition, a biochemical barrier exists which includes filaggrin, intercellular lipids and antimicrobial peptides as well as the microbial barrier, which is composed by the normal skin flora [3]. Furthermore, a barrier with innate and acquired immunity together with inflammatory cells is an important part of defense [4]. This barrier is especially altered in immunosuppressed patients.

Immunologic Epithelial Barrier

Keratinocytes produce and release not only antimicrobial peptides, but also endothelin-1 and cytokines which activate mast cells and then release TNF-α, proteases and antimicrobial peptides. Both keratinocytes and mast cells are able to kill pathogens. In addition, dendritic cells within the epidermis process microbial antigens and act against invasion of microbes.

Staphylococcus aureus, if present, adheres and grows on the epidermis. This stimulates dendritic cells but also activates T cells. Th1 cells aim to clear intracellular pathogens by interferon-γ and B cell activation. Th2 cells lead to an IgE increase by stimulation of B cells aiming at clearance of parasitic worms. All microbes, especially staphylococci, may activate Toll-like receptors, thereby increasing levels of antimicrobial peptides in the skin. In organ-transplanted patients, these mechanisms are impaired.

Langerin within the Langerhans cells functions as an antiviral receptor on Langerhans cells. Langerin for example attaches to HIV1 and internalizes the virus within Birbeck granules. After internalization the virus is degraded, preventing infection of the Langerhans cells and surrounding cells. Langerhans cells become infected by HIV1 when Langerin is inhibited or in the presence of coinfections [5]. After binding to CD4 and CCR5, the HIV1 receptors expressed on Langerhans cells, the virus integrates into the host genome and consequently new viruses are produced and transmitted to T cells.

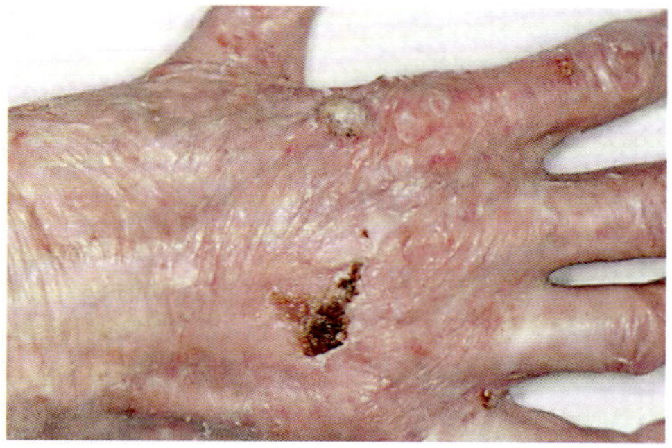

Fig. 1. Actinic keratosis and squamous cell cancer on the dorsum of the hand in an organ-transplanted patient.

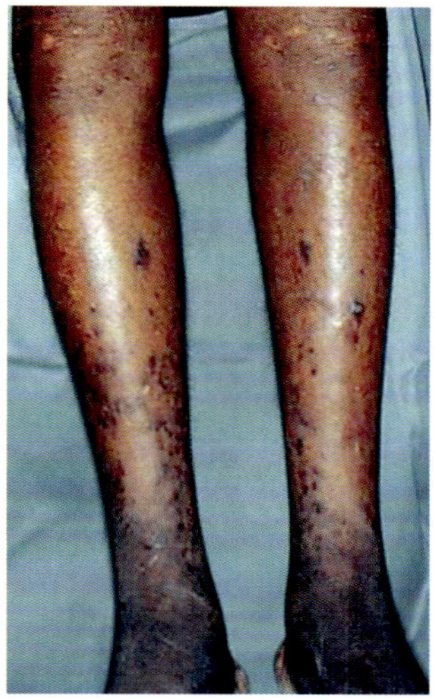

Fig. 2. Multiple Kaposi sarcomas on the legs in a renal transplant patient.

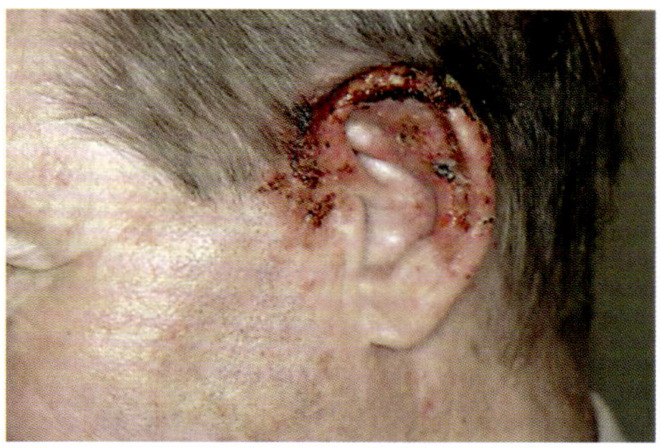

Fig. 3. Field cancerization on the ear in a renal transplant patient.

Table 2. Characteristics of mucocutaneous manifestations in severe immunosuppression

– Atypical clinical presentation
– Atypical course
– Insufficient response to conventional therapy

The EVER proteins act as a natural barrier against papillomaviruses. EVER genes are responsible for a complex with zinc which blocks β-HPV infection and virus replication. In genodermatosis epidermodysplasia verruciformis, these genes are mutated, and therefore β-HPV-infection occurs and virus replication is increased [6]. After 5 years of transplantation, the prevalence of viral warts reaches almost 90%. It has been shown repeatedly that in immunosuppressed patients squamous cell carcinomas show very often infection by β-HPV [7] (fig. 1). This illustrates the complex interplay of protective factors and its influence by genes and genetic disorders.

Type of Immunosuppression

Patients with genetic or acquired immunodeficiency have a marked increase in mucocutaneous problems compared with a control population [8, 9]. Genetic causes for immunodeficiency syndromes are rare and they may occur as combined immunodeficiency (B and T cells), isolated antibody deficiency syndrome (B cells) or isolated T cellular deficiency. In addition, there are different defects of phagocytosis and lack of different parts of the complement system. Much more common are acquired immunodeficiency syndromes such as in patients with organ transplants, who are under long-term immunosuppressive therapy. In addition, patients with malignancies and under chemotherapy are at risk. Furthermore, HIV-infected patients are characterized by marked immunodeficiency as soon as CD4 cells decrease. Importantly, quantitative immunosuppression and qualitative immunosuppression seem to play a role. This qualitative aspect of function may explain why numerous inflammatory skin diseases are found at increased rate in patients with malignancy (thymoma and lichen planus, Sweet syndrome and leukemia, granuloma anulare, myelodysplastic syndrome, etc.).

Mucocutaneous Manifestations in Immunosuppressed Patients Depending on Time Point of Transplantation (fig. 1–3; table 2)

Organ-transplanted patients are faced with acute complications such as infections, organ rejection reaction and chronic complications which include opportunistic infections and malignancies especially of the skin (fig. 4, 5). Most commonly, *S. aureus*

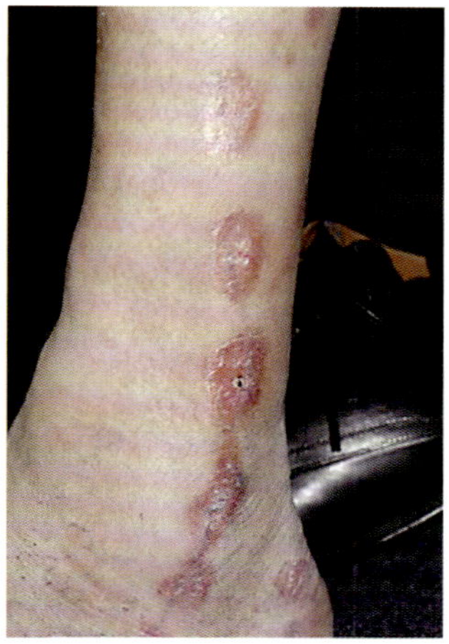

Fig. 4. Numerous granulomas in a patient with combined immunodeficiency syndrome.

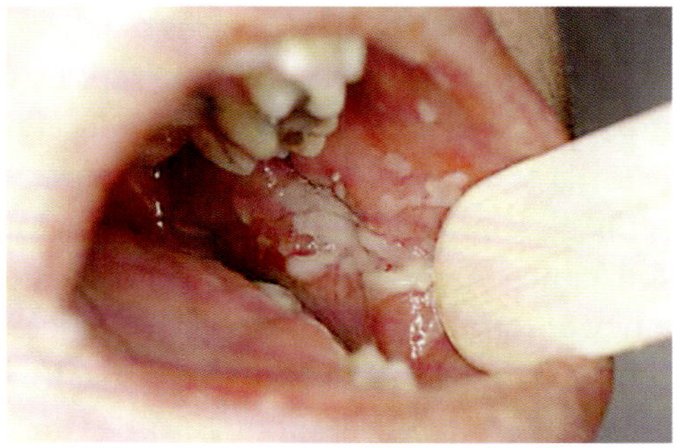

Fig. 5. Stomatitis in a patient under chemotherapy.

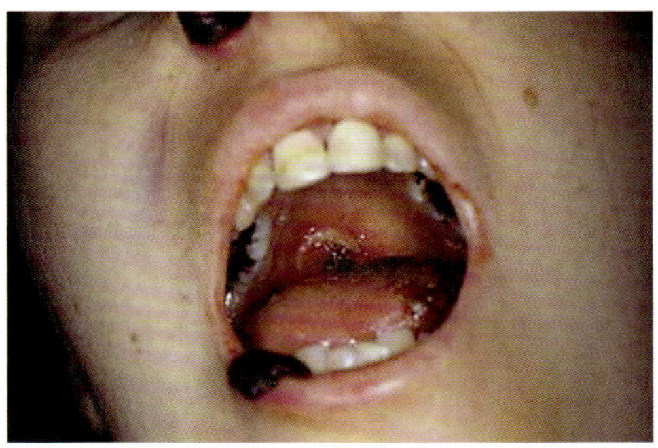

Fig. 6. Chronic herpes simplex in a patient with acute leukemia.

is causative, but a large variety of other germs may give rise to cutaneous manifestations. Viral infections include especially herpes simplex but also all the other herpes viruses (fig. 6). They can contribute to tumor formations such as herpes type 8 (Kaposi sarcoma), Merkel cell polyomavirus (Merkel cell cancer) or Epstein-Barr virus (B-cell lymphoma). Fungal infections are also quite common especially with *Candida albicans*. In 4 out of 5 organ-transplanted patients skin infections will occur. The prevalence and the spectrum of infections depend on the depth of the immunosuppression and the time with impaired immunity. Immediately after the organ transplantation, rather common wound infections may occur within the first months of transplantation, especially pyodermas caused by *S. aureus*. An increased risk for necrotizing soft tissue infections has been demonstrated in patients who have immunosuppression. Patients who are older than 50 years often have less clinical manifestations. Important clinical signs for necrotizing soft tissue infections are extreme pain, fever and systemic toxic features. These latter patients often show a reactivation of herpes type viruses 6 and 7 as well as herpes simplex. After 2 up to 5 months of the transplantation, any unusual skin infections such as nocardiosis or cryptococcosis may occur, but also herpes zoster and cytomegaly virus reactivations. In this period, increased manifestations of HPV-induced warts are observed. Later, organ-transplanted patients often develop mycosis, especially by *C. albicans*, *Aspergillus* and *Malassezia furfur* [10].

A large variety of additional benign and malignant adverse effects such as steroid acne, generalized hypertrichosis and alopecia as well as gingival hyperplasia, besides skin cancer are observed in this population [11]. Importantly, the extended life expectancy in organ transplant patients increases the risk for development of squamous cell carcinoma of the skin dramatically by approximately 65 times. Basal cell carcinomas are increased about 10 times and melanoma three times compared to a non-immunosuppressed population. In immunosuppressed patients, the oncogenic viral impact is often related to increased malignancy development. After organ transplantation, close to 40% of patients develop premalignant and malignant skin tumors. Squamous cell carcinoma is the most common skin cancer in organ-transplanted patients, whereas in the control population it is basal cell carcinoma. The longer the posttransplant period, the higher the relative risk for squamous cell carcinoma, especially in sun-exposed areas. Also, in organ transplant patients, the natural course of squamous cell carcinoma is more aggressive than in a control population.

The increased rate of Kaposi sarcoma and lymphoma as well as anogenital squamous cell cancer can be explained by the effect of oncogenic viruses such as herpes type VIII in Kaposi sarcoma and EBV in lymphoma as well as HPV in squamous cell carcinoma.

Skin Problems in HIV-Infected Patients (table 3)

HIV-infected patients have an increased chance to develop skin problems within the natural disease course. Most of the complications are a direct result of an increasing

Table 3. Most common dermatologic problems in HIV-infected patients

Xerodermia	48.1%
Tinea	43.6%
Candida stomatitis	41.7%
Seborrheic dermatitis	35.3%
Viral warts	28.8%
Folliculitis	25.3%
Herpes simplex	14.9%
Condylomata acuminata	12.4%
Mollusca contagiosa	11.0%

Data from a prospective study on skin problems in HIV-infected patients in Basel before introduction of HAART [13].

immunodeficiency. Sometimes, the occurrence of opportunistic mucocutaneous infections leads to the primary diagnosis of HIV infection.

Importantly, none of the mucocutaneous complications in HIV infections are specific for HIV itself such as oral hairy leukoplakia, oral candidiasis or the more typical erythematous variant or eosinophilic folliculitis [12]. Herpes zoster, which has a necrotizing aspect and covers more than two dermatomes is an indicator of possible HIV infection. In AIDS patients, dermatologic diseases present in atypical ways concerning the extended course and reduced success on adequate therapy. Patients with chronic immunodeficiency need a periodical complete mucocutaneous checkup because of atypical presentations. Often, biopsy needs to be performed. Nodular indurated skin lesions and pustular or erosive skin lesions need a microbiological and histological examination [9]. After the introduction of highly active antiretroviral therapy in 1996, typical HIV-associated diseases such as Kaposi sarcoma, oral hairy leukoplakia or candida stomatitis have decreased dramatically (table 4). Interestingly, HPV-associated warts have increased despite antiretroviral therapy. Anal carcinomas have increased from 35/100,000 before the introduction of antiretroviral therapy to 100/100,000 patients with current treatments against HIV. Males are 60 times more affected by anal carcinomas compared with women. Women with HIV have a 4.6 times greater risk for cervical cancer compared to the normal population.

Dry skin is very common in immunosuppressed patients, especially in HIV-infected ones. Some authors discuss early malabsorption in HIV patients with fat loss causing skin malfunction. In addition, nerve ends have been demonstrated to increase in HIV-infected patients, thereby disturbing sebum production. Dry skin commonly leads to pruritus, which can lower quality of life. Therefore, preventive moisturizing is necessary. In one study, the degree of dryness of the skin was associated with CD4 cell count. Organ-transplanted patients often develop dry skin. Itch is a common symptom, and the appearance of pruritic papules in HIV-infected patients was explained by increased reaction

Table 4. The impact of HAART on the prevalence of skin problems in HIV-infected patients [9]

	Before HAART	After HAART
Candida stomatitis	41.7%	12.0%
Oral hairy leukoplakia	34.2%	4.3%
Seborrheic dermatitis	32.5%	13.0%
Folliculitis	21.8%	10.9%
Reactive syphilis serology	18.5%	10.9%

against insect bites. The clinical normal-appearing skin in HIV-infected patients shows a clear increase in CD8 cells within the epidermis, which leads to a higher cytokine level and an increased inflammatory condition. Pruritic papules of HIV infection lead to a marked amelioration under antiretroviral therapy. Tinea corporis can often present in much larger areas. The white superficial tinea unguium is known as a marker of immunosuppression. Tinea of the skin is characterized by indurated and scaled margins with central fading and centrifugal growth. Often, tinea is associated with pustules around some follicules. Extended tinea of the skin, but also nail involvement and hair involvement as well as the dry lamellar type of tinea needs systemic treatment with terbinafine or itraconazole. Candida stomatitis can present with angular cheilitis, pseudomembranous appearance or atrophic erythematous variant. The rarest type is the hyperplastic candida infection. Local treatment with amphotericin is possible if the esophagus is not involved. For systemic treatment, fluconazole is given. In chronic or recurrent courses, patients may receive once weekly 150 mg fluconazole. Seborrheic dermatitis is quite common in the normal population, but occurrs more frequently in immunosuppressed patients. Increased density of *M. furfur* is found in HIV-positive patients with seborrheic dermatitis. Also, clinical manifestations are much more pronounced and may remind psoriasis. Therapy is always topical with antimycotics, and in case of intense inflammation 2 days with local steroids should be considered. Often, seborrheic dermatitis may increase after initiation of combined antiretroviral therapy as a result of immunoreconstitution. Viral warts are extremely resistant and are more prevalent with lower CD4 cells. Bleedless therapeutic regimens are recommended such as cryosurgery or high-percentage salicylic acid. Also, immunomodulators such as imiquimod can help to get rid of viral warts. In immunosuppressed patients, folliculitis can result most commonly from staphylococcal and pseudomonas infection but also from demodex folliculorum, herpes simplex and *M. furfur*. There is also an aseptic variant called eosinophilic folliculitis. Herpes simplex in immunosuppressed patients often manifests with chronic ulceration. A high degree of clinical suspicion is necessary to make the diagnosis and to confirm it by PCR or culture. Treatments with high-dose systemic virostatics are effective. Genital warts (condylomata acuminata) are induced by human papillomaviruses type 6 and 11 and less commonly by the oncogenic types 16 and 18. Treatments of choice against genital warts are CO_2 laser therapy and immunomodulators (imiquimod) as well as cryosurgery.

Mollusca contagiosa often present on the face. Treatment of choice is cryosurgery, and often the clinical presentation is very atypical, so that the final diagnosis is only made by histology. Kaposi sarcoma occurs with increased frequency in organ-transplanted patients and AIDS patients. Interestingly, with reduction in immunosuppression there is a marked spontaneous tendency for regression and even complete resolution. The cause is infection with herpes type 8 together with immunosuppression.

References

1 O'Reilly Zwald F, Brown M: Skin cancer in solid organ transplant recipients: advances in therapy and management. I. Epidemiology of skin cancer in solid organ transplant recipients. J Am Acad Dermatol 2011;65:253–261.

2 Bangert C, Brunner PM, Stingl G: Immune functions of the skin. Clin Dermatol 2011;29:360–376.

3 Wanke I, Steffen H, Christ C, Krismer B, Götz F, Peschel A, Schaller M, Schittek B: Skin commensals amplify the innate immune response to pathogens by activation of distinct signaling pathways. J Invest Dermatol 2011;131:382–390.

4 Gallo RL, Nakatsuji T: Microbial symbiosis with the innate immune defense system of the skin. J Invest Dermatol 2011;131:1974-1980.

5 Van der Vlist M, Geijteenbeek TB: Langerin functions as an antiviral receptor on Langerhans cells. Immunol Cell Biol 2010;88:410–415.

6 Lazarczyk M, Cassonnet P, Pons C, Jacob Y, Favre M: The EVER proteins as a natural barrier against papillomaviruses: a new insight into the pathogenesis of human papillomavirus infections. Microbiol Mol Biol Rev 2009;73:348–370.

7 Proby CM, Harwood CA, Neale RE, Green AC, Euvrard S, Naldi L, Tessari G, Feltkamp MC, de Koning MN, Quint WG, Waterboer T, Pawlita M, Weissenborn S, Wieland U, Pfister H, Stockfleth E, Nindl I, Abeni D, Ter Schegget J, Bouves Bavinck JN: A case-control study of betapapillomavirus infection and cutaneous squamous cell carcinoma in organ transplant recipients. Am J Transplant 2011;11:1498–1508.

8 Al-Herz W, Nanda A: Skin manifestations in primary immunodeficient children. Pediatr Dermatol 2011;28:494–501.

9 Beltraminelli H, Itin PH: Human immunodeficiency virus and dermatology – a focus on special diseases and a review of the literature. G Ital Dermatol Venereol 2006;141:267–277.

10 Ulrich C, Hackethal M, Meyer T, Geusau A, Nindl I, Ulrich M, Forschner T, Sterry W, Stockfleth E: Skin infections in organ transplant recipients. JDDG 2008;6:98–105.

11 Lally A, Casabonne D, Imko-Walczuk B, Newton R, Wojnarowska F: Prevalence of benign cutaneous disease among Oxford renal transplant recipients. J Eur Acad Dermatol Venereol 2011;25:462–470.

12 Itin PH, Lautenschlager S: Viral lesions of the mouth in HIV-infected patients. Dermatology 1997;194:1–7.

13 Schaub N, Gilli L, Rufli Th, Gyr N, Battegay M, Nüesch R, Itin P: Epidemiologie von Hauterkrankungen bei HIV-infizierten Patienten: eine prospektive Kohortenstudie. Schweiz Rundschau Med (PRAXIS) 1996;85:1162–1166.

Prof. Dr. Peter H. Itin
University Hospital Basel
Petersgraben 4
CH–4031 Basel (Switzerland)
Tel. +41 061 265 4084, E-Mail itinp@uhbs.ch

Häusermann P, Steiger J, Passweg J (eds): Transplantation Dermatology.
Curr Probl Dermatol. Basel, Karger, 2012, vol 43, pp 18–35

Critical Skin Cancer in Organ Transplant Recipients – A Dermatopathological View

Werner Kempf[a,b] · Kirsten D. Mertz[a,c] · Jean Kanitakis[d] · Günther F.L. Hofbauer[b]

[a]Kempf and Pfaltz, Histological Diagnostics, [b]Department of Dermatology, University Hospital Zürich, Zürich, [c]Institute of Pathology, Cantonal Hospital, Liestal, Switzerland; [d]Department of Dermatology, Ed. Herriot Hospital Group, Lyon, France

Abstract

Organ transplant recipients (OTR) are at significantly increased risk to develop a wide variety of skin cancers, particularly epithelial skin cancer, Merkel cell carcinoma and Kaposi's sarcoma. In addition, melanoma, skin adnexal neoplasm and cutaneous lymphomas are more common in OTR and may differ in their clinicopathological presentation from tumors in immunocompetent patients. The accuracy of clinical diagnosis of suspected premalignant and malignant skin lesions in OTR is modest. Therefore, histopathological diagnosis is an essential element for the diagnostic workup of skin cancers, and additionally provides important information on prognosis. This review discusses the histopathological aspects of skin cancers in OTR, the impact of dermatopathological analysis on prognosis and understanding of the pathogenesis of these neoplasms.

Organ transplant recipients (OTR) are at significantly increased risk to develop a wide variety of skin cancers, particularly epithelial skin cancer, Merkel cell carcinoma and Kaposi's sarcoma (KS) [1, 2]. Squamous cell carcinoma (SCC) and basal-cell carcinoma (BCC) account for more than 90% of all skin cancers in OTR [for review see 3]. The epidemiology of skin cancers in OTR varies depending on the grafted organ, the intensity and composition as well as the duration of the immunosuppressive therapy, UV-light exposure and genetic factors. The accuracy of clinical diagnosis of suspected premalignant and malignant skin lesions in OTR is modest [4]. Therefore, histopathological diagnosis is crucial for the diagnostic workup of skin cancers, and additionally provides important information on prognosis. In this review, the histopathological aspects of skin cancers in OTR, the impact of dermatopathological analysis on prognosis and understanding of the pathogenesis of these neoplasms will be discussed.

Squamous Cell Carcinoma and Its Precursors

SCC is the most common skin cancer in OTR. Twenty to 75% of OTR are affected by at least one SCC within 20 years after transplantation. SCC occurs 65–250 times more frequently in OTR than in the general population [2, 5, 6]. In comparison to the general population at large, where BCC is more prevalent than SCC (SCC:BCC ratio = 1:4), the SCC:BCC ratio is reversed in OTR (1.8–5:1) [3, 7]. Men are at higher risk for SCC [5, 7]. UV light-exposed body regions are the predilection sites for SCC and its precursors. Actinic or solar keratosis (AK) and Bowen's disease (BD) represent intraepidermal precursor lesions with the potential for progression into invasive SCC. Multiple AK are usually found in a skin region, a finding reflecting the phenomenon of field cancerization (fig. 1). BD is often multifocal in OTR, and arises also in UV light-protected body regions such as the trunk or in the anogenital area. Many patients develop several SCC, often within a few months or years after the first diagnosed SCC [5]. Seborrheic keratoses and warts are common in patients with SCC, and seem to be associated with the occurrence of skin cancers in OTR [3, 8]. It can be very challenging and even impossible to clinically distinguish between benign epithelial tumors, AK, BD and invasive epithelial neoplasms. Biopsies and histological workup are therefore crucial for the assessment of the patients and the choice of therapy.

Histologically, AK represent epidermal dysplasia with disarrangement of epithelial stratification of the lower part of the epidermis and keratinocytes with atypical, often hyperchromatic nuclei (fig. 2). Dysplasia may extend into the hair follicle epithelium. Small strands of atypical keratinocytes may protrude into the papillary dermis. Acantholysis and hyperparakeratosis, often alternating with orthokeratosis, as well as increased melanin deposition are common in AK. In BD, the epidermis shows full-thickness atypia with enlarged and sometimes multinucleated keratinocytes with prominent nuclear pleomorphism and atypical mitoses. Both precursors are usually accompanied by a rather dense inflammatory infiltrate composed of lymphocytes, histiocytes and plasma cells.

Clinically, SCC manifests with a hyperkeratotic or ulcerated nodule (fig. 3). The histology of SCC shows invasive growth of epithelial cells arising from the epidermis. The tumor cells show squamous differentiation with variable degrees of keratinization, mitoses and prominent nuclear pleomorphism, especially in the periphery of the epithelial proliferations and in poorly differentiated SCC (fig. 4) [9]. Ulceration is common. Perineural growth may occur. It indicates more extensive growth and a risk of recurrence, but does not seem to be more frequent in OTR [7]. Controversial data have been reported regarding the depth of tumor invasion of SCC in OTR compared with immunocompetent patients (IC). Whereas Harwood et al. [7] found no difference, another study [10] found that SCC infiltrated deeper in OTR than in IC. The peritumoral inflammatory infiltrate is significantly less intense in OTR indicating poor host response [7, 11]. Differentiation (grading) of SCC in OTR does not differ from SCC in general population [7]. SCC in OTR presents more often with spindle

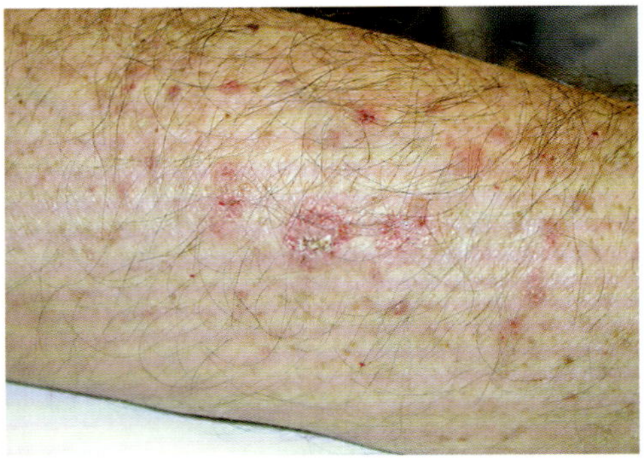

Fig. 1. Multiple erythematous and hyperkeratotic actinic keratoses on the arm. Clinical distinction from BD or invasive SCC may be challenging or even impossible in individual lesions.

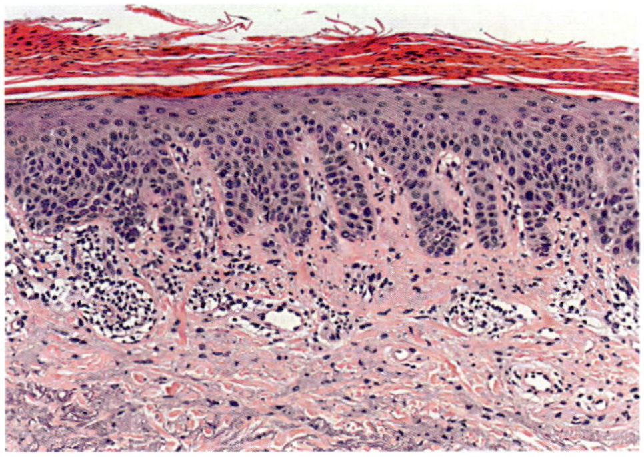

Fig. 2. AK with disarrangement of epithelial stratification of the lower part of the epidermis and keratinocytes with atypical nuclei. HE. Original magnification, ×100.

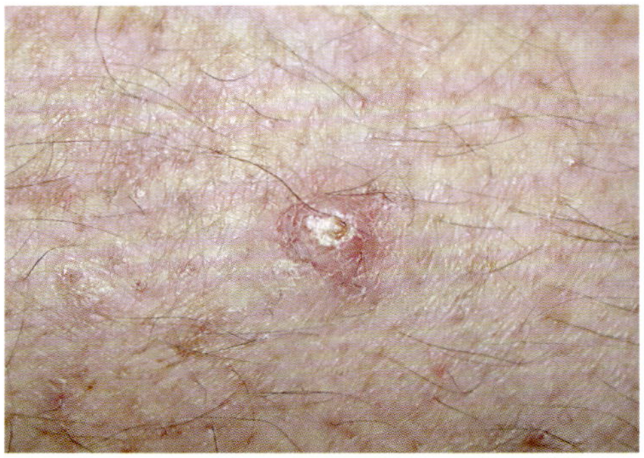

Fig. 3. SCC: nodule with central hyperkeratosis.

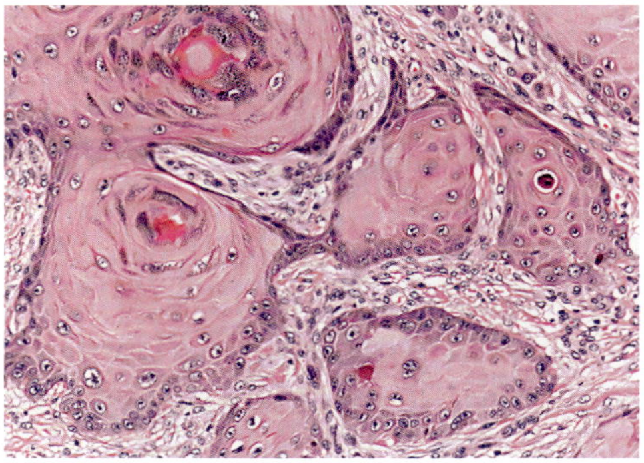

Fig. 4. SCC: proliferation of epithelial cells with squamous differentiation and nuclear pleomorphism. HE. Original magnification, ×200.

cell morphology found in 20% of the lesions, and acantholysis [7, 10]. Expression of cytokeratins (namely 5/6), p63, and CAM5.2 is particularly helpful to prove the epithelial origin of spindle-cell SCC. Verrucous SCC represents a highly differentiated SCC variant in which the malignant nature may be readily overlooked, especially in small and superficial biopsies [9]. Blunt-ended epithelial proliferations with bulbous downgrowths should raise suspicion for this SCC variant, which is more commonly observed in the anogenital area and oral mucosa. Larger and deep-reaching biopsies as well as correlation of histological findings with the clinical presentation are mandatory to establish the diagnosis of verrucous SCC. Keratoacanthoma (KA) is widely considered to represent a highly differentiated variant of SCC according to the WHO classification [9]. It manifests clinically as a rapidly growing nodule with characteristic central horn-filled crater. Histologically, KA presents as a well-circumscribed proliferation of epithelial cells with squamous differentiation and prominent central hyperparakeratosis. In IC, KA tends to regress spontaneously leaving a slightly depressed scar. In OTR, however, this spontaneous regression is uncommon. KA should therefore be treated like other forms of SCC in OTR.

Histology of SCC provides important prognostic information, which is also included in the new American Joint Committee on Cancer staging system for SCC [12]. Some localizations (ear, lip, scalp, temple as primary sites), tumor thickness (>4 mm), tumor size (>2 cm), Clark level IV, poor differentiation, spindle cell morphology, ulceration, acantholytic changes, single cell invasion, perineural growth, and bone invasion are histological indicators of an increased recurrence rate and/or poor prognosis due to subsequent metastasis [10, 12–15].

Pathogenetical studies have demonstrated the involvement of the tumor suppressor gene p53 in premalignant and malignant skin lesions of renal transplant recipients (RTR) [16]. Focusing on tumor microenvironment, a reduced number of CD123+ plasmacytoid dendritic cells and FOXP3+ T cells in the peritumoral inflammatory infiltrate is associated with progression of SCC in OTR [17].

Infection with beta human papillomaviruses (HPV) is associated with an increased risk of SCC [18]. The association between susceptibility to UV light and SCC was stronger in beta HPV-seropositive patients, suggesting a pathogenetically relevant role of HPV in the development of SCC [18]. Apart from HPV, Epstein-Barr virus (EBV) may play a role in cutaneous squamoproliferative lesions in heart transplant recipients, but not in RTR [19].

Guidelines for the management of AK, BD and SCC have been reviewed [20–22]. Surgical excision including Mohs surgery is the first-line therapy. Reduction of immunosuppressive drugs should be considered in patients with several SCC or multifocal BD, and with metastastic SCC. Conversion from calcineurin inhibitors to sirolimus reduces the thickness and vascularization of SCC in OTR [23]. Ongoing trials will provide data for the hypothesis that the switch from calcineurin inhibitors to mTOR inhibitors cuts cutaneous carcinogenesis by 50%. Several clinical trials with retinoids (acitretin) in OTR have demonstrated a reduction of new SCC [for review see 22]. In

AK, however, acitretin improved the clinical aspect via alteration of keratinization, but did not significantly change dysplasia and proliferation [24].

Basal Cell Carcinoma

BCC is the second most frequent cancer in OTR [3, 5]. The risk of BCC is 10–16 times higher among OTR compared with the general population. There are, however, only limited data on the clinicopathological features of BCC in OTR. In a retrospective study, we observed BCC in 14.5% of RTR [25]. BCC manifests with a mean delay of 5–11 years after transplantation [25, 26]. Data on the gender ratio are controversial [25, 26]. Clinically, BCC presents most commonly with a nodule undergoing central ulceration and telangiectasias at the periphery of the tumor. Occasionally, BCC may be pigmented (fig. 5). The superficial variant of BCC is characterized by a slightly infiltrated erythematous lesion, which may grow up to several centimeters in diameter. The morpheiform variant of BCC manifests with a depressed hypopigmented scar-like lesion. UV-exposed body regions, particularly the head and neck are predilection sites. Nevertheless, BCC may occur also in UV light-protected areas such as the back [25, 27]. Superficial BCC is commonly found also on the limbs. Histologically, numerous variants of BCC exist [28, 29]. Nodular BCC is the most common form seen in OTR, although there is a relatively increased proportion of superficial BCC [27]. The histology of BCC in OTR does not differ significantly from IC. Nodular BCC shows well-defined nodular proliferations of basaloid epithelial cells displaying a characteristic palisading arrangement of nuclei at the periphery of the tumor nodules (fig. 6). The tumor islands are separated from the surrounding tumor stroma by a characteristic, often mucin-containing clefts, which are also visible in vivo by reflectance confocal microscopy and therefore do not represent a retraction artifact as previously believed [30]. The stroma contains an inflammatory infiltrate composed predominantly of lymphocytes. Nodular BCC may show cystic foci, adnexal differentiation and pigmentation. In superficial BCC, the aggregates of basaloid tumor cells are attached to and bud from the interfollicular epidermis and appear to be multifocal. In horizontal sections, however, it becomes apparent that the superficial BCC form a superficial reticulated network of tumor strands. Tumor growth in superficial BCC remains restricted to the upper dermis (tumor depth <0.5 mm), although progression into nodular or morpheiform BCC can take place. A prominent tumor stroma and an inflammatory infiltrate is almost invariably present in superficial BCC, although the infiltrate is reported to be less pronounced in BCC of OTR than in the general population [15, 27]. Morpheiform (or sclerosing) BCC displays an ill-defined proliferation of small strands of basaloid tumor cells embedded in a dense, sclerotic stroma. Perineural growth is more common in this BCC type.

Basosquamous (cell) carcinoma (BSC) designates a variant with focal squamous differentiation and shows features of both, BCC and SCC [29]. In OTR, it is a rare

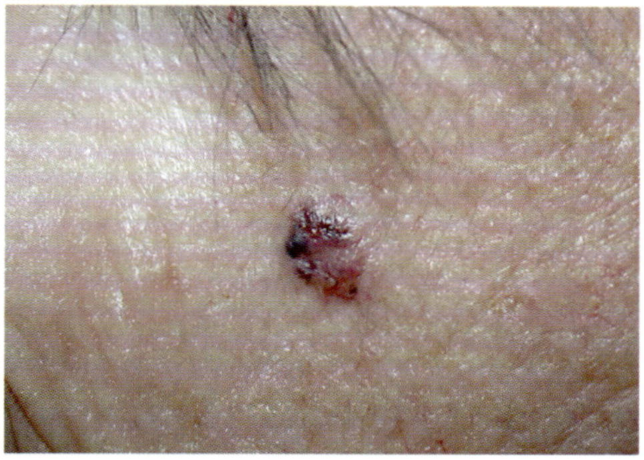

Fig. 5. Pigmented basal cell carcinoma with partly brownish pigmented nodular lesion on the right cheek.

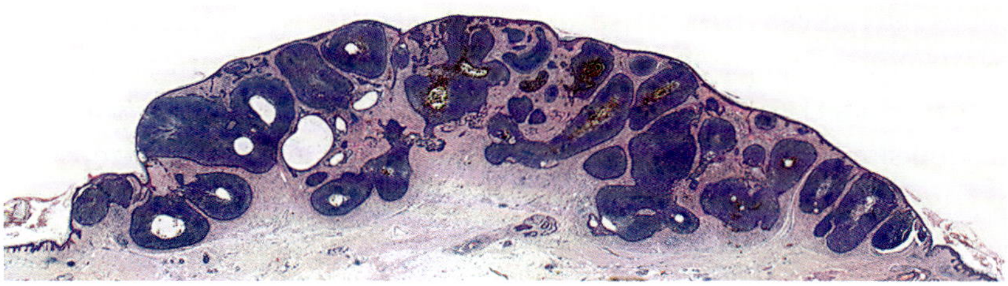

Fig. 6. Histology of pigmented nodular basal cell carcinoma with basophilic nodular proliferations extending into the deep dermis and with centrally located accumulation of melanin pigment. HE. Original magnification, ×10.

tumor with an incidence of 0.3% and develops with a long delay of 13 years after transplantation [31]. Controversial data on the prognosis have been reported. According to a recent study, BSC in OTR do not seem to behave more aggressively than other non-melanoma skin cancers (NMSC) [31].

Pathogenetically, genetic alterations in the sonic hedgehog pathway involving patched homologue 1 (PTCH1), a tumor suppressor gene, and a G-protein-coupled receptor (SMOH) play an important role [28]. Thus, inhibiting the hedgehog pathways represents a promising therapeutic approach. In addition, other genetic alterations have been found, e.g. alterations of p53 induced by UV light or chemicals (such as arsenic compounds).

Surgical excision is the first-line therapy for nodular and morpheiform BCC. Micrographically controlled excision or Mohs surgery is indicated for lesions in specific body regions (nose, eye) to limit surgical defects, for recurrent BCC, and for tumors with perineural growth. For superficial BCC, treatment with photodynamic therapy, cryosurgery or laser surgery, imiquimod and topical 5-fluorouracil are alternative treatment to surgical excision. The prognosis of BCC does not seem to be worse in OTR compared to the general population [25–27]. Recurrence after surgical excision was observed in 10% of RTR [25]. Metastasizing BCC is exceedingly rare.

Merkel Cell Carcinoma

MCC, also termed primary cutaneous neuroendocrine carcinoma, is a rare malignant neoplasm with a highly aggressive course and poor prognosis. UV light exposure, age, chronic lymphocytic leukemia and immunosuppression are risk factors for the development of MCC. Among OTR, approximately 7–8% have been reported to develop MCC, although this incidence appears to be overestimated [32]. The relative risk for OTR to develop MCC is 0.13 per 100 person-years, and is 5- to 10-fold increased compared with the general population at large [32].

MCC in OTR usually affects patients in their fifth decade, with a latency of 7.6 years after transplantation (range 5–286 months) [33]. Men are more commonly affected than women [34]. UV light-exposed skin regions, particularly the head and neck, are predilection sites. Clinically, MCC presents usually as a solitary, asymptomatic, but rapidly growing, red to bluish dome-shaped nodule which may ulcerate. A recent study showed that one third of MCC are clinically misdiagnosed as cysts [35].

Histologically, MCC manifests most commonly with nodular or diffuse infiltrates (intermediate growth pattern) of small to medium-sized basaloid appearing or blast-like cells with hyperchromatic nuclei (fig. 7, 8). Focal necrosis and mitoses are commonly found. In rare cases, foci of squamous differentiation are present. Despite its original designation as trabecular carcinoma, the trabecular growth pattern with ribbons of tumor cells is rare. At the periphery of the tumor, dissection of collagen bundles by strands of tumor cells or scattered single tumor cells is often observed. These often contain small hyperchromatic nuclei and may be misinterpreted as peritumoral lymphocytic infiltrate. Tumor cells in MCC may display pagetoid spread into the overlying epidermis [36, 37]. If present in superficial biopsies of MCC, differential diagnoses include malignant melanoma (MM), Paget's disease, BD with pagetoid growth, and sebaceous carcinoma, and have to be ruled out by immunohistochemistry. Occasionally, MCC contains a dense intra- and peritumoral lymphocytic infiltrate which may mimick lymphoma or pseudolymphoma and obscure tumor cells [38]. Collision of MCC and BD, BCC or invasive SCC has been reported [36]. Small-cell type and vascular invasion are considered as histological markers of poor prognosis. Sentinel lymph node evaluation may improve prognostic accuracy in MCC [39].

Immunohistochemistry is used to confirm the diagnosis, to exclude differential diagnoses and to assess tumor extension. Tumor cells in MCC express pan-cytokeratin (100% of the cases), CAM5.2 (100%), EMA (100%), and display expression of cytokeratin 20 in 65–93% of the cases with a characteristic perinuclear dot-like pattern (fig. 9). In addition, neuroendocrine markers such as synaptophysin (67–75%) and chromogranin (75%) as well as CD56 (N-CAM) are expressed.

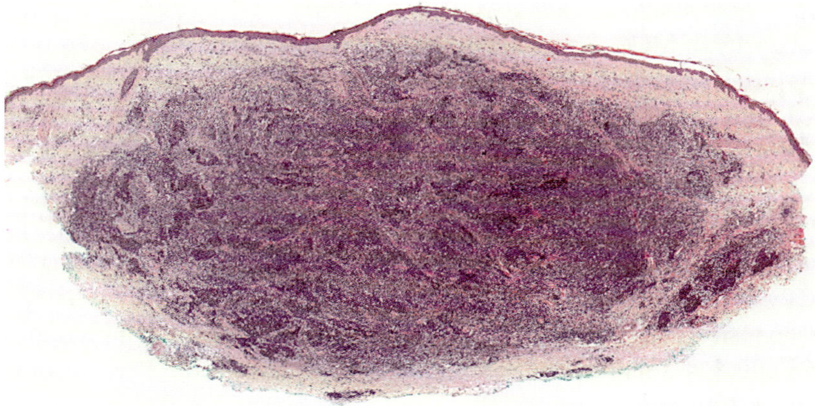

Fig. 7. Merkel cell carcinoma with dermal ill-defined nodular infiltrate of tumor cells. HE. Original magnification, ×20.

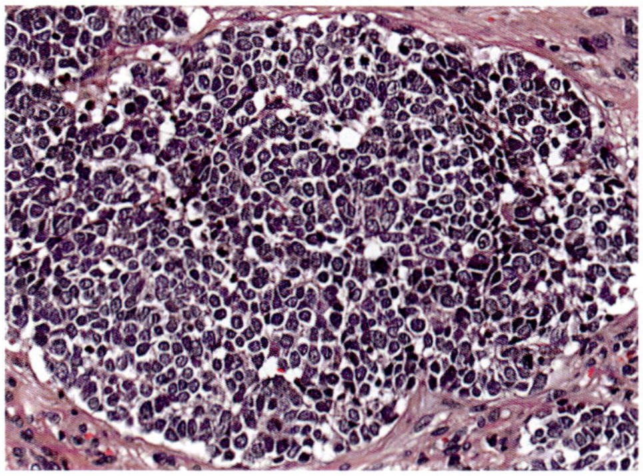

Fig. 8. Merkel cell carcinoma: blast-like tumor cells with hyperchromatic nuclei. HE. Original magnification, ×200.

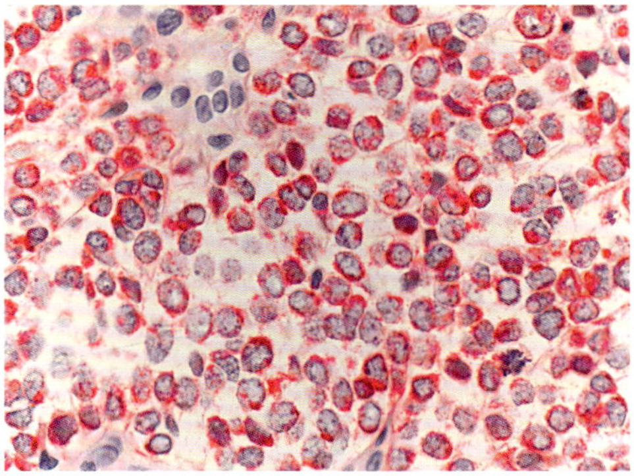

Fig. 9. Characteristic perinuclear dot-like pattern of pan-cytokeratin expression (red). Immunohistochemistry. Original magnification, ×400).

Recently, a new polyomavirus called Merkel cell polyomavirus (MCPyV) was detected in the majority of MCC cases [40]. The clonal integration of viral DNA into tumor cell DNA indicates that the virus contributes to tumor development. Viral antigens can be detected by immunohistochemistry in MCC and may be useful for diagnosis [41]. The presence of MCPyV DNA, however, is not restricted to MCC, since viral DNA has also been found in other benign and malignant neoplasms such as NMSC, seborrheic keratoses and common warts [42, 43], and may be carried to these lesions via blood-borne inflammatory CD14+ CD16– monocytes serving as reservoir for MCPyV [44].

MCC has a propensity for local and distant spread with metastasis to lymph nodes in 68% of the patients [34]. Sentinel lymph node biopsy has therefore been recommended for MCC [45]. Prognosis is generally poor with a 5-year survival rate of less than 50% [39]. Treatment includes local wide excision, radiotherapy and multiagent chemotherapy for metastatic disease.

Adnexal Skin Neoplasms

Adnexal skin neoplasms are a group of benign or malignant epithelial tumors with differentiation towards cellular components of eccrine or apocrine sweat glands, sebaceous glands or hair follicle epithelium. Retrospective analysis of OTR cohorts revealed an increased risk for the occurrence of cutaneous adnexal neoplasms with a prevalence of adnexal skin tumors in 3% of OTR [7]. Among RTR, 14% of the patients had multiple adnexal tumors with head and neck being the predilection site (74%). Benign tumors include pilomatricoma, tumor of follicular infundibulum, sebaceous adenoma, and eccrine poroma. Malignant adnexal tumors, particularly sebaceous carcinoma, seem to be more common in OTR compared with the general population. In some patients, sebaceous carcinoma may be linked to microsatellite instability as seen in the Muir-Torre syndrome [46]. Some cases have a misleading clinical presentation such as a keloid-like appearance of trichilemmal carcinoma [47]. Most OTR with adnexal skin neoplasms (71%) also suffered from other NMSC. None of the tumors recurred after complete surgical excision and none metastasized after a mean follow-up period of 3.4 years (range: 2–7 years) [7].

Malignant Melanoma

MM accounts for approximately 6% of skin cancers in OTR with a higher prevalence in pediatric (12–15%) and in Afro-American OTR (17%) [48]. MM affects young patients (mean age 36 years) with a male preponderance and develops after a median posttransplant delay of 4–5 years [3, 49, 50]. Risk factors for MM in OTR may be similar to the general population, and include intermittent exposure to UV light (and sunburns), inability to tan, multiple and dysplastic nevi as well as a family history of MM. A 2- to 8-fold increased risk for MM has been reported for OTR [2, 3, 48, 51, 52]. The clinical presentation is identical to MM in IC. Most MMs in OTR arise on the trunk and arm [50]. Histologically, MM is characterized by asymmetrical architecture, cellular atypia of melanocytes arranged as single units or in confluent nests, pagetoid spread of atypical melanocytes within the epidermis as a characteristic feature in most MM subtypes, as well as a lack of maturation of the intradermal component of the neoplasm. The diagnosis of early MM, particularly of acral lentiginous and mucosal MM, may be challenging, since only few atypical melanocytes in the junctional area may be present particularly in the marginal areas of the lesions. Histologically, lentigo maligna (LM; in situ melanoma) may be mistaken as dysplastic nevus, particularly in incisional biopsies. Therefore, melanocytic lesions displaying dysplastic features in UV-light-exposed skin particularly in elderly patients should be completely excised. Immunohistochemical stains for melanocytic markers facilitate identification of transepidermal migration as well as the vertical and horizontal extent of the lesion. MiTF is a useful nuclear marker to identify junctional melanocytes especially in sun-damaged skin, where atypical keratinocytes in AK may express other melanocytic markers such as Melan-A, and is particularly helpful for the differentiation between pigmented AK and initial LM. Desmoplastic melanoma (DM) typically arising from LM manifests with a diffuse proliferation of tumor cells with spindle-cell morphology and may completely lack pigmentation. Staining for S-100 protein and p75 is the most sensitive marker for DM, whereas other melanocytic markers are often absent in DM. Prognostic criteria in MM are tumor thickness (TT; Breslow index), mitotic index (in MM with TT less than 1 mm), and ulceration. In a series of OTR reported in 1996, MM showed TT >0.76 mm or Clark's level >III in 69% of patients [49]. In a recent study, however, the TT was <1 mm in the majority of cases [52], which may result from a closer screening of OTR for skin cancers. The 3-year overall survival rates for OTR stratified by Breslow thickness ≤0.75, 0.76–1.50, 1.51–3.00, and >3.00 mm) were 88.2, 80.8, 51.2 and 55.3%, respectively [50]. MM with Breslow thickness <2 mm in OTR has a similar prognosis like tumors in the general population, whereas MM with Breslow thickness >2 mm exhibits a worse prognosis compared to MM in IC [53].

Sentinel lymph node biopsy is recommended for MM with TT between 1 and 4 mm and MM with mitotic index >1 mm per mm^2 (representing stage pT1b according to the AJCC classification). This procedure is relevant for staging and prognosis, but its value on the overall survival of patients with MM is controversially discussed. Genetically, various genetic alterations involving BRAF, N-RAS, and PTEN have been found in the various clinical and histological MM types. Interestingly, melanocytic tumors from OTR had a lower frequency of BRAFV600E mutations than similar lesions from IC (45.4 vs. 63.5%, $p < 0.05$) [54].

Lymph node metastases occurred in 32 patients (20%) with cutaneous MM. Reduction of immunosuppressive treatment is recommended for OTR with MM [22]. Additional treatment modalities depend on tumor stage and in particular the presence of metastases.

Kaposi's Sarcoma

Kaposi's sarcoma (KS) is a rare vascular neoplasm which occurs in four epidemiological forms [classic-sporadic, iatrogenic or posttransplantation (P-KS), (African-) endemic type, and the AIDS-associated form]. KS accounts for 5.7% of all cancers in OTR, and its incidence is increased 400- to 500-fold compared to a non-transplant population of the same ethnicity [55, 56]. The male/female ratio shifts from 17:1 in classic KS to 2–3:1 in immunocompromised patients [57]. KS occurs often sooner after transplantation than NMSC with an average delay ranging from 2 months to 18 years (mean 13 months) [56, 58–60].

Clinically and histologically, three stages (patch – plaque – tumor or nodular) can be distinguished.

Early skin lesions (patch stage) show a proliferation of dilated, irregularly shaped and thin-walled vessels lined by a single layer of flattened endothelial cells lacking atypia. These surround preexisting dermal blood vessels and skin appendages (referred to as promontory sign) and dissociate dermal collagen bundles (fig. 10). Extravasated erythrocytes and hemosiderin deposits are found along with occasional spindle cells. Intra- and extracellular eosinophilic deposits (hyaline globules) are seen, most probably representing degenerated erythrocytes. The findings in early or patch stage KS are subtle and may be misinterpreted as inflammatory dermatosis. Lymphangioma and targetoid hemosiderotic hemangioma have to be differentiated from early KS. As the KS evolves to the plaque or nodular stage, a proliferation of spindle-shaped cells predominates, enclosing slit-like vessels, which are sometimes filled by erythrocytes (fig. 11). The nodular stage is characterized by a well-defined nodular proliferation of intersecting fascicles of spindle cells. An inflammatory infiltrate consisting predominantly of plasma cell, lymphocytes and histiocytes is present in all stages of KS. Cytological atypia of tumor cells is relatively subtle, contrasting with angiosarcoma. Differential diagnosis includes kaposiform hemangioendothelioma, angiosarcoma, targetoid hemosideratic hemangioma, progressive lymphangioma, and multinucleate angiohistiocytoma. Various clinical and histological variants of KS have been described including micronodular KS presenting with tiny red papules clinically resembling capillary hemangioma, hyperkeratotic (verrucous), keloidal, molluscoid, pyogenic granuloma-like, and intravascular KS [61, 62]. Immunohistochemistry demonstrates expression of endothelial markers (CD31, CD34, von Willebrand factor/factor VIII), podoplanin as well as PROX-1 by endothelial and spindle cells.

In 1994, the human herpesvirus 8 (HHV-8) was discovered as the etiologic oncogenic virus in all forms of KS. HHV-8 is a gamma-herpesvirus, and can be demonstrated by PCR or immunohistochemistry in all epidemiological forms and in all clinical and histological stages of the disease [63, 64]. The immunohistochemical staining has become a crucial diagnostic aid for the diagnosis of KS with a high sensitivity and specificity [64]. HHV-8 induces a reprogramming of CD34+ blood endothelial cells to

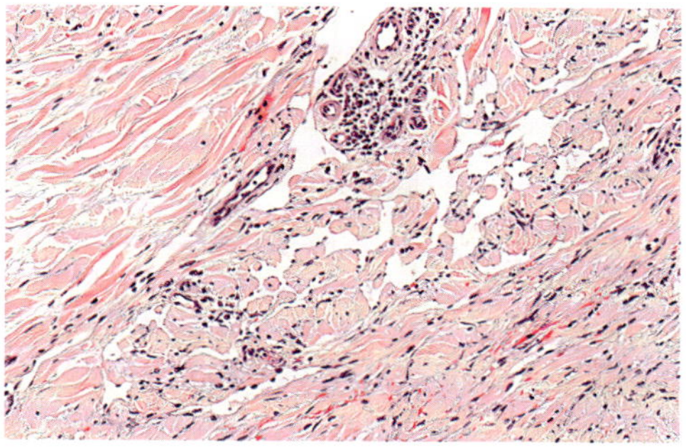

Fig. 10. KS (patch stage) with dilated, irregularly shaped and thin-walled vessels, which surround dermal blood vessels and skin appendages (so-called promontory sign) and dissociate dermal collagen bundle. HE. Original magnification, ×100.

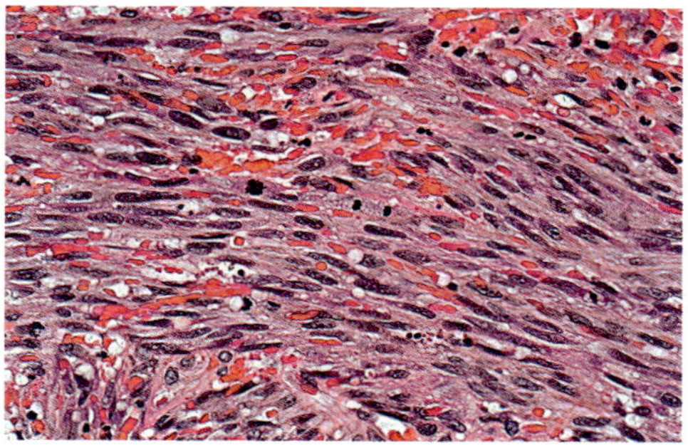

Fig. 11. KS (tumor or nodular stage) with proliferation of spindle-shaped cells enclosing slit-like vessels, which are filled by erythrocytes. HE. Original magnification, ×200.

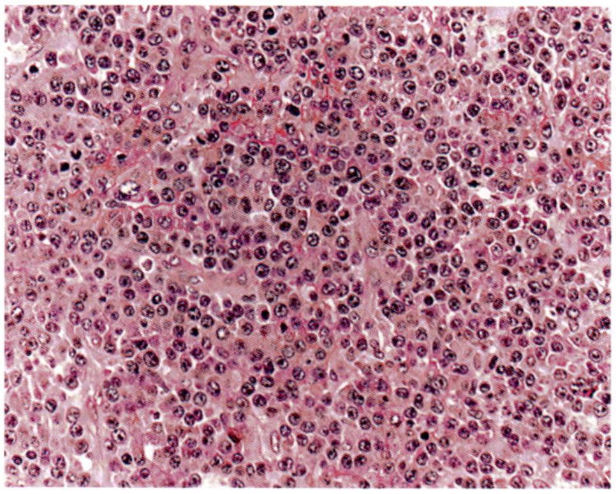

Fig. 12. Posttransplant B cell lymphoproliferative disease with monomorphic infiltrate of large lymphoid cells with predominantly centroblastic and immunoblastic differentiation. HE. Original magnification, ×200.

express a lymphatic phenotype (podoplanin, PROX-1). Moreover, viral proteins such as vIL-6 or v-Cyclin interfere with cellular functions and result in deregulation of the cell cycle, inhibition of apoptosis of tumor cells and suppression of antitumoral host immune response. The virus is usually acquired months to years before occurrence of KS. HHV-8 can be transmitted by horizontal and vertical transmission through sexual contact, blood or body fluids. In OTR, KS usually develops following HHV-8 reactivation, although transmission from the graft is not uncommon [60].

P-KS carries the risk for cutaneous and visceral dissemination and a potentially fatal outcome. OTR with KS have mucocutaneous lesions in >75% of cases, and 25–50% of them develop visceral lesions [56, 65]. The 5-year survival rate of P-KS is 69% [66, 67].

Treatment of KS in OTR primarily consists in reduction of immunosuppression, which leads to complete remission in 25–30% of patients [55]. Reduction of immunosuppression is considered as an essential and effective treatment for P-KS, since regression of tumoral lesions is typically observed in P-KS type even in the absence of additional treatment [68]. The reduction of immunosuppression, however, carries the risk for rejection of the transplanted organ. In addition, there is a high risk of relapse of P-KS after retransplantation. Apart from reduction of immunosuppressive drugs, switching the immunosuppressive medication to an mTOR inhibitor has recently shown efficacy against KS [69]. Further therapies include excision, radiotherapy, intralesional bleomycin injection, liposomal anthracyclines and interferon-α [70]. Clinical tumor regression after topical treatment does not necessarily indicate complete tumor regression as shown in a recent observation, where persisting tumor after topical treatment with imiquimod was histologically found [71]. Therefore histological confirmation is crucial to confirm a complete response.

Soft Tissue Tumors – Sarcomas

In a review on more than 8,000 OTR, sarcomas accounted for 7.4% of all cancers in OTR with KS representing the vast majority (5.7%) of cutaneous and extracutaneous ones [72]. Reports on other cutaneous forms of sarcomas in OTR are sparse and include atypical fibroxanthoma (AFX), malignant fibrous histiocytoma and cutaneous leiomyosarcoma [73–75]. AFX manifests with a nodular lesion arising on sun-exposed body regions, particularly the face and scalp, and clinically resembles BCC or SCC. Histologically, AFX is characterized by a dermal nodular proliferation of plump spindle cells and multinucleated tumor cells with prominent nuclear pleomorphism (monster cells). AFX usually occurs as single lesion, but OTR with multiple AFX have been reported [75]. AFX tends to recur locally [73]. Sarcomas should be treated with wide excision or Mohs surgery.

Cutaneous Lymphomas

Posttransplant lymphoproliferative disorders (PTLD) are lymphoid proliferations developing as a consequence of immunosuppression in a recipient of a solid organ, bone marrow or stem cell allograft [76]. PTLD affect 1–5% of solid OTR. Heart, lung and liver transplant recipients have a higher risk than RTR. PTLD are classified as early lesions, polymorphic, monorphic PTLD and classical Hodgkin lymphoma type PTLD. So far, only a few cases of primary cutaneous lymphomas (pCL) in OTR have been reported. They occur 5–8 years after transplantation [3, 77]. Seventy percent of pCLs in OTR are of T cell origin, whereas only 30% are cutaneous B-cell lymphomas (CTCL) [Seckin, in preparation]. Among primary cutaneous T-cell lymphomas, mycosis fungoides (MF) and cutaneous CD30+ lymphoproliferative disorders (CD30+ LPD) appear to be the most common forms. MF presents clinically with erythematous and slightly scaling patches and plaques mostly on the trunk. Histologically, the disease is characterized by an epidermotropic infiltrate of atypical small to medium-sized lymphocytes. Similar to other patients with MF, the disease course in OTR appears to progress slowly. Cutaneous CD30+ LPD manifest with nodular, often ulcerated lesions. In contrast to CD30+ LPD in the general population, spontaneous regression is not observed in OTR. Histologically, dense infiltrates of large pleomorphic and anaplastic lymphoid cells are seen [78]. By definition, more than 75% of tumor cells express CD30 in addition to T cell markers (CD2, CD4, CD8). Staging examinations are essential to distinguish primary cutaneous from systemic form of CD30+ LPD [78, 79]. Contrary to IC, CD30+ LPD in OTR run an aggressive course which contrasts with the excellent prognosis of cutaneous CD30+ LPD in IC. The epidemiology and composition of cutaneous B-cell lymphomas (CBCL) in OTR differ from CBCL in IC. In OTR, B-cell lymphomas are often monomorphic and of large-cell morphology (centroblastic, immunoblastic and plasmablastic; fig. 12) [77]. The vast majority of them are associated with EBV, as shown by the presence of EBV RNA transcripts (EBER) detected by in situ hybridization [Seckin, in preparation].

Conclusions

OTR are at significantly increased risk to develop a wide variety of skin cancer. Since atypical clinical manifestations are not infrequent and accuracy of clinical diagnosis is limited, dermatopathological diagnosis plays a crucial role in the diagnostic workup of skin cancer in OTR, and may also provide prognostic data. Immunohistochemical and molecular studies shed light on the pathogenesis of skin cancers in OTR decoding the complex pathogenetic pathways involving oncogenic viruses, an impaired antitumoral host response and altered cellular pathways of apoptosis and proliferation.

References

1 Euvrard S, Kanitakis J, Pouteil-Noble C, Dureau G, Touraine JL, Faure M, Claudy A, Thivolet J: Comparative epidemiologic study of premalignant and malignant epithelial cutaneous lesions developing after kidney and heart transplantation. J Am Acad Dermatol 1995;33:222–229.

2 Jensen P, Hansen S, Moller B, Leivestad T, Pfeffer P, Geiran O, Fauchald P, Simonsen S: Skin cancer in kidney and heart transplant recipients and different long-term immunosuppressive therapy regimens. J Am Acad Dermatol 1999;40:177–186.

3 Euvrard S, Kanitakis J, Claudy A: Skin cancers after organ transplantation. N Engl J Med 2003;348: 1681–1691.

4 Cooper SM, Wojnarowska F: The accuracy of clinical diagnosis of suspected premalignant and malignant skin lesions in renal transplant recipients. Clin Exp Dermatol 2002;27:436–438.

5 Lindelöf B, Sigurgeirsson B, Gabel H, Stern RS: Incidence of skin cancer in 5356 patients following organ transplantation. Br J Dermatol 2000;143: 513–519.

6 Wisgerhof HC, van der Geest LG, de Fijter JW, Haasnoot GW, Claas FH, le Cessie S, Willemze R, Bouwes Bavinck JN: Incidence of cancer in kidney-transplant recipients: a long-term cohort study in a single center. Cancer Epidemiol 2011;35:105–111.

7 Harwood CA, McGregor JM, Swale VJ, Proby CM, Leigh IM, Newton R, Khorshid SM, Cerio R: High frequency and diversity of cutaneous appendageal tumors in organ transplant recipients. J Am Acad Dermatol 2003;48:401–408.

8 Lally A, Casabonne D, Waterboer T, Imko-Walczuk B, Michael KM, Pawlita M, Newton R, Wojnarowska F: Association of seborrhoeic warts with skin cancer in renal transplant recipients. J Eur Acad Dermatol Venereol 2010;24:302–307.

9 Weedon D, Morgan MB, Gross C, Nagore E, Yu LL: Squamous cell carcinoma; in Weedon D, LeBoit P, Burg G, Sarasin A: Pathology and Genetics. Skin Tumours. Lyon, IARC, 2006, pp 20–25.

10 Smith KJ, Hamza S, Skelton H: Histologic features in primary cutaneous squamous cell carcinomas in immunocompromised patients focusing on organ transplant patients. Dermatol Surg 2004;30:634–641.

11 Hoyo E, Kanitakis J, Euvrard S, Thivolet J: Proliferation characteristics of cutaneous squamous cell carcinomas developing in organ graft recipients. Comparison with squamous cell carcinomas of nonimmunocompromised hosts by counting argyrophilic proteins associated with nucleolar organizer regions. Arch Dermatol 1993;129:324–327.

12 Farasat S, Yu SS, Neel VA, Nehal KS, Lardaro T, Mihm MC, Byrd DR, Balch CM, Califano JA, Chuang AY, Sharfman WH, Shah JP, Nghiem P, Otley CC, Tufaro AP, Johnson TM, Sober AJ, Liegeois NJ: A new American Joint Committee on Cancer staging system for cutaneous squamous cell carcinoma: creation and rationale for inclusion of tumor (T) characteristics. J Am Acad Dermatol 2011;64:1051–1059.

13 Breuninger H, Black B, Rassner G: Microstaging of squamous cell carcinomas. Am J Clin Pathol 1990; 94:624–627.

14 Petter G, Haustein UF: Histologic subtyping and malignancy assessment of cutaneous squamous cell carcinoma. Dermatol Surg 2000;26:521–530.

15 Harwood CA, Proby CM, McGregor JM, Sheaff MT, Leigh IM, Cerio R: Clinicopathologic features of skin cancer in organ transplant recipients: a retrospective case-control series. J Am Acad Dermatol 2006;54:290–300.

16 Gibson GE, O'Grady A, Kay EW, Leader M, Murphy GM: p53 tumor suppressor gene protein expression in premalignant and malignant skin lesions of kidney transplant recipients. J Am Acad Dermatol 1997;36:924–931.

17 Mühleisen B, Petrov I, Gachter T, Kurrer M, Schaerer L, Dummer R, French LE, Hofbauer GF: Progression of cutaneous squamous cell carcinoma in immunosuppressed patients is associated with reduced CD123+ and FOXP3+ cells in the perineoplastic inflammatory infiltrate. Histopathology 2009;55: 67–76.

18 Bouwes Bavinck JN, Neale RE, Abeni D, Euvrard S, Green AC, Harwood CA, de Koning MN, Naldi L, Nindl I, Pawlita M, Pfister H, Proby CM, Quint WG, ter Schegget J, Waterboer T, Weissenborn S, Feltkamp MC: Multicenter study of the association between betapapillomavirus infection and cutaneous squamous cell carcinoma. Cancer Res 2010;70: 9777–9786.

19 Ternesten-Bratel A, Kjellstrom C, Wennberg AM, Ricksten A: Cutaneous squamoproliferative lesions in kidney transplant recipients: an investigation of specific Epstein-Barr virus expression. Acta Derm Venereol 2003;83:14–17.

20 Ulrich C, Kanitakis J, Stockfleth E, Euvrard S: Skin cancer in organ transplant recipients – where do we stand today? Am J Transplant 2008;8:2192–2198.

21 Hofbauer GF, Anliker M, Arnold A, Binet I, Hunger R, Kempf W, Laffitte E, Lapointe AC, Pascual M, Pelloni F, Serra A: Swiss clinical practice guidelines for skin cancer in organ transplant recipients. Swiss Med Wkly 2009;139:407–415.

22 O'Reilly Zwald F, Brown M: Skin cancer in solid organ transplant recipients: advances in therapy and management. II. Management of skin cancer in solid organ transplant recipients. J Am Acad Dermatol 2011;65:263–279.
23 Rival-Tringali AL, Euvrard S, Decullier E, Claudy A, Faure M, Kanitakis J: Conversion from calcineurin inhibitors to sirolimus reduces vascularization and thickness of post-transplant cutaneous squamous cell carcinomas. Anticancer Res 2009;29:1927–1932.
24 Smit JV, de Sevaux RG, Blokx WA, van de Kerkhof PC, Hoitsma AJ, de Jong EM: Acitretin treatment in (pre)malignant skin disorders of renal transplant recipients: histologic and immunohistochemical effects. J Am Acad Dermatol 2004;50:189–196.
25 Mertz KD, Proske D, Kettelhack N, Kegel C, Keusch G, Schwarz A, Ambühl PM, Pfaltz M, Kempf W: Basal cell carcinoma in a series of renal transplant recipients: epidemiology and clinicopathologic features. Int J Dermatol 2010;49:385–389.
26 Moloney FJ, Comber H, O'Lorcain P, O'Kelly P, Conlon PJ, Murphy GM: A population-based study of skin cancer incidence and prevalence in renal transplant recipients. Br J Dermatol 2006;154:498–504.
27 Kanitakis J, Alhaj-Ibrahim L, Euvrard S, Claudy A: Basal cell carcinomas developing in solid organ transplant recipients: clinicopathologic study of 176 cases. Arch Dermatol 2003;139:1133–1137.
28 Saldanha G, Fletcher A, Slater DN: Basal cell carcinoma: a dermatopathological and molecular biological update. Br J Dermatol 2003;148:195–202.
29 Kossard S, Epstein Jr EH, Cerio R, Yu LL, Weedon D: Basal cell carcinoma; in Weedon D, LeBoit P, Burg G, Sarasin A: Skin Tumours. Pathology and Genetics. WHO Classification of Tumours. Lyon, IARC, 2006, pp 13–19.
30 Ulrich M, Roewert-Huber J, Gonzalez S, Rius-Diaz F, Stockfleth E, Kanitakis J: Peritumoral clefting in basal cell carcinoma: correlation of in vivo reflectance confocal microscopy and routine histology. J Cutan Pathol 2011;38:190–195.
31 Mougel F, Kanitakis J, Faure M, Euvrard S: Basosquamous cell carcinoma in organ transplant patients: a clinicopathologic study. J Am Acad Dermatol, DOI: 10.1016/j.jaad.2010.1011.1045.
32 Buell JF, Trofe J, Hanaway MJ, Beebe TM, Gross TG, Alloway RR, First MR, Woodle ES: Immunosuppression and Merkel cell cancer. Transplant Proc 2002;34:1780–1781.
33 Koljonen V, Kukko H, Tukiainen E, Bohling T, Sankila R, Pukkala E, Sihto H, Joensuu H, Kyllonen L, Makisalo H: Incidence of Merkel cell carcinoma in renal transplant recipients. Nephrol Dial Transplant 2009;24:3231–3235.
34 Penn I, First MR: Merkel's cell carcinoma in organ recipients: report of 41 cases. Transplantation 1999; 68:1717–1721.
35 Heath M, Jaimes N, Lemos B, Mostaghimi A, Wang LC, Penas PF, Nghiem P: Clinical characteristics of Merkel cell carcinoma at diagnosis in 195 patients: the AEIOU features. J Am Acad Dermatol 2008;58: 375–381.
36 Kanitakis J, Euvrard S, Chouvet B, Butnaru AC, Claudy A: Merkel cell carcinoma in organ-transplant recipients: report of two cases with unusual histological features and literature review. J Cutan Pathol 2006;33:686–694.
37 D'Agostino M, Cinelli C, Willard R, Hofmann J, Jellinek N, Robinson-Bostom L: Epidermotropic Merkel cell carcinoma: a case series with histopathologic examination. J Am Acad Dermatol 2010; 62:463–468.
38 Vazmitel M, Michal M, Kempf W, Mukensnabl P, Kazakov DV: Merkel cell carcinoma with a follicular lymphocytic infiltrate: report of 2 cases. Am J Dermatopathol 2008;30:389–391.
39 Lemos BD, Storer BE, Iyer JG, Phillips JL, Bichakjian CK, Fang LC, Johnson TM, Liegeois-Kwon NJ, Otley CC, Paulson KG, Ross MI, Yu SS, Zeitouni NC, Byrd DR, Sondak VK, Gershenwald JE, Sober AJ, Nghiem P: Pathologic nodal evaluation improves prognostic accuracy in Merkel cell carcinoma: analysis of 5823 cases as the basis of the first consensus staging system. J Am Acad Dermatol 2010;63:751–761.
40 Feng H, Shuda M, Chang Y, Moore PS: Clonal integration of a polyomavirus in human Merkel cell carcinoma. Science 2008;319:1096–1100.
41 Duncavage EJ, Le BM, Wang D, Pfeifer JD: Merkel cell polyomavirus: a specific marker for Merkel cell carcinoma in histologically similar tumors. Am J Surg Pathol 2009;33:1771–1777.
42 Ridd K, Yu S, Bastian BC: The presence of polyomavirus in non-melanoma skin cancer in organ transplant recipients is rare. J Invest Dermatol 2009;129: 250–252.
43 Mertz KD, Pfaltz M, Junt T, Schmid M, Fernandez Figueras MT, Pfaltz K, Barghorn A, Kempf W: Merkel cell polyomavirus is present in common warts and carcinoma in situ of the skin. Hum Pathol 2010;41:1369–1379.

44 Mertz KD, Junt T, Schmid M, Pfaltz M, Kempf W: Inflammatory monocytes are a reservoir for Merkel cell polyomavirus. J Invest Dermatol 2010;130:1146–1151.

45 Rao P, Balzer BL, Lemos BD, Liegeois NJ, McNiff JM, Nghiem P, Prieto VG, Smith MT, Smoller BR, Wick MR, Frishberg DP: Protocol for the examination of specimens from patients with Merkel cell carcinoma of the skin. Arch Pathol Lab Med 2010;134:341–344.

46 Harwood CA, Swale VJ, Bataille VA, Quinn AG, Ghali L, Patel SV, Dove-Edwin I, Cerio R, McGregor JM: An association between sebaceous carcinoma and microsatellite instability in immunosuppressed organ transplant recipients. J Invest Dermatol 2001;116:246–253.

47 Kanitakis J, Euvrard S, Sebbag L, Claudy A: Trichilemmal carcinoma of the skin mimicking a keloid in a heart transplant recipient. J Heart Lung Transplant 2007;26:649–651.

48 Hollenbeak CS, Todd MM, Billingsley EM, Harper G, Dyer AM, Lengerich EJ: Increased incidence of melanoma in renal transplantation recipients. Cancer 2005;104:1962–1967.

49 Penn I: Malignant melanoma in organ allograft recipients. Transplantation 1996;61:274–278.

50 Brewer JD, Christenson LJ, Weaver AL, Dapprich DC, Weenig RH, Lim KK, Walsh JS, Otley CC, Cherikh W, Buell JF, Woodle ES, Arpey C, Patton PR: Malignant melanoma in solid transplant recipients: collection of database cases and comparison with surveillance, epidemiology, and end results data for outcome analysis. Arch Dermatol 2011;147:790–796.

51 Kasiske BL, Snyder JJ, Gilbertson DT, Wang C: Cancer after kidney transplantation in the United States. Am J Transplant 2004;4:905–913.

52 Le Mire L, Hollowood K, Gray D, Bordea C, Wojnarowska F: Melanomas in renal transplant recipients. Br J Dermatol 2006;154:472–477.

53 Matin RN, Mesher D, Proby CM, McGregor JM, Bouwes Bavinck JN, del Marmol V, Euvrard S, Ferrandiz C, Geusau A, Hackethal M, Ho WL, Hofbauer GF, Imko-Walczuk B, Kanitakis J, Lally A, Lear JT, Lebbe C, Murphy GM, Piaserico S, Seckin D, Stockfleth E, Ulrich C, Wojnarowska FT, Lin HY, Balch C, Harwood CA: Melanoma in organ transplant recipients: clinicopathological features and outcome in 100 cases. Am J Transplant 2008;8:1891–1900.

54 Kanitakis J, Baldassini S, Lora V, Euvrard S: BRAF mutations in melanocytic tumors (nevi and melanomas) from organ transplant recipients. Eur J Dermatol 2010;20:167–171.

55 Pedagogos E, Nicholls K, Dowling J, Becker G: Kaposi's sarcoma post renal transplantation. Aust N Z J Med 1994;24:722–723.

56 Penn I: Cancers in renal transplant recipients. Adv Ren Replace Ther 2000;7:147–156.

57 Montagnino G, Bencini PL, Tarantino A, Caputo R, Ponticelli C: Clinical features and course of Kaposi's sarcoma in kidney transplant patients: report of 13 cases. Am J Nephrol 1994;14:121–126.

58 Frances C: Kaposi's sarcoma after renal transplantation. Nephrol Dial Transplant 1998;13:2768–2773.

59 Dreno B: Skin cancers after transplantation. Nephrol Dial Transplant 2003;18:1052–1058.

60 Frances C, Marcelin AG, Legendre C, Chevret S, Dussaix E, Lejeune J, Euvrard S, Bigorie A, Schulz TF, Agbalika F, Lebbe C: The impact of preexisting or acquired Kaposi sarcoma herpesvirus infection in kidney transplant recipients on morbidity and survival. Am J Transplant 2009;9:2580–2586.

61 Kempf W, Cathomas G, Burg G, Trüeb RM: Micronodular Kaposi's sarcoma – a new variant of classic-sporadic Kaposi's sarcoma. Dermatology 2004;208:255–258.

62 Grayson W, Pantanowitz L: Histological variants of cutaneous Kaposi sarcoma. Diagn Pathol 2008;3:31.

63 Kazakov DV, Prinz BM, Michaelis S, Schmid M, Müller B, Adams V, Burg G, Kempf W: Study of HHV-8 DNA sequences in archival biopsies from lesional skin of Kaposi's sarcoma, various mesenchymal tumors and related reactive conditions. J Cutan Pathol 2002;29:279–281.

64 Robin YM, Guillou L, Michels JJ, Coindre JM: Human herpesvirus 8 immunostaining: a sensitive and specific method for diagnosing Kaposi sarcoma in paraffin-embedded sections. Am J Clin Pathol 2004;121:330–334.

65 Antman K, Chang Y: Kaposi's sarcoma. N Engl J Med 2000;342:1027–1038.

66 Woodle ES, Hanaway M, Buell J, Gross T, First MR, Trofe J, Beebe T: Kaposi sarcoma: an analysis of the US and international experiences from the Israel Penn International Transplant Tumor Registry. Transplant Proc 2001;33:3660–3661.

67 Euvrard S, Kanitakis J, Bosshard S, Lebbe C, Garnier JL, Touraine JL, Claudy A: No recurrence of post-transplantation Kaposi's sarcoma three years after renal retransplantation. Transplantation 2002;73:297–299.

68 Brooks JJ: Kaposi's sarcoma: a reversible hyperplasia. Lancet 1986;2:1309–1311.

69 Hofbauer GF, Bouwes Bavinck JN, Euvrard S: Organ transplantation and skin cancer: basic problems and new perspectives. Exp Dermatol 2010;19:473–482.

70 Mitsuyasu RT: Update on the pathogenesis and treatment of Kaposi sarcoma. Curr Opin Oncol 2000;12:174–180.
71 Prinz BM, Hofbauer GF, Dummer R, French LE, Kempf W: Topical treatment of cutaneous Kaposi sarcoma with imiquimod 5% in renal transplant recipients – a clinico-pathological observation. Clin Exp Dermatol 2011, in press.
72 Penn I: Sarcomas in organ allograft recipients. Transplantation 1995;60:1485–1491.
73 Kanitakis J, Euvrard S, Montazeri A, Garnier JL, Faure M, Claudy A: Atypical fibroxanthoma in a renal graft recipient. J Am Acad Dermatol 1996;35: 262–264.
74 Hafner J, Kunzi W, Weinreich T: Malignant fibrous histiocytoma and atypical fibroxanthoma in renal transplant recipients. Dermatology 1999;198:29–32.
75 Kovach BT, Sams HH, Stasko T: Multiple atypical fibroxanthomas in a cardiac transplant recipient. Dermatol Surg 2005;31:467–470.
76 Swerdlow SH, Webber SA, Chadburn A, Ferry JA: Post-transplant lymphoproliferative disorders; in Swerdlow SH, Campo E, Harris NL, et al (eds): WHO Classification of Tumours of Haematopoietic and Lymphoid Tissues. Lyon, IARC, 2008, pp 343–349.
77 Beynet DP, Wee SA, Horwitz SS, Kohler S, Horning S, Hoppe R, Kim YH: Clinical and pathological features of posttransplantation lymphoproliferative disorders presenting with skin involvement in 4 patients. Arch Dermatol 2004;140:1140–1146.
78 Yurtsever H, Kempf W, Laeng RH: Posttransplant CD30+ anaplastic large cell lymphoma with skin and lymph node involvement. Dermatology 2003; 207:107–110.
79 Kempf W, Sander CA: Classification of cutaneous lymphomas – an update. Histopathology 2010;56: 57–70.

Werner Kempf, MD
Kempf and Pfaltz Histological Diagnostics
Seminarstrasse 1
CH–8042 Zürich (Switzerland)
Tel. +41 44 233 33 77, E-Mail kempf@kempf-pfaltz.ch

Häusermann P, Steiger J, Passweg J (eds): Transplantation Dermatology.
Curr Probl Dermatol. Basel, Karger, 2012, vol 43, pp 36–48

Immunosuppressive Drugs in Organ Transplant Recipients – Rationale for Critical Selection

Fabien Stucker[a] · Hans-Peter Marti[a] · Robert E. Hunger[b]

Departments of [a]Nephrology and [b]Dermatology, Inselspital, Berne University Hospital and University of Bern, Bern, Switzerland

Abstract

Transplantation is the treatment of choice for many different organ failures. Despite growing experience in surgery and immunosuppression protocols, the long-term mortality of the procedure remains much higher than in the general population. Second only to cardiovascular diseases as the cause of death in organ transplant recipients, cancer is now known to be at least partly related to the immunosuppression regimen. Nevertheless, if calcineurin inhibitors have a demonstrated pro-oncogenic effect, other classes, such as mTOR inhibitors, are antiproliferative, and even demonstrated as an efficient therapy in some advanced oncological situations. Therefore, the adaptation of the therapy protocol evolves now towards an individualized medicine based on the risk factors of each transplant recipient in terms of cardiovascular, infectious and oncological diseases. As the first organ involved by tumor is the skin, many different guidelines have been published to try and adapt the therapy to the occurrence of a new lesion. If, for example, limited actinic keratosis or the first episode of a non-melanoma skin cancer usually requires no change of the immunosuppressive therapy, but a local specialized care and frequent clinical controls, more advanced lesions imply the adaptation of the drug regimen. In any case, the collaboration between general practitioners, dermatologists and the transplantation team is mandatory.

Thanks to improving immunosuppression protocols, better surgical techniques and the availability of an increasing number of drugs, the outcome of transplantation has greatly improved in the past few decades; moreover, due to an increased number of transplantations per year (partly due to extended donor criteria), there is today more than 160,000 patients in the United States living with a transplanted organ compared with 120,000 10 years ago (ustransplant.org), and this tendency seems to grow in a similar way in Europe. This increase comes with a heavy burden: heart and vascular diseases, increased infection rates, and the higher incidence of different tumors, the first organ involved being the skin.

A Norwegian survey studied more than 2,500 transplant patients, and found a 65-fold increase in cutaneous squamous cell carcinoma (SCC), an 84-fold increase in Kaposi sarcoma, and a 3-fold increase in melanoma compared with the general population [1]. The duration of the immunosuppressive therapy seems to be decisive in the occurrence of non-melanoma skin cancer, ranging from 29.1% in the first 5 years after transplantation to 52.2% at 10 years and 82.1% of those immunosuppressed for more 20 years [2]. Compared with this Australian study, the occurrence was found to increase in a Dutch population from 10% after 10 years to 40% after 20 years of graft survival, indicating that the UV exposure also plays a significant role in the pathogenesis of skin cancer [3].

Besides the UV, the type of immunosuppressive medications is also decisive due to very different side effect profiles, including an oncogenic effect, leading to the concept of an individualized medicine, with the adaptation of the drug regimen to the immunologic and health risk profile of each patient. We will therefore review the different medications currently available, their mechanisms and side effects.

General Principles of Immunosuppression

The aim of immunosuppression is the prevention of acute and chronic allograft rejection. As this reaction is mediated through lymphocytes, immunosuppression acts by their depletion, by blocking their action, or inhibiting their proliferation.

The activation of T lymphocytes follows at least two signals: the T-cell receptor recognizes a foreign antigen presented by an antigen-presenting cell (APC), which stimulates a phosphorylation cascade, resulting in an increase in the intracellular calcium [4]. The calmodulin, loaded with calcium, stimulates the calcineurin, which in turn induces the translocation of the NFAT (nuclear factor of activated T cell) [5] to the nucleus. The NFAT is a transcription factor increasing the production of the interleukin-2, which stimulates lymphocyte proliferation. This cascade only works if a second signal, a 'costimulation', occurs. And this occurs through the binding of an APC surface protein called B7 to another T lymphocyte surface receptor called CD-28 [6]. The immunosuppressive drugs act on these different pathways, blocking the lymphocyte activation and proliferation. The molecular mechanism of action of the most important immunosuppressive drugs is schematically shown in figure 1.

As the risk of allograft rejection is highest directly after the transplantation and decreases over time, the intensity of immunosuppression is also maximal at the beginning. The typical immunosuppressive regimen therefore includes an induction phase, followed by a maintenance phase (http://tts.org/kdigo/downloads/kdigo/KDIGO_KidneyTxGuideline.pdf.).

The induction phase includes antibodies blocking T cell activation and a conventional immunosuppressive therapy, associating frequently a calcineurin inhibitor, mycophenolate mofetil and corticosteroids. The antibodies have been classified into

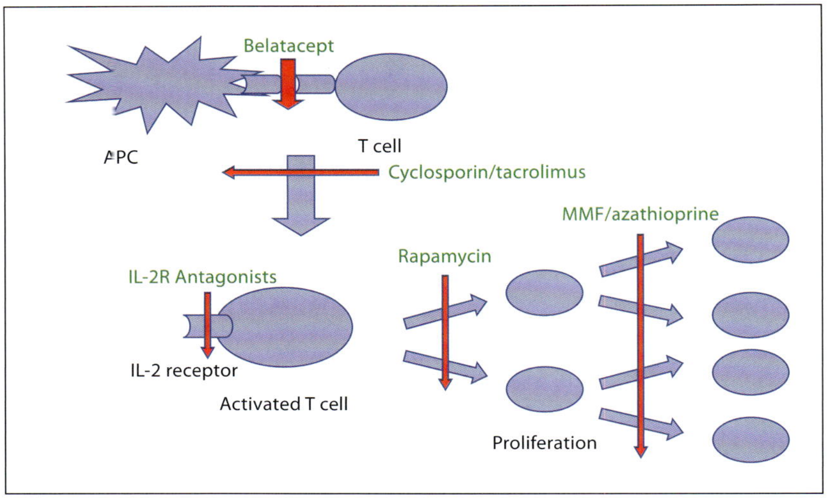

Fig. 1. Immunosuppressive drugs and their mode of action. MMF = Mycophenolate mofetil.

depleting, which destroy T or B lymphocytes, or both, and nondepleting, which block the activation of the immune system, by interacting mainly with the IL-2 receptor, the cornerstone of lymphocyte proliferation.

After this first phase, the aim of the maintenance therapy is to give an amount of immunosuppression sufficient to prevent rejection and allograft dysfunction, and associated with the lowest possible toxicity. It is mostly done by associating 2–3 drugs (depending on the association with steroids) with combinations like calcineurin inhibitors-mycophenolate, calcineurin inhibitor-mTOR inhibitors or mTOR inhibitors-mycophenolate.

Actually, despite improvement in the general management of transplant recipients, the mortality rate remains higher than in the general population. Cardiovascular diseases represent the first cause of death after transplantation. Their high occurrence derives partly from vascular damages already present before the transplantation (because of the common risk factors between kidney and cardiovascular diseases, for example hypertension, diabetes, hyperlipidemia and smoking, and because renal failure per se increases the vessel damage) and partly because of the negative effect of the immunosuppressive therapy on the metabolic disturbances [7].

Neoplasms are currently the second cause of mortality. There is now some convincing evidence confirming a 3- to 5-fold increase of the overall cancer evidence after transplantation [8]. The commonest neoplasms after transplantation involve the skin, and squamous- and basal-cell carcinomas account for more than 90% of all skin cancers.

Even if the rate of infectious complications in solid organ recipients [9] has declined rapidly, infections remain the third cause of death after transplantation. During the

1980s, about 60% of the patients developed a severe infection during the first year after transplantation, half of whom died consecutively. Thanks to new antibiotics and prevention strategies, the mortality has decreased today to about 5%. Nevertheless, urinary tract, pulmonary and cutaneous infections caused by bacteria, virus and fungi remain frequent complications associated with immune suppression, causing a significant burden to the transplant patient.

Individual Immunosuppressive Agents

Glucocorticoids

Their binding with their intracellular receptor leads to the translocation of the complex to the nucleus, where they interact with different transcriptional factors (for example NF-κB); this inhibits the production of many proinflammatory cytokines, including IL-2, inhibiting lymphocyte proliferation and inducing apoptosis.

This pleotropic effect induces a number of systemic side effects involving the cardiovascular system (hypertension, impaired glucose tolerance, hyperlipidemia, increased water and salt retention), the immune system (increased infection risk), the bone (osteoporosis), the eyes (cataract), the muscle (myopathy), the stomach (GI bleeding), the neurological system (agitation, psychosis) and the skin.

The cutaneous side effects include impaired wound healing, ulcers, striae, acne, fragile skin, atrophy, telangiectasia, hirsutism, increased number of skin infections and tumors. A Swedish study found that a higher corticosteroids dose led to a 2- to 4-fold increase in the incidence of cutaneous SCCs [10].

If the glucocorticoids remain the cornerstone of the treatment of an acute rejection, and an important piece of the maintenance therapy, many trials have tried recently to evaluate the safety of glucocorticoid withdrawal or minimizing shortly after transplantation. A prospective randomized study found no difference at 5 years in a composite primary end point of death, graft loss and moderate/severe rejection in a population comparing early (< 1 week) steroid withdrawal and a slow tapering until 5 mg per day at 6 months after transplantation. An increased number of mild rejections were observed, leading to a debate about the long-term risk of allograft dysfunction [11]. Studies are being currently conducted to assess the safety of this protocol.

Calcineurin Inhibitors

They are composed of cyclosporine A (CyA) and tacrolimus. CyA binds to cyclophilin, which is an intracellular protein, and this complex binds to calcineurin and inhibits the translocation of NFAT to the nucleus and therefore inhibits T lymphocyte proliferation. Tacrolimus is a macrolide which binds to the FK506-binding protein (FK506 being the study name of tacrolimus), and blocks the calcineurin function.

The discovery of cyclosporine and its use in organ transplantation has led to a considerable increase in the success of the procedure in the 1980s, by drastically reducing the occurrence of acute allograft rejection. Nevertheless, the long-term use of calcineurin inhibitors has a dramatic down side on the kidney, leading to a chronic vasoconstriction state through an increased production of thromboxane A2, and to an interstitial fibrosis with a hyaline arteriopathy and a focal and segmental glomerulosclerosis through an elevated production of TGF-β and other chemokines [12].

The other side effects of cyclosporine include hypertension, tremor, gingival hyperplasia and an increased incidence of infection and neoplasms. Hypertrichosis is an uncommon side effect of cyclosporine, but with cosmetic consequences, making it sometimes necessary to switch the drug to tacrolimus, which causes alopecia. Gingival hyperplasia is a dose- and time-dependent side effect affecting mostly people with bad mouth hygiene. It regresses under local therapy and drug withdrawal. As it is also a side effect of the calcium antagonists, a class of antihypertensive drug, their association is not recommended in the at-risk patients.

Several studies have demonstrated the association between calcineurin inhibitors and cancer [13]. Several mechanisms have been implicated in this pro-oncogenic effect, including the IL-2 and lymphocyte response suppression, TGF-β stimulation, VEGF and angiogenesis stimulation [14], and IL-6 increase, in particular in lymphoproliferative disorders [15].

The actual trend is therefore to minimize calcineurin inhibitor exposure to prevent the renal and systemic toxicity and to switch to another medication class (mainly mTOR inhibitors) in the presence of a neoplasm.

Azathioprine

Azathioprine is a prodrug, which needs to be metabolized into 6-mercaptopurin to block the DNA synthesis, and inhibit lymphocyte proliferation. The drug is afterwards metabolized through the xanthine oxidase. This metabolic pathway is of great clinical relevance, because this enzyme is blocked by a very frequently prescribed medication, allopurinol, and this blockage can lead to the accumulation of 6-mercaptopurin, leading to an acute toxicity.

Azathioprine has been used in association with cyclosporine in the transplantation scope, until mycophenolate mofetil was found to be superior in preventing acute rejection in renal transplantation [16].

Its side effects include nausea, pancytopenia, increased risk of developing an infection, and, mainly, various skin adverse effects ranging from warts to skin cancer. In the Swedish study cited earlier, transplant recipients under azathioprine had a 3- to 6-fold, dose-dependent, increased risk of developing an SCC, compared to transplant patients under another immunosuppressive regimen [10]. It has also been reported before that the patients having the highest risk were those who reported the highest

UV exposure [17]. It is now considered that both impaired DNA repairing capacity and increased DNA damages play an important role in the pathogenic mechanisms.

If UVB are considered to be mostly responsible for the development of skin lesions due to the higher amount of energy they are carrying, it has been described that azathioprine interacts with the UVA, inducing photosensitization and increasing DNA damage [18].

Mycophenolate Mofetil

Mycophenolate is a potent selective and reversible inhibitor of inosine monophosphate dehydrogenase, an enzyme allowing the production of guanosine monophosphate, a purine necessary for lymphocytes proliferation. Its efficacy has been demonstrated both in preventing acute rejection in transplant patients, and in the treatment of lupus nephritis through remission induction and relapse prevention, becoming therefore a commonly used drug in the field of nephrology. Other indications include myasthenia gravis and psoriasis. Its tolerance depends highly on the gastrointestinal side effects, ranging from bloating and flatulence, to diarrhea. It is available on the market either in the form of a prodrug, mycophenolate mofetil (Cellcept™) or in the form of the already active, and enteric-coated, mycophenolic acid (Myfortic™). If both formulations have the same clinical efficacy, the switch from one to the other is frequently tried to improve the intestinal tolerance. Other side effects include pancytopenia, and an increased infection risk.

The role that mycophenolate plays in the carcinogenesis is debated: if mycophenolic acid has shown to have antiproliferative and apoptotic effects in vitro and in vivo [19], and to be associated with a lower incidence of malignancies in heart-transplanted patients compared to other drug regimen [20], an increased incidence of Kaposi sarcoma following the introduction of mycophenolate mofetil in the immunosuppressive regimen of a renal transplant center raised the question of the role that the drug might play in oncogenesis [21]. But as the Kaposi sarcoma is an HHV-8-related neoplasia, it may also be argued that this higher incidence is more due to the well-described higher susceptibility to the virus-mediated diseases (including CMV) under mycophenolate, than a real pro-oncogenic effect. Until definitive answer comes, caution with the use in patients suffering from malignancy is advised.

mTOR Inhibitors

The mTOR (or mammalian target of rapamycin) inhibitor family is composed of different drugs including sirolimus (or rapamycin), temsirolimus and everolimus. Rapamycin is an antibiotic produced by *Streptomyces hygroscopicus*, a bacterium sharing many characteristics with the fungi, discovered on the island of Rapa Nui, also known as Easter Island. Everolimus is characterized by a shorter half-life than sirolimus (28 vs. 62 h). Both drugs enter the cytoplasm and bind to the FKBP (also implicated in the mechanism of action of tacrolimus), and this newly formed complex blocks the mTOR action, and modulates IL-2 secretion, which blocks lymphocyte proliferation. This action is ubiquitous, blocking the proliferation of many different cell types, resulting for example in postoperative poor wound healing or an important teratogenicity in pregnant women. Both drugs can have direct kidney toxicity, resulting in a proteinuria both through glomerular and tubular damage [22, 23]. Both drugs are also implicated in acute lung toxicity. They can induce severe hypercholesterolemia and acne.

Enthusiasm has nevertheless risen from to benefits of these new drugs over calcineurin inhibitors regarding their lower long-term kidney toxicity and their antitumoral effect.

This was best demonstrated in the advanced renal cell carcinoma, in which a treatment with high-dose everolimus improved progression-free survival [24]. Moreover, the incidence of de novo malignancies was found to be reduced in an analysis of a large kidney transplant registry under an immunosuppressive therapy with mTOR inhibitors compared with calcineurin inhibitors (0.6 vs. 1.81%). Of special interest is the fact that under a combined therapy composed of an mTOR inhibitor plus a calcineurin inhibitor, the incidence was equally low (0.6%) arguing for a protective effect of the mTOR inhibition on the oncogenesis [25]. The conversion from calcineurin inhibitors to sirolimus in the CONVERT trial was also associated with a significant lower incidence of total malignancies and skin carcinoma at 24 months. A significant increase in many other side effects under sirolimus, including aphthous stomatitis, acne, skin rash, peripheral edema, hyperlipidemia and pneumonia was also noted in the same trial [26]. It has been demonstrated in vivo that one of the possible mechanisms for this antioncogenic effect is a downregulation of the VEGF and TGF-β production [27]. This effect is to be balanced with a higher incidence of acute rejection following early conversion or direct posttransplantation treatment [28]. It is now heavily discussed if and when a conversion from calcineurin inhibitors to mTOR would be mostly beneficial in terms of kidney toxicity and cancer incidence, without endangering the transplanted organ by an increase in acute rejection.

Monoclonal and Polyclonal Anti-T Cell Antibodies

The concept of rapidly blocking or depleting the lymphocytes after an organ transplantation has gained much interest, and has been demonstrated to efficiently lower the incidence of an acute graft rejection [29]. The antibodies work through different mechanisms: either by depleting lymphocytes (OKT3, thymoglobulin, rituximab) or blocking the proliferation (anti-IL-2 receptors).

Among the depleting antibodies, if OKT3 (a mouse antibody binding to the CD3 antigen of the T-lymphocytes) is now very rarely used due to a significant toxicity (fever, lung edema), the thymoglobulins (ATG), which are animal polyclonal antibodies aiming T lymphocytes, are still used in specific immunological constellations and relapsing cellular rejections and rituximab, an anti-CD20 antibody, has become the cornerstone of the management of highly sensitized patients and of humoral rejections.

If these therapies have been reserved for specific situations, the non-depleting enzymes, which have a very favorable safety profile, are now used in almost every kidney transplantation and act by binding to the α-chain of the IL-2 receptor, blocking the lymphocyte proliferation. If the treatment with an anti-IL-2 antibody is not associated with the development of malignancies, on the contrary the OKT3 and ATG were found to be associated with a greater risk of PTLD [30].

Costimulation Blockade

Belatacept is a fusion protein composed of the Fc-part of the human immunoglobulin IgG1 and from CTLA-4, a molecule resembling CD28. This protein blocks the costimulation (see 'General Principles of Immunosuppression'), blocking the activation of T lymphocytes. This medication is now available for the induction and maintenance therapy, and has the huge advantage that it can be administrated intravenously only once a month, improving therefore patient's compliance. In a study comparing two belatacept regimens with cyclosporin in kidney transplantation, it has been shown that belatacept had significantly fewer side effects than calcineurin inhibitors, and that the kidney function one year after kidney transplantation was significantly improved by this medication. It also had a better cardiovascular safety profile, in terms of blood pressure, glucose intolerance and dyslipidemia. The concern regards the increased incidence of biopsy-proven acute rejections, and an unexpectedly high number of posttransplantation lymphoproliferative disorders, an especially aggressive type of lymphoma occurring in transplant patients, in the belatacept-treated patients [31, 32]. This peculiar type of lymphoma is closely linked to EBV infection, which is clinically relevant mostly in patients who were not previously immunized (EBV serology IgG negative). The incidence of PTLD in the belatacept study was mostly high in patients who were EBV negative (i.e. not immunized) before the transplantation, which makes this drug highly inappropriate in this population.

The 2-year results of this study have been recently published, and confirm the better kidney function [33].

The general incidence of malignancy, including skin cancers, was similar in the belatacept 'less intensive' group and in the group treated with calcineurin inhibitor. A higher dose of belatacept seems nevertheless to be associated with more neoplasms.

Rationale for Selection with Respect to Occurrence of Skin Lesions

There is for the time being no perfect drug combination. The choice of the best immunosuppressive regimen has to be adapted to each patient, depending of his/her immunological risk of developing an acute rejection, and the occurrence of cardiovascular, infectious or neoplastic side effects.

The occurrence of severe drug-related side effects, for example a creatinine rise with biopsy-proven signs of calcineurin inhibitor toxicity, warrants usually a switch to another immunosuppressant. The apparition of a pneumonitis in a patient under sirolimus, with a bronchoalveolar lavage excluding an infection and evocating a sirolimus toxicity also requires the immediate stopping of the drug.

Other reasons to undergo a drug change are recurrent infections, or appearance of hematological disorders (for example neutropenia under mycophenolate) or cosmetic issues, like hypertrichosis or gingival hyperplasia under cyclosporine.

As mTOR inhibitors are antiproliferative, any transplant recipient who has to undergo a major surgery is usually switched to calcineurin inhibitors, to favor postoperative scar healing.

But one of the most important situations in which a change is required is the occurrence of a malignancy: as there are now many lines of evidence that calcineurin inhibitors are pro-oncogenic, and mTOR inhibitors antiproliferative, the apparition of a neoplasm encourages either a reduction or a switch of the immunosuppressive drugs.

As 50% of kidney transplant patients develop some kind of skin cancer, and about 5% of them die of their neoplasm, different guidelines have been published recently to help the clinicians deal with the immunosuppression in skin cancer [34, 35].

It seems already important before the transplantation to establish the 'risk profile' of each patient, depending on his/her skin type (Fitzpatrick classification), his/her immunosuppression status (for example HIV) and the presence of infectious or neoplastic lesion, which have to be treated prior to the transplantation. After immunosuppression, UV exposure is the second greatest risk factor, and the first easily avoidable. Careful and comprehensive information about UV protection through appropriate closing, regular sunscreen application and avoidance of sun exposure is therefore of great interest. A specialized monitoring in a dermatological clinic has been shown to provide higher UV awareness than previously reported [36]. A yearly control by a dermatologist and regular self-examinations should also be encouraged.

Actinic Keratosis and Non-Melanoma Skin Cancer

The prevention of development of more invasive tumors relies on early recognition and frequent monitoring of the actinic keratosis lesions. Local non-surgical therapy is recommended, and avoidance of radiotherapy to prevent further DNA damages is mandatory. Most experts agree that a switch of immunosuppressant at this stage is not necessary [34].

The first occurrence of a squamous cell carcinoma is usually best treated by an early surgical removal, and followed by very frequent clinical controls. A reduction in the immunosuppression to prevent relapse and help healing outweighs the risk of acute rejections only in the very aggressive forms of SCC.

By relapsing skin viral infections and any moderate or severe skin carcinogenesis, the avoidance of azathioprine is to be recommended and to be replaced by mycophenolate mofetil, which is associated with a lower rate of both acute rejections and dermatological complications.

By good graft function, no history of acute rejections and the absence of contraindications (moderate to severe proteinuria, previous episode of pneumonitis under mTOR inhibitors), a progressive switch from calcineurin inhibitors to mTOR inhibitors is generally safe and effective and can be recommended in these situations.

A patient suffering from a chronic graft dysfunction without proven chronic rejection in the case of aggressive forms of SCC can also benefit from this switch.

In the more complex situations associating graft rejections and several neoplastic relapses, a reduction in calcineurin inhibitor blood levels, and the association of low-dose mTOR inhibitors while maintaining the other immunosuppressants may be discussed.

Malignant Melanoma

Contradictory results have been published about the occurrence of malignant melanoma after solid organ transplantation, and it is still not clear if its favored by immunosuppression. Two recent studies analyzing the outcome of melanoma patients under immunosuppression found no difference for patients with early melanoma (Breslow level <2 mm). For thicker melanoma, however, the authors of one study reported a worse outcome for patients under immunosuppression [37], whereas the authors of another study found no difference for high-risk melanoma [38]. Nevertheless, as it is known that melanoma can be more aggressive in other classes of immunosuppressed patients, for example HIV patients [39], we would encourage a clear reduction in the immunosuppressive therapy in subjects with metastatic melanoma.

Currently, there is no hard clinical evidence to switch or to reduce an immunosuppressive regimen in the presence of a malignant melanoma. However, on the experimental level [40] and for instance based on a recently published early phase 2 trial [41], there is growing evidence that mTOR inhibitors show a favorable effect on the progression of melanoma. Therefore, along with the reduction in immunosuppression, the use of an mTOR inhibitor in patients with melanoma can be considered or even advocated.

Kaposi Sarcoma

This neoplasm occurs 400–500 times more often in solid organ transplant recipients than in the general population [42] and is related to HHV-8 reactivation. Conversion to sirolimus [43] and reduction in immunosuppression [44] have both been described as efficient in these situations, but leading sometimes to allograft loss due to rejection. Careful switch or reduction in therapy is therefore recommended in those cases.

Other Types of Cancer

Other rare types of cancer including Merkel cell carcinoma have been described in transplant recipients. As they seem to occur more commonly and behave in a more aggressive way, adaptation of the immunosuppressive therapy may be required.

Conclusions

The better outcome of transplant recipients has led to an increase in drug-related complications including cardiovascular diseases, recurrent infections and malignancies, among others.

Skin-related side effects are also frequent, making the prevention through patient information, sun avoidance strategies and regular specialized controls mandatory. If a skin lesion appears, its early recognition and a narrow collaboration between dermatologists, general practitioners and the transplantation team is necessary to establish a treatment plan to treat the current lesion and prevent the apparition of others.

References

1 Jensen P, Hansen S, Moller B, Leivestad T, Pfeffer P, Geiran O, Fauchald P, Simonsen S: Skin cancer in kidney and heart transplant recipients and different long-term immunosuppressive therapy regimens. J Am Acad Dermatol 1999;40:177–186.

2 Ramsay HM, Fryer AA, Hawley CM, Smith AG, Harden PN: Non-melanoma skin cancer risk in the Queensland renal transplant population. Br J Dermatol 2002;147:950–956.

3 Hartevelt MM, Bavinck JN, Kootte AM, Vermeer BJ, Vandenbroucke JP: Incidence of skin cancer after renal transplantation in the Netherlands. Transplantation 1990;49:506–509.

4 Nel AE, Slaughter N: T-cell activation through the antigen receptor. 2. Role of signaling cascades in T-cell differentiation, anergy, immune senescence, and development of immunotherapy. J Allergy Clin Immunol 2002;109:901–915.

5 Wesselborg S, Fruman DA, Sagoo JK, Bierer BE, Burakoff SJ: Identification of a physical interaction between calcineurin and nuclear factor of activated T cells (NFATP). J Biol Chem 1996;271:1274–1277.

6 Felix NJ, Suri A, Salter-Cid L, Nadler SG, Gujrathi S, Corbo M, Aranda R: Targeting lymphocyte co-stimulation: from bench to bedside. Autoimmunity 2010;43:514–525.

7 Marcen R: Immunosuppressive drugs in kidney transplantation: impact on patient survival, and incidence of cardiovascular disease, malignancy and infection. Drugs 2009;69:2227–2243.

8 Wong G, Chapman JR: Cancers after renal transplantation. Transplant Rev (Orlando) 2008;22:141–149.

9 Simon DM, Levin S: Infectious complications of solid organ transplantations. Infect Dis Clin North Am 2001;15:521–549.

10 Ingvar A, Smedby KE, Lindelof B, Fernberg P, Bellocco R, Tufveson G, Hoglund P, Adami J: Immunosuppressive treatment after solid organ transplantation and risk of post-transplant cutaneous squamous cell carcinoma. Nephrol Dial Transplant 2010;25:2764–2771.

11 Woodle ES, First MR, Pirsch J, Shihab F, Gaber AO, Van Veldhuisen P: A prospective, randomized, double-blind, placebo-controlled multicenter trial comparing early (7 day) corticosteroid cessation versus long-term, low-dose corticosteroid therapy. Ann Surg 2008;248:564–577.

12 Vitko S, Viklicky O: Cyclosporine renal dysfunction. Transplant Proc 2004;36:243S–247S.

13 Doesch AO, Muller S, Konstandin M, Celik S, Kristen A, Frankenstein L, Ehlermann P, Sack FU, Katus HA, Dengler TJ: Malignancies after heart transplantation: incidence, risk factors, and effects of calcineurin inhibitor withdrawal. Transplant Proc 2010;42:3694–3699.
14 Guba M, von Breitenbuch P, Steinbauer M, Koehl G, Flegel S, Hornung M, Bruns CJ, Zuelke C, Farkas S, Anthuber M, Jauch KW, Geissler EK: Rapamycin inhibits primary and metastatic tumor growth by antiangiogenesis: involvement of vascular endothelial growth factor. Nat Med 2002;8:128–135.
15 Tanner JE, Menezes J: Interleukin-6 and Epstein-Barr virus induction by cyclosporine A: potential role in lymphoproliferative disease. Blood 1994;84: 3956–3964.
16 A blinded, randomized clinical trial of mycophenolate mofetil for the prevention of acute rejection in cadaveric renal transplantation. The Tricontinental Mycophenolate Mofetil Renal Transplantation Study Group. Transplantation 1996;61:1029–1037.
17 Bottomley WW, Ford G, Cunliffe WJ, Cotterill JA: Aggressive squamous cell carcinomas developing in patients receiving long-term azathioprine. Br J Dermatol 1995;133:460–462.
18 O'Donovan P, Perrett CM, Zhang X, Montaner B, Xu YZ, Harwood CA, McGregor JM, Walker SL, Hanaoka F, Karran P: Azathioprine and UVA light generate mutagenic oxidative DNA damage. Science 2005;309:1871–1874.
19 Vegso G, Sebestyen A, Paku S, Barna G, Hajdu M, Toth M, Jaray J, Kopper L: Antiproliferative and apoptotic effects of mycophenolic acid in human B-cell non-Hodgkin lymphomas. Leuk Res 2007;31: 1003–1008.
20 O'Neill JO, Edwards LB, Taylor DO: Mycophenolate mofetil and risk of developing malignancy after orthotopic heart transplantation: analysis of the transplant registry of the International Society for Heart and Lung Transplantation. J Heart Lung Transplant 2006;25:1186–1191.
21 Eberhard OK, Kliem V, Brunkhorst R: Five cases of Kaposi's sarcoma in kidney graft recipients: possible influence of the immunosuppressive therapy. Transplantation 1999;67:180–184.
22 Cai Y, Chen Y, Zheng S, Chen B, Yang Y, Xia P: Sirolimus damages podocytes in rats with protein overload nephropathy. J Nephrol 2011;24:307–312.
23 Straathof-Galema L, Wetzels JF, Dijkman HB, Steenbergen EJ, Hilbrands LB: Sirolimus-associated heavy proteinuria in a renal transplant recipient: evidence for a tubular mechanism. Am J Transplant 2006;6:429–433.
24 Motzer RJ, Escudier B, Oudard S, Hutson TE, Porta C, Bracarda S, Grunwald V, Thompson JA, Figlin RA, Hollaender N, Urbanowitz G, Berg WJ, Kay A, Lebwohl D, Ravaud A: Efficacy of everolimus in advanced renal cell carcinoma: a double-blind, randomised, placebo-controlled phase III trial. Lancet 2008;372:449–456.
25 Kauffman HM, Cherikh WS, Cheng Y, Hanto DW, Kahan BD: Maintenance immunosuppression with target-of-rapamycin inhibitors is associated with a reduced incidence of de novo malignancies. Transplantation 2005;80:883–889.
26 Schena FP, Pascoe MD, Alberu J, del Carmen Rial M, Oberbauer R, Brennan DC, Campistol JM, Racusen L, Polinsky MS, Goldberg-Alberts R, Li H, Scarola J, Neylan JF: Conversion from calcineurin inhibitors to sirolimus maintenance therapy in renal allograft recipients: 24-month efficacy and safety results from the convert trial. Transplantation 2009; 87:233–242.
27 Luan FL, Ding R, Sharma VK, Chon WJ, Lagman M, Suthanthiran M: Rapamycin is an effective inhibitor of human renal cancer metastasis. Kidney Int 2003;63:917–926.
28 Ekberg H, Tedesco-Silva H, Demirbas A, Vitko S, Nashan B, Gurkan A, Margreiter R, Hugo C, Grinyo JM, Frei U, Vanrenterghem Y, Daloze P, Halloran PF: Reduced exposure to calcineurin inhibitors in renal transplantation. N Engl J Med 2007;357:2562–2575.
29 Webster AC, Playford EG, Higgins G, Chapman JR, Craig JC: Interleukin 2 receptor antagonists for renal transplant recipients: a meta-analysis of randomized trials. Transplantation 2004;77:166–176.
30 Opelz G, Dohler B: Lymphomas after solid organ transplantation: a collaborative transplant study report. Am J Transplant 2004;4:222–230.
31 Vincenti F, Charpentier B, Vanrenterghem Y, Rostaing L, Bresnahan B, Darji P, Massari P, Mondragon-Ramirez GA, Agarwal M, Di Russo G, Lin CS, Garg P, Larsen CP: A phase III study of belatacept-based immunosuppression regimens versus cyclosporine in renal transplant recipients (BENEFIT study). Am J Transplant 2010;10:535–546.
32 Durrbach A, Pestana JM, Pearson T, Vincenti F, Garcia VD, Campistol J, Rial Mdel C, Florman S, Block A, Di Russo G, Xing J, Garg P, Grinyo J: A phase III study of belatacept versus cyclosporine in kidney transplants from extended criteria donors (BENEFIT-EXT study). Am J Transplant 2010;10: 547–557.

33 Larsen CP, Grinyo J, Medina-Pestana J, Vanrenterghem Y, Vincenti F, Breshahan B, Campistol JM, Florman S, Rial Mdel C, Kamar N, Block A, Di Russo G, Lin CS, Garg P, Charpentier B: Belatacept-based regimens versus a cyclosporine A-based regimen in kidney transplant recipients: 2-year results from the benefit and BENEFIT-EXT studies. Transplantation 2010;90:1528–1535.
34 Hofbauer GF, Anliker M, Arnold A, Binet I, Hunger R, Kempf W, Laffitte E, Lapointe AC, Pascual M, Pelloni F, Serra A: Swiss clinical practice guidelines for skin cancer in organ transplant recipients. Swiss Med Wkly 2009;139:407–415.
35 Morelon E, Mahe E, Touraine JL: The role of the transplant physician in the management of skin cancers after organ transplantation. Cancer Treat Res 2009;146:377–390.
36 Ismail F, Mitchell L, Casabonne D, Gulati A, Newton R, Proby CM, Harwood CA: Specialist dermatology clinics for organ transplant recipients significantly improve compliance with photoprotection and levels of skin cancer awareness. Br J Dermatol 2006;155:916–925.
37 Matin RN, Mesher D, Proby CM, McGregor JM, Bouwes Bavinck JN, del Marmol V, Euvrard S, Ferrandiz C, Geusau A, Hackethal M, Ho WL, Hofbauer GF, Imko-Walczuk B, Kanitakis J, Lally A, Lear JT, Lebbe C, Murphy GM, Piaserico S, Seckin D, Stockfleth E, Ulrich C, Wojnarowska FT, Lin HY, Balch C, Harwood CA: Melanoma in organ transplant recipients: clinicopathological features and outcome in 100 cases. Am J Transplant 2008;8:1891–1900.
38 Dapprich DC, Weenig RH, Rohlinger AL, Weaver AL, Quan KK, Keeling JH, Walsh JS, Otley CC, Christenson LJ: Outcomes of melanoma in recipients of solid organ transplant. J Am Acad Dermatol 2008;59:405–417.
39 Rodrigues LK, Klencke BJ, Vin-Christian K, Berger TG, Crawford RI, Miller JR 3rd, Ferreira CM, Nosrati M, Kashani-Sabet M: Altered clinical course of malignant melanoma in HIV-positive patients. Arch Dermatol 2002;138:765–770.
40 Werzowa J, Koehrer S, Strommer S, Cejka D, Fuereder T, Zebedin E, Wacheck V: Vertical inhibition of the mTORC1/mTORC2/PI3K pathway shows synergistic effects against melanoma in vitro and in vivo. J Invest Dermatol 2010;131:495–503.
41 Hainsworth JD, Infante JR, Spigel DR, Peyton JD, Thompson DS, Lane CM, Clark BL, Rubin MS, Trent DF, Burris HA, 3rd: Bevacizumab and everolimus in the treatment of patients with metastatic melanoma: a phase 2 trial of the Sarah Cannon Oncology Research Consortium. Cancer 2010;116:4122–4129.
42 Harwood AR, Osoba D, Hofstader SL, Goldstein MB, Cardella CJ, Holecek MJ, Kunynetz R, Giammarco RA: Kaposi's sarcoma in recipients of renal transplants. Am J Med 1979;67:759–765.
43 Campistol JM, Gutierrez-Dalmau A, Torregrosa JV: Conversion to sirolimus: a successful treatment for posttransplantation kaposi's sarcoma. Transplantation 2004;77:760–762.
44 Duman S, Toz H, Asci G, Alper S, Ozkahya M, Unal I, Celik A, Ok E, Basci A: Successful treatment of post-transplant Kaposi's sarcoma by reduction of immunosuppression. Nephrol Dial Transplant 2002;17:892–896.

Dr. F. Stucker
Department of Nephrology
Inselspital
University of Bern
CH–3010 Bern (Switzerland)
Tel. +41 31 632 3116, E-Mail fabadt@gmail.com

Häusermann P, Steiger J, Passweg J (eds): Transplantation Dermatology.
Curr Probl Dermatol. Basel, Karger, 2012, vol 43, pp 49–56

Human Papillomavirus and Squamous Cell Cancer of the Skin – Epidermodysplasia Verruciformis-Associated Human Papillomavirus Revisited

Andreas W. Arnold[a,c] · Günther F.L. Hofbauer[b]

[a]Dermatology Department, University Hospital Basel, Basel, Switzerland; [b]Dermatology Department, University Hospital Zürich, Zürich, Switzerland; [c]Dermatology Department, Freiburg University Medical Center, Freiburg, Germany

Abstract

As squamous cell cancer (SCC) is the most common malignancy in organ transplant recipients, a viral etiology has been proposed. Human papillomavirus (HPV) is found more often in organ transplant recipients than in the general population, but its role in cancer development has been debated for years. As a model of susceptibility of HPV the inherited disease epidermodysplasia verruciformis (EV) has been investigated intensively. EV is an autosomal-recessive skin disease leading to multiple flat warts and pityriasis versicolor-like macules in early youth. EV patients are at great risk of developing skin cancer due to a lack of defense against beta HPV. Beta HPV are causally involved in the formation of skin cancer in patients afflicted with EV. Beta HPV has frequently been detected in SCC and its early lesions such as actinic keratoses. Depending on the methods used, a prevalence of 30–90% has been reported for beta HPV for SCC in organ transplant recipients, while this prevalence in the general population is lower, but still considerable at 50%. Epidemiologic studies in the general population seem to suggest that beta HPV plays a role in the formation of SCC, both for invasive and in situ lesions.

As squamous cell cancer (SCC) is the most common malignancy in organ transplant recipients, a viral etiology has been proposed in the last decade, notably because the incidence of the majority of human cancers like lung, breast or prostate cancer is not greater than in the normal population. However, the incidence of SCC is about 100-fold greater compared to the general population [1, 2]. Human papillomavirus (HPV) is found more often in organ transplant recipients (OTRs) than in the general population, but its role in cancer development has been debated for years. As a model of susceptibility to HPV, the inherited disease epidermodysplasia verruciformis (EV) has been investigated intensively.

Beta HPV

The papillomaviruses are part of the family Papillomaviridae [3]. The classification is based on a comparison of the nucleotide sequence of the major capsid L1. A genotype is defined by sequence homology below 90% [4]. Alpha and beta HPV are the most common genera. Alpha HPV comprises genital and mucosal HPV and some cutaneous genotypes causing skin warts. Beta HPV causes mainly unapparent skin infections in immunocompetent individuals but potentially plays a role in developing skin cancer in immunocompromised patients. Beta HPV are causally involved in the formation of skin cancer in patients afflicted with EV. Currently, 41 types of completely sequenced beta HPV are known. These types are grouped into 5 species. High-risk genotypes are mainly HPV 5 and HPV 8, since they are associated with skin cancer in EV patients. All classic EV-associated beta HPV belong to species beta 1 and beta 2. All beta HPV show the typical genome organization of HPV. This means a noncoding region, responsible for the control of the viral transcription, an early region (E) and a late region (L), which are responsible for the viral structure proteins. The open reading frame E1, E2 and E4 encode for proteins important for viral replication, transcription and release of virus. E6 and E7 have transforming activity and are known to be oncogenes [5, 6]. The structure of beta HPV is remarkable because they do not express E5 as alpha HPV do [7].

With the highly sensitive method of polymerase chain reaction, beta HPV DNA has frequently been detected in healthy skin of immunocompetent individuals [8, 9]. In OTRs, the percentage of positively tested patients ranges from 87 to 98% in comparison to immunocompetent persons with 84–91% of plucked eyebrows [9]. The types of beta HPV are comparable in the two groups. Because the viral load is generally low, seroprevalence is low as well and rises continuously after the age of 15 years [10]. A high seroprevalence is found in psoriasis patients, suggesting a more efficient multiplication in comparison to healthy individuals in proliferating keratinocytes. In OTRs without skin cancer, 86% were seropositive to at least one HPV, 56% to beta HPV [11]. According to other studies, environmental factors are probably more important for susceptibility to HPV than the immune status of patients [11–14]. Beta-HPV could be regulated by genetic factors as it has been demonstrated in patients with EV lacking an inherited defense against beta HPV.

Epidermodysplasia Verruciformis

EV is an autosomal-recessive skin disease leading to multiple flat warts and pityriasis versicolor-like macules in early youth. It has been recently classified as a primary immunodeficiency [15]. EV patients are at great risk of developing skin cancer due to a lack of defense against beta HPV [16], and therefore serve as a model to study susceptibility to beta HPV and their carcinogenesis. EV patients cannot appropriately control beta HPV replication, and therefore have a strong antibody response against a broad variety of beta HPV types [17]. No unusual susceptibility is noted to HPVs other than beta HPV. Whereas patients are usually infected with more than one beta HPV, only some of the genotypes, mainly HPV 5 and 8 are detected in skin carcinomas [18]. The skin cancer occurs usually in the fourth or fifth decade, and is localized mainly in sun exposed areas indicating an important role of environmental factors, notably UV irradiation [19, 20].

The gene locus has been mapped on chromosome 17q25.3 [21]. *EVER1* and *EVER2* are two genes responsible for disease [22]. They are transcribed in numerous tissues including the skin. *EVER1* and *EVER2* belongs to a gene family, known as TMC (transmembrane channel like), whereas EVER1 is TMC6 and EVER2 is TMC8. EVER1 and EVER2 interact with the zinc transporter 1 (ZnT-1) forming a complex. ZnT-1 is a protein which is responsible for the zinc efflux and resistance against zinc therefore being responsible for intracellular the zinc homeostasis [23]. EVER/ZnT-1 complex participates in the regulation of cellular zinc fluxes and allows the maintenance of the zinc balance in keratinocytes [24]. Zinc is known to modify signal transduction, but its excess might be toxic for the cell and can induce apoptosis [25]. Zinc is an element which is needed by HPV being a cofactor of viral proteins and a constituent of intracellular signaling network of the virus [18].

EVER and ZnT-1 are suppressors of transcription factors like AP-1, a factor important for the proliferation of HPV [24]. This effect is likely to be indirect by influencing the zinc balance [18]. The downregulation of AP-1 also takes place when AP-1 is activated by other stimulating factors like epidermal growth factor or TGF-α [24]. AP-1 levels have been found to be significantly higher in EVER2 defect keratinocytes than in the wild-type EVER2 cells [24]. The increased level of AP-1 in EVER2–/– keratinocytes could be responsible for the high proliferation rate of HPV and promote persistence of HPV in those cells leading to malignant transformation through a permanent overexpression [18]. Although the contribution of HPV 5 and 8 to skin carcinogenesis is evident, it has been proposed that EVER2 deficiency alone can promote skin cancer without HPV infection [24, 26]. Indeed continuously uncontrolled AP-1 overexpression may lead to a malignant transformation of cells [26].

The fact that non-sense mutations in EV subject patients to skin cancer elicited the discussion whether single nucleotide polymorphisms (SNPs) could influence skin carcinogenesis in the general population. While UV light as a cause of skin cancer is accepted, HPV could serve as a cocarcinogen. Even though SNPs may not lead to EV-like lesions, it could be supposed that through a deficient defense against HPV, viral oncogene expression is facilitated. Such continued replication of viral oncogenes might promote skin carcinogenesis. A common SNP of EVER2 gene has recently been correlated with seropositivity for beta HPV and a risk of squamous cell carcinoma [27]. Whether there is a similar correlation with EVER1 SNP remains to be established.

Organ Transplant Recipients, Beta HPV and Squamous Cell Cancer

Continued immunosuppression in OTRs allows virally driven neoplasms to occur at a higher rate than in the general population [28]. Beta HPV has frequently been detected in SCC and its early lesions such as actinic keratoses [29–34]. Depending on the methods used, a prevalence of 30–90% has been reported for beta HPV for SCC in OTRs [30, 31, 35, 36], while this prevalence in the general population is lower, but still considerable at 50% [37]. Typically, multiple beta HPV types are isolated on single skin biopsies from OTRs [30, 32], where hair bulbs form the reservoir for beta HPV. Eyebrow hairs show persistent beta HPV colonization [9, 38]. Focusing on highly sensitive DNA detection techniques, a prevalence approaching 100% for beta HPV in humans with high prevalence in plucked hairs could be demonstrated [38].

Epidemiologic studies in the general population seem to suggest that beta HPV play a role in the formation of SCC, both for invasive and in situ lesions [36, 39]. An association between the DNA of beta-HPV and SCC has been supported by several studies [40–43]. Seroreactivity to beta HPV and antibodies to the major capsid protein L1 as markers for HPV exposure have been reported in association with SCC [43–48].

A straightforward link between HPV and carcinogenesis requires the presence of viral DNA in high numbers in the cancer, the expression of viral oncogenes in cancer cells and the persistence of viral DNA in the progression of cancer. A connection as clear cut as for HPV16 and HPV18 in cervical cancer has to date not been established for beta HPV in cutaneous SCC. While beta HPV clearly is found in a wide variety of HPV types in human skin and SCC, a direct influence has been hard to establish for beta HPV.

As discussed above, there is a widespread presence of HPV in human skin both in the general population and in particular in OTRs. Such HPV presence is not short lived, but rather persists over prolonged periods of time [38]. Still, the absolute number of beta HPV copies detectable in normal skin and SCC is very low [49, 50]. Some have raised the question whether hitherto unknown HPV family members might be involved in the development of cutaneous SCC and have escaped notice to this point. Recent transcriptome sequencing, however, has denied any support for an unknown HPV type to be involved in SCC formation [50]. While the possibility persists that an unknown virus with low similarity to known viral sequences may be involved, the role of HPV as a direct causative agent in SCC remains doubtful at best.

As no permanent and continued HPV persistence in SCC could be demonstrated, the possibility remains that HPV may contribute to SCC development by transient rather than permanent infection. Beta HPV counts seem higher in actinic keratoses than in invasive SCC [49]. UV radiation may be potentiated in its carcinogenicity by a hit-and-run phenomenon or a direct interaction of HPV with UV [36, 51]. At least in vitro, the E6 protein of beta HPVs impairs the repair of DNA damage induced by UV at the G1 cell cycle stage and by inhibition of UV induced apoptosis [52–56]. These observations support the concept that cells with beta-HPV infection sustain DNA damage which persists even when HPV is cleared from cells. Such DNA-damaged cells may then progress to actinic keratosis and invasive SCC [36, 39, 57]. While such a hit-and-run mechanism has been shown for bovine papillomavirus type 4 where alimentary tract papillomas are induced after viral infection which progress to cancer in cattle in experimental conditions where the final cancer no longer harbors HPV DNA [58], no such direct proof has been recorded yet for beta HPV in cutaneous SCC in humans, in particular OTRs.

Voices more critical of HPV involvement have raised their concern that beta HPV detection at high frequency may be an expression of general immunosuppression in OTRs rather than of a causal role of HPV in SCC in OTRs. Beta HPV would thus be innocent bystanders to SCC formation, just reflecting a general state of immunosuppression allowing among many other consequences also the increased occurrence of cutaneous SCC due to non-HPV-related driving factors. Besides this rather plain interpretation, others have pointed out that new viral agents are discovered continuously and may turn out to be the ones responsible for SCC formation in OTRs [59]. Recent examples of such newly discovered viral agents include Merkel cell polyomavirus [60], HPvV6 and HPvV7 [61], and trichodysplasia spinulosa-associated polyomavirus [62].

Conclusion

HPV are viral agents clearly associated with malignant transformation of cells. In human skin, the hereditary disease of EV provides a clear model where beta HPV, in particular types 5 and 8, contribute to SCC of the skin. The extrapolation of findings from this genetic disease model has not been achieved yet. OTRs do show a high prevalence of beta HPV, but no particular HPV type at convincingly high copy numbers has been identified.

Current thinking encompasses a hit-and-run mechanism for beta HPV, hitherto undiscovered viral agents or simply general immunosuppression reflected by a high prevalence of beta HPV as driving factors in the greatly increased incidence of SCC in OTRs.

References

1 Lindelof B, Sigurgeirsson B, Gabel H, Stern RS: Incidence of skin cancer in 5356 patients following organ transplantation. Br J Dermatol 2000;143:513–519.

2 Jensen AO, Svaerke C, Farkas D, Pedersen L, Kragballe K, Sorensen HT: Skin cancer risk among solid organ recipients: a nationwide cohort study in Denmark. Acta Derm Venereol 2010;90:474–479.

3 Bernard HU: The clinical importance of the nomenclature, evolution and taxonomy of human papillomaviruses. J Clin Virol 2005;32(suppl 1):S1–S6.

4 de Villiers EM, Fauquet C, Broker TR, Bernard HU, zur Hausen H: Classification of papillomaviruses. Virology 2004;324:17–27.

5 Pfefferle R, Marcuzzi GP, Akgul B, Kasper HU, Schulze F, Haase I, Wickenhauser C, Pfister H: The human papillomavirus type 8 E2 protein induces skin tumors in transgenic mice. J Invest Dermatol 2008;128:2310–2315.

6 Pfister H, Fuchs PG, Majewski S, Jablonska S, Pniewska I, Malejczyk M: High prevalence of epidermodysplasia verruciformis-associated human papillomavirus DNA in actinic keratoses of the immunocompetent population. Arch Dermatol Res 2003;295:273–279.

7 Pfister H: Biology of epidermodysplasia verruciformis-associated HPV (in German). Hautarzt 2011; 62:17–21.

8 Astori G, Lavergne D, Benton C, Hockmayr B, Egawa K, Garbe C, de Villiers EM: Human papillomaviruses are commonly found in normal skin of immunocompetent hosts. J Invest Dermatol 1998; 110:752–755.

9 Boxman IL, Berkhout RJ, Mulder LH, Wolkers MC, Bouwes Bavinck JN, Vermeer BJ, ter Schegget J: Detection of human papillomavirus DNA in plucked hairs from renal transplant recipients and healthy volunteers. J Invest Dermatol 1997;108:712–715.

10 Michael KM, Waterboer T, Sehr P, Rother A, Reidel U, Boeing H, Bravo IG, Schlehofer J, Gartner BC, Pawlita M: Seroprevalence of 34 human papillomavirus types in the German general population. PLoS Pathog 2008;4:e1000091.

11 Casabonne D, Waterboer T, Michael KM, Pawlita M, Lally A, Mitchell L, Imko-Walczuk B, Wojnarowska F, Newton R, Proby C, Harwood C: The sero-epidemiology of human papillomavirus among Caucasian transplant recipients in the UK. Infect Agent Cancer 2009;4:13.

12 Weissenborn SJ, Neale R, de Koning MN, Waterboer T, Abeni D, Bouwes Bavinck JN, Wieland U, Pfister HJ: Prevalence and multiplicity of cutaneous beta papilloma viruses in plucked hairs depend on cellular DNA input. J Virol Methods 2009;161:280–283.

13 Weissenborn SJ, De Koning MN, Wieland U, Quint WG, Pfister HJ: Intrafamilial transmission and family-specific spectra of cutaneous betapapillomaviruses. J Virol 2009;83:811–816.

14 Casabonne D, Waterboer T, Michael KM, Pawlita M, Mitchell L, Newton R, Harwood C, Proby C: The seroprevalence of human papillomavirus by immune status and by ethnicity in London. Infect Agent Cancer 2009;4:14.

15 Notarangelo L, Casanova JL, Fischer A, Puck J, Rosen F, Seger R, Geha R: Primary immunodeficiency diseases: an update. J Allergy Clin Immunol 2004;114:677–687.

16 Arnold AW, Burger B, Kump E, Rufle A, Tyring SK, Kempf W, Hausermann P, Itin PH: Homozygosity for the c.917A–>T (p.N306l) polymorphism in the EVER2/TMC8 gene of two sisters with epidermodysplasia verruciformis Lewandowsky-Lutz originally described by Wilhelm Lutz. Dermatology 2011;222:81–86.

17 Dell'Oste V, Azzimonti B, De Andrea M, Mondini M, Zavattaro E, Leigheb G, Weissenborn SJ, Pfister H, Michael KM, Waterboer T, Pawlita M, Amantea A, Landolfo S, Gariglio M: High beta-HPV DNA loads and strong seroreactivity are present in epidermodysplasia verruciformis. J Invest Dermatol 2009;129:1026–1034.

18 Lazarczyk M, Cassonnet P, Pons C, Jacob Y, Favre M: The ever proteins as a natural barrier against papillomaviruses: a new insight into the pathogenesis of human papillomavirus infections. Microbiol Mol Biol Rev 2009;73:348–370.

19 Gewirtzman A, Bartlett B, Tyring S: Epidermodysplasia verruciformis and human papilloma virus. Curr Opin Infect Dis 2008;21:141–146.

20 Orth G: Genetics of epidermodysplasia verruciformis: insights into host defense against papillomaviruses. Semin Immunol 2006;18:362–374.

21 Ramoz N, Rueda LA, Bouadjar B, Favre M, Orth G: A susceptibility locus for epidermodysplasia verruciformis, an abnormal predisposition to infection with the oncogenic human papillomavirus type 5, maps to chromosome 17qter in a region containing a psoriasis locus. J Invest Dermatol 1999;112:259–263.

22 Ramoz N, Rueda LA, Bouadjar B, Montoya LS, Orth G, Favre M: Mutations in two adjacent novel genes are associated with epidermodysplasia verruciformis. Nat Genet 2002;32:579–581.
23 Palmiter RD, Findley SD: Cloning and functional characterization of a mammalian zinc transporter that confers resistance to zinc. EMBO J 1995;14:639–649.
24 Lazarczyk M, Pons C, Mendoza JA, Cassonnet P, Jacob Y, Favre M: Regulation of cellular zinc balance as a potential mechanism of ever-mediated protection against pathogenesis by cutaneous oncogenic human papillomaviruses. J Exp Med 2008;205:35–42.
25 Haase H, Maret W: Intracellular zinc fluctuations modulate protein tyrosine phosphatase activity in insulin/insulin-like growth factor-1 signaling. Exp Cell Res 2003;291:289–298.
26 Lazarczyk M, Favre M: Role of Zn^{2+} ions in host-virus interactions. J Virol 2008;82:11486–11494.
27 Patel AS, Karagas MR, Pawlita M, Waterboer T, Nelson HH: Cutaneous human papillomavirus infection, the EVER2 gene and incidence of squamous cell carcinoma: a case-control study. Int J Cancer 2008;122:2377–2379.
28 Grulich AE, van Leeuwen MT, Falster MO, Vajdic CM: Incidence of cancers in people with HIV/AIDS compared with immunosuppressed transplant recipients: a meta-analysis. Lancet 2007;370:59–67.
29 de Jong-Tieben LM, Berkhout RJ, ter Schegget J, Vermeer BJ, de Fijter JW, Bruijn JA, Westendorp RG, Bouwes Bavinck JN: The prevalence of human papillomavirus DNA in benign keratotic skin lesions of renal transplant recipients with and without a history of skin cancer is equally high: a clinical study to assess risk factors for keratotic skin lesions and skin cancer. Transplantation 2000;69:44–49.
30 Berkhout RJ, Bouwes Bavinck JN, ter Schegget J: Persistence of human papillomavirus DNA in benign and (pre)malignant skin lesions from renal transplant recipients. J Clin Microbiol 2000;38: 2087–2096.
31 de Jong-Tieben LM, Berkhout RJ, Smits HL, Bouwes Bavinck JN, Vermeer BJ, van der Woude FJ, ter Schegget J: High frequency of detection of epidermodysplasia verruciformis-associated human papillomavirus DNA in biopsies from malignant and premalignant skin lesions from renal transplant recipients. J Invest Dermatol 1995;105:367–371.
32 Harwood CA, Surentheran T, McGregor JM, Spink PJ, Leigh IM, Breuer J, Proby CM: Human papillomavirus infection and non-melanoma skin cancer in immunosuppressed and immunocompetent individuals. J Med Virol 2000;61:289–297.
33 Stockfleth E, Nindl I, Sterry W, Ulrich C, Schmook T, Meyer T: Human papillomaviruses in transplant-associated skin cancers. Dermatol Surg 2004;30: 604–609.
34 Nindl I, Rosl F: Molecular concepts of virus infections causing skin cancer in organ transplant recipients. Am J Transplant 2008;8:2199–2204.
35 Barr BB, Benton EC, McLaren K, Bunney MH, Smith IW, Blessing K, Hunter JA: Human papilloma virus infection and skin cancer in renal allograft recipients. Lancet 1989;1:124–129.
36 Feltkamp MC, de Koning MN, Bavinck JN, Ter Schegget J: Betapapillomaviruses: innocent bystanders or causes of skin cancer. J Clin Virol 2008;43: 353–360.
37 Asgari MM, Kiviat NB, Critchlow CW, Stern JE, Argenyi ZB, Raugi GJ, Berg D, Odland PB, Hawes SE, de Villiers EM: Detection of human papillomavirus DNA in cutaneous squamous cell carcinoma among immunocompetent individuals. J Invest Dermatol 2008;128:1409–1417.
38 De Koning M N, Struijk L, Bavinck J N, Kleter B, ter Schegget J, Quint WG, Feltkamp MC: Betapapillomaviruses frequently persist in the skin of healthy individuals. J Gen Virol 2007;88:1489–1495.
39 Bouwes Bavinck JN, Plasmeijer EI, Feltkamp MC: Beta-papillomavirus infection and skin cancer. J Invest Dermatol 2008;128:1355–1358.
40 Forslund O: Genetic diversity of cutaneous human papillomaviruses. J Gen Virol 2007;88:2662–2669.
41 Struijk L, Bouwes Bavinck JN, Wanningen P, van der Meijden E, Westendorp RG, Ter Schegget J, Feltkamp MC: Presence of human papillomavirus DNA in plucked eyebrow hairs is associated with a history of cutaneous squamous cell carcinoma. J Invest Dermatol 2003;121:1531–1535.
42 Forslund O, Lindelof B, Hradil E, Nordin P, Stenquist B, Kirnbauer R, Slupetzky K, Dillner J: High prevalence of cutaneous human papillomavirus DNA on the top of skin tumors but not in 'Stripped' Biopsies from the same tumors. J Invest Dermatol 2004;123: 388–394.
43 Struijk L, Hall L, van der Meijden E, Wanningen P, Bavinck JN, Neale R, Green AC, Ter Schegget J, Feltkamp MC: Markers of cutaneous human papillomavirus infection in individuals with tumor-free skin, actinic keratoses, and squamous cell carcinoma. Cancer Epidemiol Biomarkers Prev 2006;15: 529–535.

44 Feltkamp MC, Broer R, di Summa FM, Struijk L, van der Meijden E, Verlaan BP, Westendorp RG, ter Schegget J, Spaan WJ, Bouwes Bavinck JN: Seroreactivity to epidermodysplasia verruciformis-related human papillomavirus types is associated with nonmelanoma skin cancer. Cancer Res 2003;63: 2695–2700.

45 Karagas MR, Nelson HH, Sehr P, Waterboer T, Stukel TA, Andrew A, Green AC, Bavinck JN, Perry A, Spencer S, Rees JR, Mott LA, Pawlita M: Human papillomavirus infection and incidence of squamous cell and basal cell carcinomas of the skin. J Natl Cancer Inst 2006;98:389–395.

46 Dang C, Koehler A, Forschner T, Sehr P, Michael K, Pawlita M, Stockfleth E, Nindl I: E6/E7 expression of human papillomavirus types in cutaneous squamous cell dysplasia and carcinoma in immunosuppressed organ transplant recipients. Br J Dermatol 2006;155:129–136.

47 Casabonne D, Michael KM, Waterboer T, Pawlita M, Forslund O, Burk RD, Travis RC, Key TJ, Newton R: A prospective pilot study of antibodies against human papillomaviruses and cutaneous squamous cell carcinoma nested in the Oxford component of the European prospective investigation into cancer and nutrition. Int J Cancer 2007;121:1862–1868.

48 Waterboer T, Abeni D, Sampogna F, Rother A, Masini C, Sehr P, Michael KM, Pawlita M: Serological association of beta and gamma human papillomaviruses with squamous cell carcinoma of the skin. Br J Dermatol 2008;159:457–459.

49 Weissenborn SJ, Nindl I, Purdie K, Harwood C, Proby C, Breuer J, Majewski S, Pfister H, Wieland U: Human papillomavirus-DNA loads in actinic keratoses exceed those in non-melanoma skin cancers. J Invest Dermatol 2005;125:93–97.

50 Arron ST, Ruby JG, Dybbro E, Ganem D, Derisi JL: Transcriptome sequencing demonstrates that human papillomavirus is not active in cutaneous squamous cell carcinoma. J Invest Dermatol 2011; 131:1745–1753.

51 Bouwes Bavinck JN, Feltkamp MC: Milk of human kindness?–hamlet, human papillomavirus, and warts. N Engl J Med 2004;350:2639–2642.

52 Jackson S, Storey A: E6 proteins from diverse cutaneous HPV types inhibit apoptosis in response to UV damage. Oncogene 2000;19:592–598.

53 Jackson S, Harwood C, Thomas M, Banks L, Storey A: Role of BAK in UV-induced apoptosis in skin cancer and abrogation by HPV E6 proteins. Genes Dev 2000;14:3065–3073.

54 Iftner T, Elbel M, Schopp B, Hiller T, Loizou JI, Caldecott KW, Stubenrauch F: Interference of papillomavirus E6 protein with single-strand break repair by interaction with XRCC1. EMBO J 2002;21: 4741–4748.

55 Leverrier S, Bergamaschi D, Ghali L, Ola A, Warnes G, Akgul B, Blight K, Garcia-Escudero R, Penna A, Eddaoudi A, Storey A: Role of HPV E6 proteins in preventing UVB-induced release of pro-apoptotic factors from the mitochondria. Apoptosis 2007;12: 549–560.

56 Struijk L, van der Meijden E, Kazem S, ter Schegget J, de Gruijl FR, Steenbergen RD, Feltkamp MC: Specific betapapillomaviruses associated with squamous cell carcinoma of the skin inhibit UVB-induced apoptosis of primary human keratinocytes. J Gen Virol 2008;89:2303–2314.

57 Hofbauer GF, Bouwes Bavinck JN, Euvrard S: Organ transplantation and skin cancer: basic problems and new perspectives. Exp Dermatol 2010;19:473–482.

58 Campo MS, O'Neil BW, Barron RJ, Jarrett WF: Experimental reproduction of the papilloma-carcinoma complex of the alimentary canal in cattle. Carcinogenesis 1994;15:1597–1601.

59 Schiller JT, Buck CB: Cutaneous squamous cell carcinoma: a smoking gun but still no suspects. J Invest Dermatol 2011;131:1595–1596.

60 Feng H, Shuda M, Chang Y, Moore PS: Clonal integration of a polyomavirus in human Merkel cell carcinoma. Science 2008;319:1096–1100.

61 Schowalter RM, Pastrana DV, Pumphrey KA, Moyer AL, Buck CB: Merkel cell polyomavirus and two previously unknown polyomaviruses are chronically shed from human skin. Cell Host Microbe 2010;7:509–515.

62 van der Meijden E, Janssens RW, Lauber C, Bouwes Bavinck JN, Gorbalenya AE, Feltkamp MC: Discovery of a new human polyomavirus associated with trichodysplasia spinulosa in an immunocompromized patient. PLoS Pathog 2010;6:e1001024.

Dr. Andreas W. Arnold
Universitätsspital Basel
Petersgraben 4
CH–4031 Basel (Switzerland)
Tel. +41 61 265 40 95, E-Mail aarnold@uhbs.ch

Häusermann P, Steiger J, Passweg J (eds): Transplantation Dermatology.
Curr Probl Dermatol. Basel, Karger, 2012, vol 43, pp 57–70

Pre- and Posttransplant Management of Solid Organ Transplant Recipients: Risk-Adjusted Follow-Up

Bahar Shafaeddin Schreve[a] · Mark Anliker[b] · Andreas W. Arnold[c] · Werner Kempf[a] · Emmanuel Laffitte[d] · Anne-Karine Lapointe[e] · Carlo Mainetti[f] · Francesco Pelloni[g] · Patrick Oberholzer[h] · Andreas Serra[a] · Markus Streit[i] · Günther F.L. Hofbauer[a]

For the working group Organ Transplantation of the Swiss Society for Dermatology and Venerology
[a]Universitätsspital Zürich, [b]Kantonsspital St. Gallen, [c]Universitätsspital Basel, [d]Hopitaux Universitaires de Genève, [e]Centre Hopitalier Universitaire Vaudois, Lausanne, [f]Ospedale San Giovanni, Bellinzona, [g]Studio di Dermatologie, Lugano, [h]Inselspital Bern, and [i]Kantonsspital Aarau, Switzerland

Abstract

Solid organ transplant recipients (SOTR) have an increased risk of skin cancer due to their long-term immunosuppressive state. As the number of these patients is increasing, as well as their life expectancy, it is important to discuss the screening and management of skin cancer in this group of patients. The role of the dermatologist, in collaboration with the transplant team, is important both before transplantation, where patients are screened for skin lesions and the individual risk for skin cancer development is assessed, and after transplantation. Posttransplant management consists of regular dermatological consultations (the frequency depends on different factors discussed below), where early skin cancer screening and management, as well as patient education on sun protective behavior is taught and enforced. Indeed, SOTR are very sensitive to sun damage due to their immunosuppressive state, leading to cumulative sun damage which results in field cancerization with numerous lesions such as in situ squamous cell carcinoma, actinic keratosis and Bowen's disease. These lesions should be recognized and treated as early as possible. Therapeutic options discussed will involve topical therapy, surgical management, adjustment of the patient's immunosuppressive therapy (i.e. reduction of immunosuppression and/or switch to mammalian target of rapamycin inhibitors) and chemoprevention with the retinoid acitretin, which reduces the recurrence rate of squamous cell carcinoma. The dermatological follow-up of SOTR should be integrated into the comprehensive posttransplant care.

Pretransplant Screening

Recommendations on skin care for organ transplant recipients will be discussed based on the joint American and European guidelines for the prevention and treatment of skin cancers in solid organ transplant recipients (SOTR) [1], as well as on the collective clinical experience of the Swiss Society of Transplantation, Nephrology and Dermatology network. These recommendations will be graded following the Oxford Centre for Evidence-Based Medicine.

A dermatological consultation is recommended before receiving a transplant to screen and treat skin disease, in particular for warts, actinic keratosis (AK), Bowen's disease (BD), and squamous cell carcinoma of the skin (SCC). The patient's risk for developing skin cancer (level D recommendation) should be assessed (level D recommendation) [2]. The quantity and intensity of exposure to UV rays, the frequency of sunburns in the past, and the personal and family history for skin cancer should be documented. Presence of specific skin diseases must be noted such as HPV-associated verruca, AK, BD, and invasive skin cancer such as SCC, basal cell carcinoma (BCC), melanoma, Kaposi's sarcoma (KS), and Merkel cell carcinoma. Melanoma history should be evaluated, especially if the primary melanoma measured >1 mm Breslow tumor thickness and/or the diagnosis was made less than 5 years before (recommendation D) [3, 4]. Systemic diseases and/or an immunosuppressive state in the patient's history or current state should be noted, such as immunosuppressive medications, viral infections (e.g. HIV), or carcinomas. In particular, a history of SCC and BCC is associated with a higher risk of developing these tumors after transplantation (recommendation D). Further risk factors for nonmelanoma skin cancers in SOTR are fair skin, male gender, older age, sun-damaged skin and previous radiation treatment [5].

Besides immunosuppression, UV exposure is the main factor in skin carcinogenesis [6]. There is room for improvement in the sun protection education and compliance in SOTR [3, 4] both immediately after transplantation, and during the long run of follow-up consultations by a dermatologist (recommendation D). Patients must be informed on how to recognize appearance of common benign, premalignant and malignant skin lesions (recommendation D) and encouraged to perform monthly self-skin examinations to detect any changing growths including pink patches or spots, scaly growths, bleeding spots, or changing moles. In addition, for high-risk patients (i.e. history of high-risk SCC, melanoma or metastatic disease) self-examination of the lymph nodes every month is recommended [7]. A growth occurring for >4 weeks or a wound without healing >4 weeks deserves dermatological evaluation (recommendation D).

After completing the patient consultation with a complete skin examination including oral and anogenital regions, UV protection advice and skin cancer preventive measures should be explained thoroughly. These include sun avoidance (recommendation D) especially between 11 am and 3 pm, avoidance of tanning beds, protective clothing (wide-brim hat, sunglasses, long sleeved-tops and trousers when possible), and high SPF factor sun screen application with UVA protection (COLIPA norm preferably over Australian norm) and UBV protection (SPF 50+) on chronically exposed skin: face, ears, neck, hand [8]. Regular sun cream application must be performed in sunny weather as well as cloudy/rainy weather, as this significantly reduces the risk of developing precancerous and cancerous lesions, i.e. 365 days a year. Phototherapy treatments must be avoided. Patient education sessions regarding sun protection and self-skin examination should be repeated at the recommended yearly dermatological consultation. Written information should also be provided (recommendation D) [9].

Management of skin cancer is discussed separately. In brief, invasive skin cancer should be removed surgically, and high-risk SCC should be discussed with the transplant team, as it may require an observation period before transplantation. Metastatic skin cancer is generally an exclusion criterion for transplantation.

Standard Management after Transplantation

Management of skin cancer in SOTR involves both the transplant physician and the dermatologist. We shall discuss the importance of the dermatologist in transplant patients, as well as skin-cancer screening, education, and interdisciplinary coordination. Topical and systemic management will be reviewed.

Management of Skin Cancer

Skin cancers in SOTR require a multidisciplinary team consisting of the transplant team, dermatologist, surgeon, oncologist, and radio-oncologist. The presence of a specialized dermatologist for transplant patients within a specialty transplant center allows a better follow-up of transplant patients at risk [2]. The role of the dermatologist is to raise awareness of increased skin cancer risk in these patients, and to provide education for photoprotection. Previous studies have shown poor compliance regarding sun protection and sunscreen use within these patients [10], particularly in patients who never attended a dermatology clinic [2], suggesting the importance of a dermatological follow-up and care of transplant patients. Regular screening by a dermatologist has shown to not only reduce the risk of associated skin cancer in the posttransplant period, but to improve the general quality of life of the patient [7].

Skin care education should comprise teaching self-examination for suspicious lesions (palpation of draining lymph nodes for high-risk patients, counseling on sun protection (protective clothing, use of sunscreen) and advice against the use of tanning salons.

The use of sun screen has been shown to protect against ultraviolet damage to the skin and development of AK and invasive SCC in these patients [11]. Only under very strict conditions can vitamin D deficiency be observed in sun screen users [12]. Vitamin D deficiency should be still be searched and corrected due to associated risks described in SOTR [9]. The American Academy of Dermatology has recommended considering administration of 1,000 U of daily vitamin D in adults who regularly practice photoprotection and may be at risk for vitamin D insufficiency [9, 13].

Table 1. Recommended dermatological examination intervals for SOTR

Patient characteristics	Interval for total body skin examination (months)
No previous skin cancer/no field cancerization	12
Field cancerization	6
One SCC of the skin	3–6
Multiple SCC of the skin	3
High-risk SCC or melanoma	1–3
Metastatic SCC or melanoma	1–3

Recommended dermatological follow-up would ideally start before transplantation, in order to determine the presence of preexisting lesions before transplant, followed by a post-transplant consultation. According to the development of skin cancer, follow-up varies between once a month to once a year (table 1).

In situ Squamous Cell Carcinoma (Actinic Keratosis and Bowen's Disease)

Nonmelanoma skin cancer is the most frequent malignancy in SOTR, causing a negative impact on patients' posttransplantation quality of life [14]. It is important to recognize and treat these lesions at an early stage in order to prevent progression into invasive tumors. AKs are generally characterized by hyperkeratosis and macular erythema, and may be diagnosed without histological examination. Biopsy should be performed whenever a lesion is suspicious, indurated, progressive or refractory (recommendation D) [15].

All low-risk SCC proven by biopsy should benefit from Mohs micrographic surgery (MMS) or excision with clear surgical margins. It is recommended to perform a skin biopsy at an early stage, especially in areas of 'field cancerization', where it is tricky to distinguish multiple keratotic lesions from skin cancer. Field cancerization is a concept of large areas of sun-damaged skin having a higher incidence of in situ and invasive skin cancer [16, 17] such as AK, BD, and SCC, which are associated with extensive areas of actinic damage, representing clinical and subclinical lesions of epidermal dysplasia [18]. Early handling of field cancerization by treatments such as topical 5-fluoracil (5-FU), imiquimod, and photodynamic therapy (PDT) may delay subsequent tumor development [19–22].

If skin lesions do not respond to treatment, a biopsy should be obtained without delay for histologic evaluation. As the treatment of an isolated lesion does not prevent appearance of new lesions, we recommend combining surgical therapy with topical therapies on the clinical and subclinical lesions in the large sun-damaged fields (field therapy) [18]. SOTR usually require a longer course of treatment with more frequent applications and use of occlusive dressings to reach clinical responses compared to the general population.

Radiotherapy is contraindicated for therapy of in situ skin cancer in SOTR and to be preferably avoided in invasive SCC, as radiation causes supplementary DNA damage and decreases the time lag of radiation-induced cancer, while radiation-induced dermatitis, a needed reaction for efficacy of radiation therapy is not sufficiently induced in SOTR.

Topical Therapy in Field Disease and Prevention of Squamous Cell Carcinoma

Topical therapies are alterative noninvasive measures that may be applied on large areas. Such therapies include imiquimod, 5-FU, and PDT. 5-FU may be used alone or in combination with topical alpha/beta hydroxyacids in order to decrease the number and size of the lesions. It is especially used on arms and hands.

Topical use of diclofenac has shown to be an effective and tolerated option for the treatment of AK in immunocompetent patients, but its safety and efficacy in SOTR was not evaluated. A recent study showed that the treatment of AKs (patients with 3 more AKs) with 3% diclofenac in 2.5% hyaluronic acid twice daily during 16 weeks demonstrated a greater lesion clearance rate of AKs compared to the placebo group. Although a 55% recurrence of AK lesions was noted in the previously cleared patients, a 24-month follow-up showed no invasive SCC, suggesting that diclofenac 3% gel (also known as Solaraze®) is an efficient and well-tolerated treatment for multiple AKs in SOTR, but may also prevent invasive SCC in these high-risk patients [23].

Imiquimod is an immunomodulator used in treatment of genital condylomas, actinic keratoses on the head and neck, trunk and extremities, and BCCs of the upper extremities, head and neck. A recent review of the use of imiquimod in SOTR indicates that this is safe in transplant patients with no observed adverse effects on graft function [24].

PDT consists in the application of a topical photosensitizer on the patient's skin (such as 5-ALA or 5-FU cream), which is subsequently activated by light to destroy tumor cells, especially in AK and superficial BCC. It is particularly useful in the treatment of multiple lesions on a large surface area. PDT in SOTR has been shown to be more efficient [25] and cosmetically acceptable than 5-FU for the treatment of post-transplant epidermal dysplasia. Another study showed that scalp/facial AK lesions respond better to acral surfaces using MAL-PDT with red light, in SOTR not responsive to conventional treatments (cryotherapy, topical 5-FU, CO_2 laser, curettage, electrosurgery) [26]. The efficacy of PDT in reducing the risk of new SCC lesions in SOTR is still debated, with conflicting data [19–21].

SOTR with SCC are recommended to benefit from surgical excision and MMS. However, in case of multiple lesions or where electrodessication and curettage is easier, these techniques may be used instead of multiple surgery [27] for appropriately selected low-risk, i.e. small and superficial, SCC.

High-Risk Squamous Cell Carcinoma

High-risk SCC is defined by multiple SCCs, or SCCs developing in a high-risk location (ears, perioral, periorbital, temple region), of large size (>2 cm diameter), rapidly growing, recurring, in transit to metastasis, or of specific histological criteria (poorly differentiated, perineural invasion, deep invasion beyond 5 mm Breslow thickness).

Management of these tumors involves evaluation of nodal involvement by ultrasound and distant metastasis by positron emission tomography (PET)-computed tomography (CT), followed by early aggressive surgical treatment, as well as reduction of immunosuppression, and possibly adjuvant radiation therapy of the primary site and draining lymph nodes [28, 29].

Recommended surgical therapy for invasive SCC consists in surgical excision with margins of 4–6 mm beyond any surrounding erythema [30]. MMS is preferred in sites where tissue conservation is needed [29]. Risk of metastasis or local recurrences must be evaluated by histologic examination of resected tumors. Risk factors for metastatic and local recurrences have been described to be: SCCs >2 cm and in particular 6 mm of thickness, desmoplastic growth, a context of immunosuppression, and poor differentiation [31].

Locally extensive tumors or tumors spreading to lymph nodes or distant organs require individual treatment with a multidisciplinary approach. There are no clear guidelines on the elective treatment of at-risk lymph nodes by radiotherapy or surgery to prevent regional relapse. Risk of resection of first-echelon nodes must be weighed against the risk of metastatic nodal SCC. Tumors which may be considered for this would be high-risk tumors, even if lymphadenopathy is not clinically detectable, such as patients with SCC near the parotid gland [32], and patients with clinical involvement of cervical nodes (lymphadenopathy). Radiotherapy should be applied to the ipsilateral neck if more than 2 nodes are involved or extranodal spread is present in a single node [33].

Staging and additional prognostic information may be obtained through surgical staging of the first-echelon lymph node. This may be obtained through sentinel lymph node biopsy (SLNB) or elective lymph node dissection, allowing early therapeutic lymphadenectomy if positive for metastasis. SLNB in patients with high-risk SCC allows detection of subclinical nodal disease with minimal risk and morbidity [34], and a 2006 review showed that SLNB detects subclinical lymph node metastasis accurately in patients with high-risk SCC [35]. However, prospective studies are necessary to determine which patients should benefit from an SNLB.

Keratoacanthoma is an entity histologically indistinguishable from highly differentiated SCC, characterized by rapid growth over weeks, dome-shaped appearance with a central keratin-filled crater and should be handled as SCC in SOTR; therefore, also to be removed by complete excision. Complete tumor removal at early stages efficiently prevents subsequent metastasis, which is a significant problem in SOTR. After SCC occurrence and treatment, SOTR should be followed at closer intervals. Chemoprevention is possible against SCC, and discussed separately.

Primary radiotherapy is only used for patients who cannot benefit from surgery. Adjuvant or postoperative radiotherapy may be used after incomplete tumor resection, especially when there is extensive lymph node or perineural involvement, which has been described to lower recurrence and improve 5-year disease-free survival in SCCs of the head and neck [36].

Basal Cell Carcinoma

BCC treatment in SOTR follows the same recommendations as for the general population [13]. Radiotherapy is not recommended in these patients (recommendation D) due to risks of additional DNA damage and reduced time lag to radiation-induced cancer development.

Melanoma

There are conflicting data regarding the increase in melanoma incidence in SOTR compared to the general population. Some data report up to an 8-fold increase in this tumor [37], other studies did not observe an increased incidence [38]. Recently, a study reported similar outcomes of melanoma in SOTR as compared to prognostically matched non-immunosuppressed patients [39] for melanoma <2 mm Breslow thickness, but a worse outcome for melanoma >2 mm Breslow in these patients compared to the general population [40, 41].

Due to the limited number of reports concerning this tumor, we recommend that SOTR with a history of melanoma or at high risk for developing melanoma be monitored closely with dermatological consultations every 3 months. Patients presenting melanoma should be treated according to the general applicable guidelines (recommendation C) [41, 42]. This entails wide local excision with margins based on Breslow thickness, as in non-immunosuppressed patients (0.5 cm for in situ disease up to 2 cm for deeper invasive disease, i.e. 4 mm) [37]. Evaluation of the lymph node status is also important for management, as patients with positive lymph nodes require supplementary staging investigations in the form of PET, PET/CT, or directed CT or MRI.

The benefit of reducing or switching immunosuppression in metastatic melanoma remains unclear and should be weighed on an individual basis [29].

Kaposi Sarcoma

The iatrogenic form of KS related to long-term immunosuppressive drugs occurs with a 400- to 500-fold increase in cumulative incidence in SOTR [43], with a prevalence of 0.4% in US and European SOTR [44–46].

KS prevalence after transplantation is influenced by the prevalence of HHV8 infection in the general population. Indeed, most cases of posttransplant KS develop due to a viral reactivation [47] of HHV8. However, screening and measure of HHV8 viral load is not an appropriate test in a clinical setting for monitoring KS or predicting its occurrence in transplant patients due to low interval variations of this test [47].

Due to its variable clinical appearance, KS diagnosis should be sought early with careful examination of whole skin including mucosa (especially the palate) and be confirmed by biopsy. Multiple KS lesions are an indication of a higher likelihood of visceral involvement [48]. Workup for detection of potential visceral involvement should be discussed with a multidisciplinary transplant team.

Reduction of immunosuppressive therapy generally leads to resolution of iatrogenic KS [49, 50–55]. Several studies report maintaining immunosuppression by switching from calcineurin inhibitors to mammalian target of rapamycin (mTOR) inhibitors in renal transplant patients to resolve or stabilize KS [48]. Consequently, the current first-line recommendation for KS management in SOTR is a switch from calcineurin inhibitors to mTOR inhibitors (recommendation C). It must be noted that this recommendation particularly applies to renal transplant recipients, as this regimen has been described in these types of patients, and published data are lacking for other transplant recipients – this recommendation may not apply to the same extent to other SOTR. Second-line recommendation for the transplant physician is a reduction in immunosuppressive regimen (recommendation D).

Rare Types of Skin Cancers

Merkel cell carcinoma appeared increased in SOTR [56], and case reports for atypical fibroxanthoma, angiosarcoma, leiomyosarcoma, cutaneous T and B cell lymphoma are found. These tumors are very rare, even in SOTR, and no special recommendations have been phrased.

Choice and Modification of Immunosuppressive Regimen

SOTR patients have an increased risk of skin cancer, resulting from the long-term immunosuppression necessary for preventing graft rejection. The increase in incidence of skin cancer is related to the intensity of the treatment, the duration of immunosuppressive therapy, and the type of therapy. Reduction of this immunosuppressive state should be considered in patients at high risk for recurrent or aggressive skin cancer, especially in SCC with a high risk for metastasis or rapidly developing SCC (more than 1–3 high-risk SCCs per year) [57]. The best evidence of the impact of reduction of immunosuppression on the course of disease has been shown in KS, while this is less well described in other cancers. A likely benefit in reducing immunosuppressive therapy has been shown in SCC and should thus be carefully evaluated by transplant physicians in moderate and aggressive forms of SCC. For all other forms of skin cancer, benefits stemming from the reduction of immunosuppression may not necessarily exceed the advantages and quality of life resulting in maintaining an immunosuppression and preventing graft rejection. This decision should thus be considered on an individual basis (recommendation D) [12]. The following factors should be assessed when deciding whether or not to adjust immunotherapy, patient age, medication levels, HLA match, history of allograft rejection, time after transplantation, organ grafted [33].

Adjustment of immunosuppressive therapy may consist in decreasing the dosage, or reducing a triple therapy regimen to a dual immunosuppressive therapy. Another possibility is to switch a calcineurin inhibitor-based immunosuppression to mTOR inhibition by sirolimus or everolimus. Indeed, increased skin cancer risk has been shown in patients receiving triple immunosuppression compared to a dual therapy [58, 59], as well as in patients receiving induction therapy with OKT3 (antithymocyte globulin) or monoclonal anti-IL-2R antibodies [59]. Minimization of immunosuppressive therapy is therefore preferred in transplant recipients to reduce cutaneous malignancy.

When simplifying a triple regimen to a dual one, commonly azathioprine is discontinued. Azathioprine is a UVA photosensitizer leading to increased photocarcinogenesis [9, 45], which is why our current recommendation to transplant physicians is to consider a switch from azathioprine to another antimetabolite such as mycophenolate mofetil in SOTR with stable transplant function with moderate to severe cutaneous carcinogenesis of SCC (recommendation D) [16]. Cyclosporine A is known to increase levels of TGFβ and VEGF which potentially can contribute to cutaneous carcinogenesis and to directly upregulate ATF3 as a driver of carcinogenesis [17]. The class of mTOR inhibitors on the other side has shown antiproliferative effects in vitro and in vivo. Several studies have shown that once mTOR inhibitors were either added to regimens with calcineurin inhibitors or were substituted for calcineurin inhibitors, the rate of cutaneous malignancies decreased considerably [44]. These findings were not part of these studies' primary hypotheses, though, and there are currently multi-center trials in France, the Netherlands and Germany underway to validate the observation that mTOR inhibitors may decrease the incidence of SCC in SOTR. With results from these confirmatory trials pending, our current recommendation to transplant physicians is to consider a switch from calcineurin inhibitors to mTOR inhibitors in SOTR with stable transplant function in either (a) KS (recommendation C), or (b) moderate to severe cutaneous carcinogenesis of SCC (recommendation C).

Voriconazole is a second-generation antifungal approved for treatment of invasive aspergillosis in transplant recipients. It has been associated with accelerated skin cancer development [60–62]; particularly multifocal SCC in susceptible individuals, probably through a synergistic immunosuppressive and photosensitizing effect. Until the true population at risk for SCC associated with voriconazole is clearly determined, we suggest to carefully evaluate the need for long-term use in transplant recipients at risk [33].

Systemic Chemoprevention

Systemic Retinoid Therapy

Acitretin is a systemic retinoid shown to be beneficial in the prevention of SCC in the general population, and also in SOTR, where the benefit in SCC reduction may reach 85% [63–65]. We recommend evaluating the introduction of acitretin in SOTR with stable transplant function, especially in patients with moderate or severe forms of SCC, patients with significant SCC development (1–3 SCC per year), multiple SCC lesions in high-risk locations (neck and head), eruptive keratoacanthomas, patients with SCC and a history of lymphoma/leukemia, patients with SCC and a high metastatic risk or with presence of metastasis or field AK (recommendation A) [63–67].

This treatment is not a substitute for surgical therapy; rather it is a life-long chemoprevention-accompanying treatment. Patients who cannot benefit from surgery may receive systemic retinoid therapy to reduce morbidity and mortality associated with high-risk tumor [18] and metastatic disease [68]. This is a long-term continuous treatment at a typical dose of 0.4 mg/kg once per day (Neotigason®). We recommend starting at 10 mg every other day, and increasing to 10 mg per day after 2–4 weeks. After 2–4 weeks at this regimen, dosage can then be increased to 10 and 25 mg on alternating days during 2–4 weeks until achieving a daily regimen of 25 mg/day. In case this is not tolerated, doses may be reduced to the last dosage tolerable by the patient (recommendation D). Typical dose-dependent side effects are dryness of the lips, mouth, hair loss. These are reversible upon dose reduction or cessation. Liver transaminases, creatinine and lipids should be monitored twice a week during the first 2 months, then every month. Contraindicated medications are tetracyclines, methotrexate and other vitamin A derivatives. This highly teratogenic medication requires adequate contraception before treatment initiation, and maintained 2 years after end of therapy.

Isotretinoin is preferred for women who are of childbearing potential, as it is rapidly eliminated and contraception needs to be maintained only for one month after discontinuation. Should the medication be discontinued, we recommend to taper the dosage gradually as rebound effects have been reported with multiple and rapidly growing, aggressive SCC.

Capecitabine

Orally applied capecitabine, which converts systematically to 5-FU, is used for the treatment of metastatic breast cancer and metastatic colon cancer [69]. It has been described to have beneficial effects on chemoprevention for SOTR in small case series, at doses lower than those used for colorectal cancer [70]. Use of this drug is limited by its renal toxicity, side effects such as diarrhea and neutropenic fever, and intolerance in patients with dihydropyrimidine dehydrogenase deficiency. Further studies are required to evaluate efficacy and safety of this treatment which may be an optional off-label use in the future.

Integrated Care

The numbers of SOTR experiencing cutaneous adverse events in relation to transplantation, in particular skin cancer, are increasing. For optimal care of this frequently polymorbid population, a close collaboration between dermatologists and the transplant team is recommended both for patient education in prevention and for early treatment of evolving skin cancer. This should take place in secondary and tertiary medical centers where specialized organ transplant recipient clinics have been set up within many dermatology departments. Here, a standard of care can be defined and maintained along with transplant physicians, while medical residents can be trained focused on the special aspects of skin care in SOTR, and lastly clinical as well as laboratory studies can be conducted. On the other hand, the increasing number of SOTR implies that all dermatologists should at some point be involved and educated in the particular needs of this patient group, because an increasing amount of care will also have to be provided in a peripheral setting outside the transplant center. Exchange of individual clinical information should thus not only take place between dermatologists and transplant physicians within large centers, but also between dermatologists at centers and those in the periphery. The main objectives of such an integrated care should be to recognize and communicate to all transplant physicians involved the current state of cutaneous carcinogenesis in a given SOTR. It is crucial that an occurrence of SCC is not seen as isolated event, but rather as one in a chain of events that may influence transplant decisions such as the choice of immunosuppressive regimen, the treatment of field cancerization, systemic chemoprevention (recommendation D) and decisions regarding retransplantation.

Future Trends

Skin cancer development in SOTR is a significant problem requiring multidisciplinary care involving the transplant team and the dermatologist. Key points are early and regular patient education on sun protection, early therapeutic intervention, frequent and regular follow-up to monitor disease evolution and eventual recurrence. Recent developments such as switching calcineurin inhibitors to mTOR inhibitors, applying α-MSH analogue for systemic photoprotection and the use of EGFR inhibitors in advanced SCC are being investigated.

References

1 Stasko T, Brown MD, Carucci JA, Euvrard S, Johnson TM, Sengelmann RD, et al: Guidelines for the management of squamous cell carcinoma in organ transplant recipients. Dermatol Surg 2004;30:642–650.

2 Christenson LJ, Geusau A, Ferrandiz C, Brown CD, Ulrich C, Stockfleth E, Berg D, Orengo I, Shaw JC, Carucci JA, Euvrard S, Pacheco T, Stasko T, Otley CC: Specialty clinics for the dermatologic care of solid-organ transplant recipients. Dermatol Surg 2004;30:598–603.

3 Donovan JC, Rosen CF, Shaw JC: Evaluation of sunprotective practices of organ transplant recipients. Am J Transplant 2004;4:1852–1858.

4 Firooz A, Amin-Nejad R, Bouzari N, Nafar M, Firoozan A, Mahdavi-Mazdeh M: Sun protection in Iranian kidney transplant recipients: knowledge, attitude and practice. J Eur Acad Dermatol Venereol 2007;21:754–757.

5 Lapointe AK, Hofbauer G, Anliker M, Arnold A, Binet I, Hunger R, Kempf W, Pascual M, Pelloni F, Serra A, Laffitte E: Swiss clinical practice guidelines for skin cancer in organ transplant recipients (in French). Rev Med Suisse 2010;6:854–859.

6 Berg D, Otley CC: Skin cancer in organ transplant recipients: epidemiology, pathogenesis, and management. J Am Acad Dermatol 2002;47:1–17, quiz 18–20.

7 O'Reilly F TC, Pennie ML, Foster JK, Chen SC: Baseline quality of life and anxiety in solid organ transplant recipients: a pilot study. Dermatol Surg 2006;32:1480–1485.

8 Whitmore SE, Morison WL: Prevention of UVB-induced immunosuppression in humans by a high sun protection factor sunscreen. Arch Dermatol 1995;131: 1128–1133.

9 Ducloux D, Courivaud C, Bamoulid J, Kazory A, Dumoulin G, Chalopin JM: Pretransplant serum vitamin D levels and risk of cancer after renal transplantation. Transplantation 2008;85:1755–1759.

10 Seukeran DC, Newstead CG, Cunliffe WJ: The compliance of renal transplant recipients with advice about sun protection measures. Br J Dermatol 1998;138:301–303.

11 Ulrich C, Jurgensen JS, Degen A, Hackethal M, Ulrich M, Patel MJ, Eberle J, Terhorst D, Sterry W, Stockfleth E: Prevention of non-melanoma skin cancer in organ transplant patients by regular use of a sunscreen: a 24 months, prospective, case-control study. Br J Dermatol 2009;161(suppl 3):78–84.

12 Norval M, Wulf HC: Does chronic sunscreen use reduce vitamin D production to insufficient levels? Br J Dermatol 2009;161:732–736.

13 Reichrath J NB: Solar UV-radiation, vitamin D and skin cancer surveillance in organ transplant recipients (SOTRs). Adv Exp Med Biol 2008;624:203–214.

14 Zwald FO, Brown M: Skin cancer in solid organ transplant recipients: advances in therapy and management. I. Epidemiology of skin cancer in solid organ transplant recipients. J Am Acad Dermatol 2011;65:253–261, quiz 262.

15 Hofbauer GF, Anliker M, Arnold A, Binet I, Hunger R, Kempf W, Laffitte E, Lapointe AC, Pascual M, Pelloni F, Serra A: Swiss clinical practice guidelines for skin cancer in organ transplant recipients. Swiss Med Wkly 2009;139:407–415.

16 Hofbauer GF, Attard NR, Harwood CA, McGregor JM, Dziunycz P, Iotzova-Weiss G, Straub G, Meyer R, Kamenisch Y, Berneburg M, French LE, Wuthrich RP, Karran P, Serra AL: Reversal of UVA skin photosensitivity and DNA damage in kidney transplant recipients by replacing azathioprine. Am J Transplant 2012;12:218–225.

17 Wu X, Nguyen BC, Dziunycz P, Chang S, Brooks Y, Lefort K, Hofbauer GF, Dotto GP: Opposing roles for calcineurin and ATF3 in squamous skin cancer. Nature 2010;465:368–372.

18 Zwald FO, Brown M: Skin cancer in solid organ transplant recipients: advances in therapy and management. II. Management of skin cancer in solid organ transplant recipients. J Am Acad Dermatol 2011;65:263–279, quiz 280.

19 Wulf HC, Pavel S, Stender I, Bakker-Wensveen CA: Topical photodynamic therapy for prevention of new skin lesions in renal transplant recipients. Acta Derm Venereol 2006;86:25–28.

20 de Graaf YG, Kennedy C, Wolterbeek R, Collen AF, Willemze R, Bouwes Bavinck JN: Photodynamic therapy does not prevent cutaneous squamous-cell carcinoma in organ-transplant recipients: results of a randomized-controlled trial. J Invest Dermatol 2006;126:569–574.

21 Wennberg AM, Stenquist B, Stockfleth E, Keohane S, Lear JT, Jemec G, Mork C, Christensen E, Kapp A, Solvsten H, Talme T, Berne B, Forschner T: Photodynamic therapy with methyl aminolevulinate for prevention of new skin lesions in transplant recipients: a randomized study. Transplantation 2008;86:423–429.

22 Willey A, Mehta S, Lee PK: Reduction in the incidence of squamous cell carcinoma in solid organ transplant recipients treated with cyclic photodynamic therapy. Dermatol Surg 2009;36:652–658.

23 Ulrich C, Johannsen A, Rowert-Huber J, Ulrich M, Sterry W, Stockfleth E: Results of a randomized, placebo-controlled safety and efficacy study of topical diclofenac 3% gel in organ transplant patients with multiple actinic keratoses. Eur J Dermatol 2010; 20:482–488.

24 Kovach BT, Stasko T: Use of topical immunomodulators in organ transplant recipients. Dermatol Ther 2005;18:19–27.

25 Perrett CM, McGregor JM, Warwick J, Karran P, Leigh IM, Proby CM, Harwood CA: Treatment of post-transplant premalignant skin disease: a randomized intrapatient comparative study of 5-fluorouracil cream and topical photodynamic therapy. Br J Dermatol 2007;156:320–328.

26 Piaserico S, Belloni Fortina A, Rigotti P, Rossi B, Baldan N, Alaibac M, Marchini F: Topical photodynamic therapy of actinic keratosis in renal transplant recipients. Transplant Proc 2007;39: 1847–1850.

27 de Graaf YG, Basdew VR, van Zwan-Kralt N, Willemze R, Bavinck JN: The occurrence of residual or recurrent squamous cell carcinomas in organ transplant recipients after curettage and electrodessication. Br J Dermatol 2006;154:493–497.

28 Leibovitch I, Huilgol SC, Selva D, Hill D, Richards S, Paver R: Cutaneous squamous cell carcinoma treated with Mohs micrographic surgery in Australia II. Perineural invasion. J Am Acad Dermatol 2005; 53:261–266.

29 Stasko T, Brown MD, Carucci JA, Euvrard S, Johnson TM, Sengelmann RD, Stockfleth E, Tope WD: Guidelines for the management of squamous cell carcinoma in organ transplant recipients. Dermatol Surg 2004;30:642–650.

30 Dinehart SM: The treatment of actinic keratoses. J Am Acad Dermatol 2000;42:25–28.

31 Brantsch KD, Meisner C, Schonfisch B, Trilling B, Wehner-Caroli J, Rocken M, Breuninger H: Analysis of risk factors determining prognosis of cutaneous squamous-cell carcinoma: a prospective study. Lancet Oncol 2008;9:713–720.

32 Veness MJ, Palme CE, Morgan GJ: High-risk cutaneous squamous cell carcinoma of the head and neck: results from 266 treated patients with metastatic lymph node disease. Cancer 2006;106:2389–2396.

33 O'Reilly Zwald F, Brown M: Skin cancer in solid organ transplant recipients: Advances in therapy and management. II. Management of skin cancer in solid organ transplant recipients. J Am Acad Dermatol 2011;65:263–279.

34 Wagner JD, Evdokimow DZ, Weisberger E, Moore D, Chuang TY, Wenck S, Coleman JJ 3rd: Sentinel node biopsy for high-risk nonmelanoma cutaneous malignancy. Arch Dermatol 2004;140:75–79.

35 Ross AS, Schmults CD: Sentinel lymph node biopsy in cutaneous squamous cell carcinoma: a systematic review of the English literature. Dermatol Surg 2006;32:1309–1321.

36 Veness MJ, Porceddu S, Palme CE, Morgan GJ: Cutaneous head and neck squamous cell carcinoma metastatic to parotid and cervical lymph nodes. Head Neck 2007;29:621–631.

37 Tsao H, Atkins MB, Sober AJ: Management of cutaneous melanoma. N Engl J Med 2004;351:998–1012.

38 Lindelöf B, Sigurgeirsson B, Gäbel H, Stern RS: Incidence of skin cancer in 5356 patients following organ transplantation. Br J Dermatol 2000;143:513–519.

39 Dapprich DC, Weenig RH, Rohlinger AL, Weaver AL, Quan KK, Keeling JH, Walsh JS, Otley CC, Christenson LJ: Outcomes of melanoma in recipients of solid organ transplant. J Am Acad Dermatol 2008;59:405–417.

40 Matin RN, Mesher D, Proby CM, McGregor JM, Bouwes Bavinck JN, del Marmol V, Euvrard S, Ferrandiz C, Geusau A, Hackethal M, Ho WL, Hofbauer GF, Imko-Walczuk B, Kanitakis J, Lally A, Lear JT, Lebbe C, Murphy GM, Piaserico S, Seckin D, Stockfleth E, Ulrich C, Wojnarowska FT, Lin HY, Balch C, Harwood CA: Melanoma in organ transplant recipients: clinicopathological features and outcome in 100 cases. Am J Transplant 2008;8:1891–1900.

41 Dummer R, Hauschild A, Jost L: Cutaneous malignant melanoma: ESMO clinical recommendations for diagnosis, treatment and follow-up. Ann Oncol 2008;19(suppl 2):ii86–ii88.

42 Wulf HC, Pavel S, Stender I, Bakker-Wensveen CA: Topical photodynamic therapy for prevention of new skin lesions in renal transplant recipients. Acta Derm Venereol 2006;86:25–28.

43 Zavos G, Bokos J, Papaconstantinou I, Boletis J, Gazouli M, Kakisis J, Zografidis A, Kostakis A: Clinicopathological aspects of 18 Kaposi's sarcoma among 1055 Greek renal transplant recipients. Artif Organs 2004;28:595–599.

44 Farge D: Kaposi's sarcoma in organ transplant recipients. The Collaborative Transplantation Research Group of Ile de France. Eur J Med 1993;2:339–343.

45 Penn I: Kaposi's sarcoma in organ transplant recipients: report of 20 cases. Transplantation 1979;27: 8–11.

46 Penn I: Cancers following cyclosporine therapy. Transplant Proc 1987;19:2211–2213.

47 Lebbe C, Legendre C, Frances C: Kaposi sarcoma in transplantation. Transplant Rev (Orlando) 2008;22: 252–261.

48 Schwartz RA, Micali G, Nasca MR, Scuderi L: Kaposi sarcoma: a continuing conundrum. J Am Acad Dermatol 2008;59:179–206, quiz 207–178.

49 Brenner B, Weissmann-Brenner A, Rakowsky E, Weltfriend S, Fenig E, Friedman-Birnbaum R, Sulkes A, Linn S: Classical Kaposi sarcoma: prognostic factor analysis of 248 patients. Cancer 2002;95:1982–1987.

50 Campistol JM, Gutierrez-Dalmau A, Torregrosa JV: Conversion to sirolimus: a successful treatment for posttransplantation Kaposi's sarcoma. Transplantation 2004;77:760–762.

51 Duman S, Toz H, Asci G, Alper S, Ozkahya M, Unal I, Celik A, Ok E, Basci A: Successful treatment of post-transplant Kaposi's sarcoma by reduction of immunosuppression. Nephrol Dial Transplant 2002; 17:892–896.

52 Kaplan L, Abrams D, Volberding P: Treatment of Kaposi's sarcoma in acquired immunodeficiency syndrome with an alternating vincristine-vinblastine regimen. Cancer Treat Rep 1986;70:1121–1122.

53 Marcelin AG, Roque-Afonso AM, Hurtova M, Dupin N, Tulliez M, Sebagh M, Arkoub ZA, Guettier C, Samuel D, Calvez V, Dussaix E: Fatal disseminated Kaposi's sarcoma following human herpesvirus 8 primary infections in liver-transplant recipients. Liver Transpl 2004;10:295–300.

54 Moray G, Basaran O, Yagmurdur MC, Emiroglu R, Bilgin N, Haberal M: Immunosuppressive therapy and Kaposi's sarcoma after kidney transplantation. Transplant Proc 2004;36:168–170.

55 Zavos G, Bokos J, Papaconstantinou J, Boletis J, Gazouli M, Pappas P, Kostakis A: Study of 'de novo' malignancies among Greek renal transplant recipients. Transplant Proc 2003;35:1399–1403.

56 Penn I, First MR: Merkel's cell carcinoma in organ recipients: report of 41 cases. Transplantation 1999; 68:1717–1721.

57 Otley CC, Berg D, Ulrich C, Stasko T, Murphy GM, Salasche SJ, Christenson LJ, Sengelmann R, Loss GE Jr, Garces J: Reduction of immunosuppression for transplant-associated skin cancer: expert consensus survey. Br J Dermatol 2006;154:395–400.

58 Campistol JM, Eris J, Oberbauer R, Friend P, Hutchison B, Morales JM, Claesson K, Stallone G, Russ G, Rostaing L, Kreis H, Burke JT, Brault Y, Scarola JA, Neylan JF: Sirolimus therapy after early cyclosporine withdrawal reduces the risk for cancer in adult renal transplantation. J Am Soc Nephrol 2006;17:581–589.

59 Geusau A, Dunkler D, Messeritsch E, Sandor N, Heidler G, Rodler S, Ankersmit J, Zuckermann A, Tschachler E: Non-melanoma skin cancer and its risk factors in an Austrian population of heart transplant recipients receiving induction therapy. Int J Dermatol 2008;47:918–925.

60 Mabruk MJ, Toh LK, Murphy M, Leader M, Kay E, Murphy GM: Investigation of the effect of UV irradiation on DNA damage: comparison between skin cancer patients and normal volunteers. J Cutan Pathol 2009;36:760–765.

61 Laing ME, Dicker P, Murphy GM: Toll-like receptor 4, 7 and 8 polymorphisms have no association with nonmelanoma skin cancer in renal transplant patients. Br J Dermatol 2009;161:715–717.

62 Tuttleton Arron S, Jennings L, Nindl I, Rosl F, Bouwes Bavinck JN, Seckin D, Trakatelli M, Murphy GM: Viral oncogenesis and its role in nonmelanoma skin cancer. Br J Dermatol 2011;164:1201–1213.

63 Bavinck JN, Tieben LM, Van der Woude FJ, Tegzess AM, Hermans J, ter Schegget J, Vermeer BJ: Prevention of skin cancer and reduction of keratotic skin lesions during acitretin therapy in renal transplant recipients: a double-blind, placebo-controlled study. J Clin Oncol 1995;13:1933–1938.

64 George R, Weightman W, Russ GR, Bannister KM, Mathew TH: Acitretin for chemoprevention of nonmelanoma skin cancers in renal transplant recipients. Australas J Dermatol 2002;43:269–273.

65 Harwood CA, Leedham-Green M, Leigh IM, Proby CM: Low-dose retinoids in the prevention of cutaneous squamous cell carcinomas in organ transplant recipients: a 16-year retrospective study. Arch Dermatol 2005;141:456–464.

66 DiGiovanna JJ: Retinoid chemoprevention in the high-risk patient. J Am Acad Dermatol 1998;39: S82–S85.

67 McKenna DB, Murphy GM: Skin cancer chemoprophylaxis in renal transplant recipients: 5 years of experience using low-dose acitretin. Br J Dermatol 1999;140:656–660.

68 Martinez JC, Otley CC, Stasko T, Euvrard S, Brown C, Schanbacher CF, Weaver AL: Defining the clinical course of metastatic skin cancer in organ transplant recipients: a multicenter collaborative study. Arch Dermatol 2003;139:301–306.

69 Peramiquel L, Dalmau J, Puig L, Roe E, Fernandez-Figueras MT, Alomar A: Inflammation of actinic keratoses and acral erythrodysesthesia during capecitabine treatment. J Am Acad Dermatol 2006; 55:S119–S120.

70 Endrizzi BT, Lee PK: Management of carcinoma of the skin in solid organ transplant recipients with oral capecitabine. Dermatol Surg 2009;35:1567–1572.

PD Dr. Günther Hofbauer
Dermatologische Klinik, Universitätsspital Zürich
Gloriastrasse 31
CH–8091 Zürich (Switzerland)
Tel. +41 44 255 46 20, E-Mail hofbauer@usz.ch

Häusermann P, Steiger J, Passweg J (eds): Transplantation Dermatology.
Curr Probl Dermatol. Basel, Karger, 2012, vol 43, pp 71–80

Future Trends in Organ Transplant Recipients – Important Issues for Dermatologists

Daniel Zecher · Jürg Steiger

Clinic for Transplantation Immunology and Nephrology, University Hospital Basel, Basel, Switzerland

Abstract

It is on the tip of everyone's tongue in the transplant community that recent improvements in short-term survival of solid organ allografts have not translated into the expected increase in long-term survival. Besides chronic immune-mediated damage to the transplanted organ, the poor long-term survival of allografts has been attributed to the nephrotoxic effects of the calcineurin inhibitors. Moreover, the immunosuppressive burden and metabolic side effects of the current anti-rejection drugs are clearly related to increased rates of malignancies, infections and accelerated atherosclerosis, all of which make up for the premature death of a considerable proportion of transplant recipients with a functioning allograft. Therefore, attempts have been made over the last decade to either reduce or withdraw both steroids and calcineurin inhibitors from maintenance regimens. Furthermore, there is an ongoing intensive search for new less toxic and more specific drugs which would ideally selectively impair the alloimmune response while preserving the immune system's capacity to fight infection and malignancy (i.e. induce tolerance). Moreover, new concepts have emerged to individualize a patient's immunosuppressive therapy based on an improved pretransplant risk assessment. With the causes of chronic allograft damage being increasingly well defined, better and more personalized long-term follow-up strategies are being developed to ultimately prevent late allograft loss. These aspects will be reviewed here with a focus on kidney transplantation and the possible impact of these new approaches on the incidence of skin cancer.

The introduction of the calcineurin inhibitors (CNIs) cyclosporine (CsA) in the 1980s and tacrolimus (FK) and the anti-metabolite mycofenolate-mofetil (MMF) in the 1990s into clinical transplantation has dramatically improved short-term survival of all transplanted solid organ allografts. Despite excellent 1-year graft survival rates exceeding 90% for kidney transplants and reaching 85% for heart and lung grafts, long-term graft survival rates have remained almost unchanged over recent years with a median survival of kidney, heart and lung allografts of 8.8 (deceased donors only), 11.2 and 5.2 years, respectively [1, 2]. Besides chronic immune-mediated damage to the transplanted organ, the poor long-term survival of kidney grafts has been attributed to the nephrotoxic effects of the CNIs [3]. Moreover, the immunosuppressive burden and metabolic side effects of the anti-rejection drugs are clearly related to increased rates of malignancies, infections and accelerated atherosclerosis, all of which make up for the premature death of up to 40% of transplant recipients with a functioning allograft [2]. Therefore, attempts have been made over the last decade to either reduce or withdraw both steroids and CNIs from maintenance regimens following transplantation. There is also an ongoing intensive search for new less toxic and more specific immunosuppressive drugs. Moreover, new concepts have emerged to reduce the immunosuppressive burden by individualizing patients' induction and maintenance immunosuppressive therapy based on an improved pretransplant risk assessment. With the causes of chronic allograft damage being increasingly well defined, better and more personalized long-term follow-up strategies are being developed to ultimately prevent late allograft loss. These aspects will be reviewed here with a focus on kidney transplantation and the possible impact of these strategies on the incidence of skin cancer.

Steroid Avoidance or Withdrawal

Due to their potent immunosuppressive effects, corticosteroids (CS) have been used for induction and maintenance therapy as well as treatment of acute cellular rejection episodes since the early days of solid organ transplantation. Given their well-known side effects associated with long-term administration (new-onset diabetes after transplantation, hypertension, hyperlipidemia, osteoporosis, avascular necrosis), the aim of reducing CS exposure is compelling. Different strategies have been used for patients considered at low risk for acute allograft rejection: steroid-free protocols were compared with early (before day 7 after transplantation) vs. late (3–6 months after transplantation) steroid withdrawal vs. standard dose regimens. Most trials found a higher rate of acute rejection episodes in patients whose regimens were either steroid free or who had discontinued CS early [4, 5]. The only long-term follow-up data available today came from a trial that compared early CS cessation with standard therapy. Notably, this trial found a doubling in chronic allograft nephropathy after 5 years in those patients that had stopped steroids within 7 days after transplantation (9.9 vs. 4.1%) [6]. This trial also reported an increased risk of non-melanoma skin cancer in those patients that were still on CS at 5 years (9.2 vs. 5.2%), likely reflecting the higher burden of immunosuppression in those patients. Despite some controversy with regard to the best time point of CS withdrawal [7], recent meta-analyses concluded that CS withdrawal is safe, particularly in those patients receiving FK as immunosuppressive backbone as opposed to those taking CsA [8]. Until today, however, there has been a lack of studies that clearly show a long-term survival benefit, preserved allograft function and a reduction in cardiovascular events and mortality following CS withdrawal.

Calcineurin Inhibitor Sparing

CNIs are the backbone of all current maintenance immunosuppressive regimens. Due to their metabolic side effects and renal toxicity, efforts have been made to reduce exposure either by dose reduction or replacement by other agents, most notably the mTOR inhibitors sirolimus (SRL) and everolimus. Three recent prospective, randomized, multi-center trials exemplify these efforts: the ELITE-Symphony trial compared standard dose CsA in combination with MMF and CS with either low-dose CsA, low-dose FK or low-dose SRL, all three in combination with daclizumab (anti-IL2Rβ) induction, MMF and CS [9]. Biopsy-confirmed acute rejection and allograft survival at 12 months were best in the low-dose FK and worst in the SRL group (12.3 and 94.2% vs. 37.2 and 89.3%, respectively). Rates of infections and cancers tended to be higher in the groups containing a CNI. The CAESAR study compared discontinuation of CsA 6 months after transplantation with standard- and low-dose CsA [10]. All groups received daclizumab induction together with MMF and CS maintenance. At 12 months, patients who had stopped CsA had a significantly higher rate of biopsy-confirmed rejection compared to those patients still on CsA (38 vs. 25.4 vs. 27.5% for withdrawal, low- or standard dose, respectively). None of these trials showed the anticipated improvement in glomerular filtration rate (GFR) after reducing CNI exposure. In an attempt to avoid long-term CNI toxicity, replacement of CNIs by mTOR inhibitors has been considered a promising strategy. This is of particular interest as the use of mTOR inhibitors has consistently been associated with reduced rates of both skin and non-dermal malignancies [11, 12]. The CONVERT trial switched maintenance renal transplant recipients from CNI to standard-dose SRL at variable times following transplantation [13]. This study identified a subset of stable patients with preserved renal function (GFR>40 ml/min and proteinuria <100 mg/day) that could successfully be switched without an increased rate of biopsy-confirmed acute rejection 12 and 24 months after the intervention. However, side effects including proteinuria, bone marrow suppression and hyperlipidemia were found to be significantly increased in those patients switched to SRL, raising doubts about the safety of this drug. The overall incidence of de novo malignancy as well as non-melanoma skin cancer was significantly lower in those patients that had switched to SRL (3.8 vs. 11% and 2.2 vs. 8.1%, respectively). Interestingly, 75% of those patients on SRL that were found to have non-melanoma skin cancer during the 24 months' observation period had a similar diagnosis prior to inclusion in the study, arguing that SRL reduces de novo skin cancer more than recurrence of the disease [14]. In conclusion, the above-mentioned trials confirm the efficacy but also the superiority of CNI-containing maintenance regimens over alternative strategies with a potential advantage of FK over CsA. Despite initial enthusiasm with the use of mTOR inhibitors to replace CNIs and the well-documented reduced incidence of malignancy with SRL, the risk-benefit ratio clearly argues against a generalized use of these agents.

Future Concepts of Immunosuppression and New Immunosuppressive Drugs

Allospecific tolerance, i.e. the achievement of donor-specific unresponsiveness to a transplanted organ while preserving the capacity of the recipient's immune system to fight infection and cancer, still remains the Holy Grail in transplantation. Despite much progress in basic research in identifying key cellular players and pathways relevant for tolerance induction in small animals, none of these strategies has so far been successfully applied in clinical transplantation. One of the major aims therefore still remains to identify drugs or strategies that are potent enough to replace long-term CNI administration without an increased risk-benefit ratio. Moreover, B cells have recently received much attention due to the implementation of blood group-incompatible renal transplantation into clinical practice and the recognition of antibody-mediated rejection (AMR) as a major risk factor for long-term allograft loss [15]. Finally, the introduction of monoclonal antibodies into clinical transplantation bears the promise to shift today's unspecific immunosuppression strategies with their inherent side effect profiles towards a more specific targeting of individual molecules or signaling pathways that are central to the alloimmune response. Most antibody preparations have so far been used in the context of short-term induction therapy in patients at high risk for graft rejection. Progress in biotechnology has led to the generation of humanized antibodies with reduced immunogenicity, which will pave the way for some of these molecules to be used as maintenance immunosuppression.

Rituximab

Rituximab is a lytic chimeric monoclonal antibody targeting the surface molecule CD20 on premature and naïve B cells (fig. 1). In combination with immunoadsorption or plasmapheresis protocols and application of polyclonal immunoglobulin preparations (IVIG), rituximab has completely replaced splenectomy prior to ABO-incompatible transplantation. Rates of acute rejection and patient as well as graft survival are now equivalent to ABO-matched kidney recipients [16]. Interestingly, there is increasing evidence that ABO-incompatible transplantation might even be possible without rituximab, suggesting that better removal and monitoring strategies of the isoagglutinins in the peritransplant period is actually the main reason for the recent success in ABO-incompatible transplantation [17]. Rituximab has also been used for desensitization in patients with either high titers of human leukocyte antigen (HLA) antibodies [18, 19] or donor-specific HLA antibodies (HLA-DSA) [20], patients at high risk for AMR and allograft loss. Results were quite variable with acute rejection rates between 20 and 50%; therefore, caution is warranted regarding the long-term outcome of these patients. The partial success of rituximab when used for the above indications is particularly interesting given that it is thought to spare mature, antibody-producing plasma cells. These findings are highly suggestive for additional B cell functions such

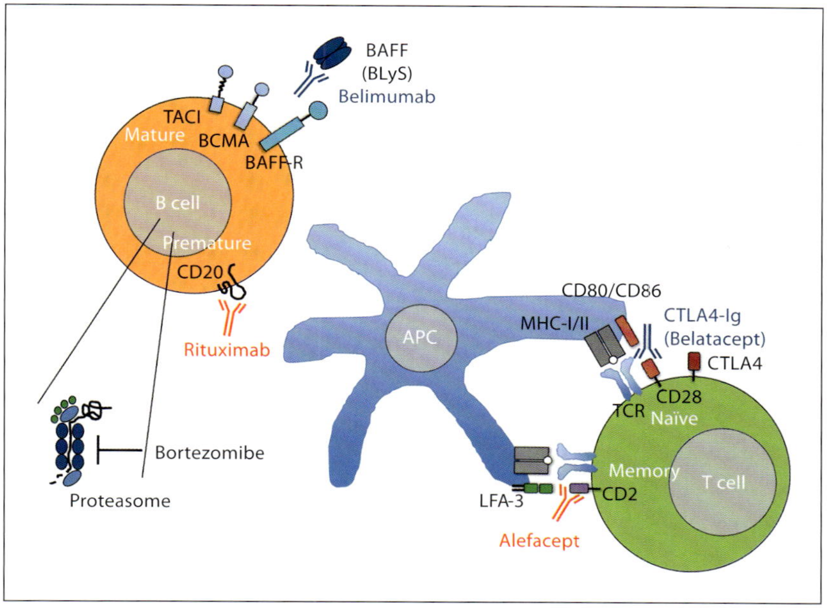

Fig. 1. Cellular targets of the novel immunosuppressive drugs. For simplicity, fusion proteins (belatacept, alefacept) and monoclonal antibodies (all others) are depicted with an antibody symbol. Depleting agents are shown in red whereas blocking agents are in blue. APC = antigen-presenting cell; CD = cluster of differentiation; TCR = T-cell receptor; MHC I/II = major histocompatibility complex I or II; LFA-3 = lymphocyte function-associated antigen 3; CTLA4 = cytotoxic T-lymphocyte-associated antigen; BAFF = B cell activation factor; TACI = transmembrane activator and calcium modulator and cyclophilin ligand interactor; BCMA = B cell maturation protein; BAFF-R = BAFF receptor.

as antigen presentation, cytokine production or T cell help, and have brought B cells back in the focus of both clinical and basic research. However, they also clearly underline the need for more efficient therapies targeting the humoral alloimmune response.

Belimumab

Another promising agent to target humoral immunity is belimumab. This fully human monoclonal antibody impairs B cell activation and maturation by targeting the anti-apoptotic B cell survival factors BAFF (B cell activation factor, also known as B lymphocyte stimulator BLyS) and APRIL (a proliferation inducing ligand) (fig. 1). Belimumab has been used for the treatment of systemic lupus erythematodes where it has proven efficacious in the treatment of active disease [21]. A phase II study is currently under way to test the efficacy of belimumab as a desensitization agent in highly sensitized patients awaiting kidney transplantation (clinicaltrials.gov NCT01025193).

Belatacept

The interaction of CD80 or CD86 on antigen-presenting cells with CD28 on T cells provides costimulatory signals that are germane for effective activation of naïve T cells. Belatacept, a recombinant fusion protein containing the extracellular domain of cytotoxic T lymphocyte-associated antigen 4 (CTLA4-Ig) selectively inhibits binding of CD80/86 to CD28 and thereby prevents costimulation (fig. 1). Belatacept was FDA-approved in June 2011 as first-line agent to prevent rejection of kidney allografts. Approval was based on the results of two phase III studies that showed similar patient and graft survival at 12 months in patients receiving one of two doses of belatacept versus a group that received standard-dose CsA. All patients received additionally MMF and low-dose CS [22, 23]. Notably, patients in the belatacept groups had significantly better renal function as measured by calculated GFR at 12 [22, 23] and 24 months [24]. These results render belatacept probably the most promising new agent in renal transplantation at the moment. However, several aspects need to be considered. Belatacept treatment also resulted in significantly more and more severe acute rejection episodes (22 vs. 17 vs. 7% for more intensive vs. low intensive belatacept vs. CsA at 12 months). Acute rejection still being one of the most important risk factors for late allograft loss, long-term follow-up data will reveal the efficacy of belatacept in preserving renal allograft function. Importantly, there have been major concerns about the safety of belatacept. Until June 2009, a total of 14 cases of EBV-associated posttransplant lymphoproliferative disease have been reported among 949 patients that had received belatacept for a minimum of 12 months compared to 2/476 cases in CsA-treated patients [25]. Of particular concern was the high percentage of posttransplant lymphoproliferative disease localized to the central nervous system (9/14) in belatacept-treated patients [25]. The incidence of non-melanoma skin cancer showed subtle differences among the groups, with no clear benefit for those patients on belatacept (3.1 vs. 1.3 vs. 2.3% for more intensive vs. low intensive vs. CsA, respectively) [25].

Alefacept

Memory T cells play a major role in acute and chronic allograft rejection. One major obstacle in translating basic research into clinical practice is the presence of a large repertoire of memory cells in humans that is absent in small animals most often used for experimental studies. Memory cells do not require costimulation for efficient activation, and therefore do not respond to belatacept. Alefacept is a dimeric fusion protein consisting of the CD2-binding portion of the human lymphocyte function-associated antigen 3 linked to the Fc portion of human IgG1 (fig. 1). CD2 is more densely expressed on memory as compared to naïve T cells, and therefore alefacept preferentially depletes memory T cells. It is currently used for the treatment of psoriasis [26]. Simultaneous administration of costimulation blockade with CTLA4-Ig and alefacept has recently been shown to prevent renal allograft rejection and formation of alloantibodies in a non-human primate model [27], rendering this a promising strategy to be applied in clinical transplantation.

Bortezomibe

Bortezomibe, a proteasome inhibitor used for the treatment of multiple myeloma, induces apoptosis of rapidly dividing cells, and has been used experimentally in desensitization protocols prior to ABO-incompatible kidney transplantation [28] and for the treatment of AMR [29]. A recent study by Trivedi et al. [30] described the use of bortezomibe together with transfusion of donor-derived peripheral stem cells and a conditioning regimen including cyclophosphamide, ATG and rituximab in 18 young living-related kidney transplant recipients. This approach was intended to achieve a state of operational tolerance by clonal deletion of allospecific cells allowing no maintenance immunosuppression. Albeit conceptually intriguing, evidence for clonal deletion was not provided, and 22% of patients developed donor-specific anti-HLA-antibodies (HLA-DSA). During a median follow-up of 264 days, acute rejection rate was 22% with only 4/18 patients being indeed free of maintenance immunosuppression.

Due to their potent immunosuppressive properties and widespread expression, the major concern of many of these new molecules is their safety profile, and a thorough risk-benefit analysis will have to be done prior to their widespread introduction into clinical practice. So far, data are not available for any of these agents (except rituximab and belatacept) regarding their impact on skin malignancies.

Strategies to Improve Pretransplant Risk Assessment

Current risk assessment strategies in the US classify more than 50% of all kidney transplant recipients to be at high risk for rejection. The current algorithms have resulted in an increase rather than a decrease in administration of depleting antibodies over the last 10 years (11% in 1998 vs. 53% in 2009) [31]. An alternative approach to reduce the overall immunosuppressive burden of transplant recipients therefore is to improve the pretransplant risk assessment. The primary goal of this strategy would be to allow for the reduction in immunosuppression in those individuals identified to be at low risk for rejection. Allocation of both living and deceased donor allografts is based on donor and recipient matching for the major HLA molecules A, B (class I) and DR, DQ (class II). The strongest predictor for acute allograft rejection and allograft loss is the presence of HLA-DSA in a recipient's serum reflecting prior sensitization to donor alloantigens [32]. Various strategies have been proposed to better define the risk of rejection prior to transplantation: expansion of donor HLA typing (HLA DP, Cw) as well as screening for DSA targeting non-HLA molecules (e.g. MICA, endothelial cell, angiotensin II antibodies [33–35]). Traditionally, the presence of HLA-DSA has been identified by cell-based crossmatch assays (i.e. by complement-dependent cytotoxicity, CDC-XM, or flow cytometry). These methods have considerable limitations in both sensitivity and specificity. In recent years, the development of microparticles coated with single HLA molecules has allowed the precise determination of the specificity of the recipient's HLA antibodies with high sensitivity [36]. By comparing the recipient's HLA antibodies with the HLA antigens of the donor, the presence of HLA-DSA can be determined virtually (= virtual crossmatch; virtual-XM). Due to the increased sensitivity of the method, a subset of patients with a negative CDC-XM can be identified, in which a positive virtual-XM indicates the presence of low-level HLA-DSA. Several retrospective studies have shown that these patients have a significantly higher incidence of early rejection, especially AMR, and that this translates into a significantly higher allograft loss at 5 years [37, 38]. Recently, Amico et al. [39] prospectively studied the impact of virtual-XM risk stratification and subsequent allocation of higher initial immunosuppression to virtual-XM-positive compared to XM-negative patients on graft and patient outcome. Virtual-XM-positive patients (18%) received ATG and IVIG induction, whereas XM-negative patients (82%) were treated with the less potent basiliximab. Both groups received standard triple immunosuppression. The cumulative incidence of AMR at 1 year was significantly higher in the former compared to the latter group despite the higher immunosuppressive load (42 vs. 8%, respectively). After a median follow-up of 2.6 years, allograft loss because of AMR occurred less often in the negative virtual-XM group (1 vs. 7%). The results of this study indicate that pretransplant risk assessment by virtual-XM can identify a relevant subset of patients (82%) at very low risk for rejection. In these patients, a further reduction of long-term maintenance immunosuppression might therefore be safe. However, this study also shows that, despite more potent induction therapy, virtual-XM-positive patients still have a high risk of AMR that translates into an increased rate of late allograft loss. This underscores the need for new therapeutic strategies or agents that are effective once sensitization to the allograft has already occurred.

Strategies to Improve Long-Term Outcome

Another key aspect to address in the years to come is the improvement of long-term follow-up. It is increasingly recognized that chronic allograft damage is due to a variety of different and identifiable causes. Depending on the period after transplantation, the most frequent etiologies are acute and chronic rejection, infection (e.g. polyoma nephropathy) and recurrence of disease. Therefore, strategies involving serial protocol biopsies and serologic monitoring (occurrence of de novo HLA-DSA, viral PCR) will have to be implemented into clinical practice to identify specific patients at increased risk of allograft loss. Moreover, serial monitoring strategies will also allow to more specifically tailor immunosuppression. Lastly, new drugs will have to be developed that aim at preventing or treating late causes of allograft failure.

Conclusions

Various strategies have been explored in recent years to reduce the overall burden of immunosuppression, i.e. steroid minimization and CNI-free protocols. Several promising new drugs with more specificity and potentially less toxicity are currently under study. At the same time, better pretransplant risk stratification strategies as well as improvements in long-term follow-up will allow individualization of immunosuppression. It is tempting to speculate that all these efforts will not only result in better long-term outcomes but also in a decrease in therapy-related side effects and skin and overall malignancy rates in the transplant population.

References

1 Lodhi SA, Lamb KE, Meier-Kriesche HU: Solid organ allograft survival improvement in the United States: the long-term does not mirror the dramatic short-term success. Am J Transplant 2011;11:1226–1235.

2 Lamb KE, Lodhi S, Meier-Kriesche HU: Long-term renal allograft survival in the United States: a critical reappraisal. Am J Transplant 2011;11:450–462.

3 Nankivell BJ, Borrows RJ, Fung CL, O'Connell PJ, Allen RD, Chapman JR: The natural history of chronic allograft nephropathy. N Engl J Med 2003;349:2326–2333.

4 Vincenti F, Schena FP, Paraskevas S, Hauser IA, Walker RG, Grinyo J: A randomized, multicenter study of steroid avoidance, early steroid withdrawal or standard steroid therapy in kidney transplant recipients. Am J Transplant 2008;8:307–316.

5 Knight SR, Morris PJ: Steroid avoidance or withdrawal after renal transplantation increases the risk of acute rejection but decreases cardiovascular risk. A meta-analysis. Transplantation 2010;89:1–14.

6 Woodle ES, First MR, Pirsch J, Shihab F, Gaber AO, Van Veldhuisen P: A prospective, randomized, double-blind, placebo-controlled multicenter trial comparing early (7 day) corticosteroid cessation versus long-term, low-dose corticosteroid therapy. Ann Surg 2008;248:564–577.

7 Sprangers B, Vanrenterghem Y: Steroid avoidance or withdrawal after kidney transplantation: a balancing act. Transplantation 2010;90:350–352.

8 Pascual J, Galeano C, Royuela A, Zamora J: A systematic review on steroid withdrawal between 3 and 6 months after kidney transplantation. Transplantation 2010;90:343–349.

9 Ekberg H, Tedesco-Silva H, Demirbas A, Vitko S, Nashan B, Gurkan A, et al: Reduced exposure to calcineurin inhibitors in renal transplantation. N Engl J Med 2007;357:2562–2575.

10 Ekberg H, Grinyo J, Nashan B, Vanrenterghem Y, Vincenti F, Voulgari A, et al: Cyclosporine sparing with mycophenolate mofetil, daclizumab and corticosteroids in renal allograft recipients: the CAESAR Study. Am J Transplant 2007;7:560–570.

11 Campistol JM, Eris J, Oberbauer R, Friend P, Hutchison B, Morales JM, et al: Sirolimus therapy after early cyclosporine withdrawal reduces the risk for cancer in adult renal transplantation. J Am Soc Nephrol 2006;17:581–589.

12 Kauffman HM, Cherikh WS, Cheng Y, Hanto DW, Kahan BD: Maintenance immunosuppression with target-of-rapamycin inhibitors is associated with a reduced incidence of de novo malignancies. Transplantation 2005;80:883–889.

13 Schena FP, Pascoe MD, Alberu J, del Carmen Rial M, Oberbauer R, Brennan DC, et al: Conversion from calcineurin inhibitors to sirolimus maintenance therapy in renal allograft recipients: 24-month efficacy and safety results from the CONVERT trial. Transplantation 2009;87:233–242.

14 Alberu J, Pascoe MD, Campistol JM, Schena FP, Rial MD, Polinsky M, et al: Lower malignancy rates in renal allograft recipients converted to sirolimus-based, calcineurin inhibitor-free immunotherapy: 24-month results from the CONVERT Trial. Transplantation 2011;92:303–310.

15 Webber A, Hirose R, Vincenti F: Novel strategies in immunosuppression: issues in perspective. Transplantation 2011;91:1057–1064.

16 Genberg H, Kumlien G, Wennberg L, Berg U, Tyden G: ABO-incompatible kidney transplantation using antigen-specific immunoadsorption and rituximab: a 3-year follow-up. Transplantation 2008;85:1745–1754.

17 Segev DL, Simpkins CE, Warren DS, King KE, Shirey RS, Maley WR, et al: ABO incompatible high-titer renal transplantation without splenectomy or anti-CD20 treatment. Am J Transplant 2005;5:2570–2575.

18 Vo AA, Lukovsky M, Toyoda M, Wang J, Reinsmoen NL, Lai CH, et al: Rituximab and intravenous immune globulin for desensitization during renal transplantation. N Engl J Med 2008;359:242–251.

19 Vo AA, Peng A, Toyoda M, Kahwaji J, Cao K, Lai CH, et al: Use of intravenous immune globulin and rituximab for desensitization of highly HLA-sensitized patients awaiting kidney transplantation. Transplantation 2010;89:1095–1102.

20 Loupy A, Suberbielle-Boissel C, Zuber J, Anglicheau D, Timsit MO, Martinez F, et al: Combined post-transplant prophylactic IVIg/anti-CD 20/plasmapheresis in kidney recipients with preformed donor-specific antibodies: a pilot study. Transplantation 2010;89:1403–1410.

21 Navarra SV, Guzman RM, Gallacher AE, et al: Efficacy and safety of belimumab in patients with active systemic lupus erythematosus: a randomised, placebo-controlled, phase 3 trial. Lancet 2011;377:721–731.

22 Durrbach A, Pestana JM, Pearson T, Vincenti F, Garcia VD, Campistol J, et al: A phase III study of belatacept versus cyclosporine in kidney transplants from extended criteria donors (BENEFIT-EXT study). Am J Transplant 2010;10:547–557.

23 Vincenti F, Charpentier B, Vanrenterghem Y, Rostaing L, Bresnahan B, Darji P, et al: A phase III study of belatacept-based immunosuppression regimens versus cyclosporine in renal transplant recipients (BENEFIT study). Am J Transplant 2010;10: 535–546.

24 Larsen CP, Grinyo J, Medina-Pestana J, Vanrenterghem Y, Vincenti F, Breshahan B, et al: Belatacept-based regimens versus a cyclosporine A-based regimen in kidney transplant recipients: 2-year results from the BENEFIT and BENEFIT-EXT studies. Transplantation 2010;90:1528–1535.

25 FDA's Cardiovascular and Renal Drugs Advisory Committee Briefing Document for March 2010 Meeting.

26 Ellis CN, Krueger GG: Treatment of chronic plaque psoriasis by selective targeting of memory effector T lymphocytes. N Engl J Med 2001;345:248–255.

27 Weaver TA, Charafeddine AH, Agarwal A, Turner AP, Russell M, Leopardi FV, et al: Alefacept promotes co-stimulation blockade based allograft survival in nonhuman primates. Nat Med 2009;15: 746–749.

28 Lonze BE, Dagher NN, Simpkins CE, Locke JE, Singer AL, Segev DL, et al: Eculizumab, bortezomib and kidney paired donation facilitate transplantation of a highly sensitized patient without vascular access. Am J Transplant 2010;10:2154–2160.

29 Walsh RC, Everly JJ, Brailey P, Rike AH, Arend LJ, Mogilishetty G, et al: Proteasome inhibitor-based primary therapy for antibody-mediated renal allograft rejection. Transplantation 2010;89:277–284.

30 Trivedi HL, Terasaki PI, Feroz A, Vanikar AV, Trivedi VB, Khemchandani SI, et al: Clonal deletion with bortezomib followed by low or no maintenance immunosuppression in renal allograft recipients. Transplantation 2010;90:221–222.

31 2009 Annual report of the U.S. Organ Procurement and Transplantation Network and the Scientific Registry of Transplant Recipients: transplant data 1999–2008. Rockville, Health Resources and Services Administration HSB, Division of Transplantation, 2009.

32 Lefaucheur C, Loupy A, Hill GS, Andrade J, Nochy D, Antoine C, et al: Preexisting donor-specific HLA antibodies predict outcome in kidney transplantation. J Am Soc Nephrol 2010;21:1398–1406.

33 Breimer ME, Rydberg L, Jackson AM, Lucas DP, Zachary AA, Melancon JK, et al: Multicenter evaluation of a novel endothelial cell crossmatch test in kidney transplantation. Transplantation 2009;87: 549–556.

34 Dragun D, Muller DN, Brasen JH, Fritsche L, Nieminen-Kelha M, Dechend R, et al: Angiotensin II type 1-receptor activating antibodies in renal-allograft rejection. N Engl J Med 2005;352:558–569.

35 Amico P, Honger G, Bielmann D, Lutz D, Garzoni D, Steiger J, et al: Incidence and prediction of early antibody-mediated rejection due to non-human leukocyte antigen-antibodies. Transplantation 2008; 85:1557–1563.

36 Pei R, Lee JH, Shih NJ, Chen M, Terasaki PI: Single human leukocyte antigen flow cytometry beads for accurate identification of human leukocyte antigen antibody specificities. Transplantation 2003;75:43–49.

37 Gupta A, Iveson V, Varagunam M, Bodger S, Sinnott P, Thuraisingham RC: Pretransplant donor-specific antibodies in cytotoxic negative crossmatch kidney transplants: are they relevant? Transplantation 2008; 85:1200–1204.

38 Amico P, Honger G, Mayr M, Steiger J, Hopfer H, Schaub S: Clinical relevance of pretransplant donor-specific HLA antibodies detected by single-antigen flow-beads. Transplantation 2009;87:1681–1688.

39 Amico P, Hirt-Minkowski P, Honger G, Gurke L, Mihatsch MJ, Steiger J, et al: Risk stratification by the virtual crossmatch: a prospective study in 233 renal transplantations. Transpl Int 2011;24:560–569.

Daniel Zecher, MD
Transplantation Immunology and Nephrology
University Hospital Basel
Petersgraben 4, CH–4031 Basel (Switzerland)
Tel. +41 61 328 6730,E-Mail daniel.zecher@unibas.ch

Häusermann P, Steiger J, Passweg J (eds): Transplantation Dermatology.
Curr Probl Dermatol. Basel, Karger, 2012, vol 43, pp 81–90

History of Hematopoietic Stem Cell Transplantation: Evolution and Perspectives

Alois Gratwohl[a] · Dietger Niederwieser[b]

[a]Hematology, University Hospital, Basel, Switzerland; [b]Hematology-Oncology Department, University Hospital, Leipzig, Germany

Abstract

Hematopoietic stem cell transplantation (HSCT) has evolved over the last half century from experimental bone marrow transplantation for patients with incurable leukemia or bone marrow failure to standard of care for a broad range of patients with congenital or acquired disorders of the hematopoietic system or radio-, chemo- or immune-sensitive malignancies. More than 60,000 such transplants are currently carried out annually worldwide with increasing frequency. HSCT has always been closely linked to Dermatology from its very beginning through its main and most devastating complication graft-versus-host disease. Treatment complications of HSCT have provided a great deal of insight into basic mechanisms of immunology, clinical medicine and networking in general. It remains a challenge to turn this knowledge from the two disciplines into benefit for the future patients with disturbed immune function and skin diseases.

Treatment with stem cells in general is today considered by many as *the* medical treatment form of the 21st century. It is expected that one day failed organs or failed organ function will be replaced or restored by new healthy functioning stem cells. Organogenesis, this fine-tuned process from a few cells to a fully established functioning organ during ontogenesis should become reproducible in adult life [1]. Understanding the process and access to 'stem cells' appear as key prerequisites. So far, transplantation of hematopoietic stem cells (hematopoietic stem cell transplantation, HSCT) provides proof of principle for such a concept [2]. Indeed, a failed hematopoietic system can be replaced reproducibly today with reasonable success rate and at reasonable expenses. Lessons learned from HSCT form a basis for better understanding of stem cell development as well as for future stem cell therapies.

The Beginning

The basic idea to restore failed bone marrow function is not a product of modern transplantation medicine. It dates far back to history and old mythology with concepts such as 'to purge bad blood' by the use of blood or bone marrow from healthy individuals or animals. Richard Lower was one of the first to postulate in public that blood from one individual could be replaced by blood from another individual: he connected the carotid artery of a lamb with the elbow vein of a volunteer. Only now can we value the courage of his undertaking and the many painstaking individual steps required on the long journey to today's transfusion medicine and stem cell transplantation. Melnikoff provided the first rational basis for HSCT at the beginning of the last century. He stipulated that all circulating corpuscular blood elements, erythrocytes, leukocytes and platelets were derived from one single cell, a mother stem cell. He suspected, quite correctly, this stem cell to hide amongst the population of lymphocytes.

The recognition of late bone marrow failure after atomic bomb exposure in Hiroshima and Nagasaki provided the initial massive trigger for today's HSCT. Substantial military research funds were allotted to find ways to overcome this lethal complication of high-dose radiation exposure. Results did fall in rapidly. Jacobson described in his pioneering work as early as 1949 the protecting effects of spleen shielding during otherwise lethal total body irradiation. Spleen-derived humoral factors were believed to be the protective agent. Two years later, Lorenz provided evidence that cellular factors were responsible. He demonstrated that bone marrow cells from healthy mice could abrogate radiation-induced bone marrow aplasia. Ford confirmed a few years later in mice that indeed donor-derived bone marrow cells were responsible for the repopulation of the recipient's hematopoiesis [3, 4]. The debate whether humoral or cellular factors were key elements to protect bone marrow from the early sequelae of total body irradiation was considered closed. It is of interest to note that 40 years later combinations of growth factors were proven to be radioprotective for the bone marrow after total body irradiation as well, even though this approach never gained clinical application [5].

These early animal data confirmed the concept of a hematopoietic stem cell and its potential to restore a destroyed hematopoietic system. At the same time, clinicians realized the unique potential of the marrow lethal effects of radiation. For the first time it became possible to remove a diseased bone marrow; total body irradiation was the tool. It was only necessary to replace the removed organ with healthy donor cells. Treatment of leukemia, a malignant transformation of the hematopoietic system and hitherto incurable disease, became possible. It was only a question of time to find out the adequate doses of total body irradiation, sufficient enough to kill leukemia but low enough not to induce irreversible organ damage outside the bone marrow. The idea was swiftly explored in patients. Bone marrow transplantation (BMT) spread rapidly as a promising tool and more than 60 such transplants were reported to the

International Bone Marrow Transplant Registry in 1962. Results however were frustrating. Complications tempered enthusiasm and BMT came to a halt for nearly a decade. Despite successful engraftment and complete remissions of leukemia in some patients, none survived for more than a few months. Early complications associated with bone marrow aplasia were high including bleeding as a consequence of thrombocytopenia and severe infections as a consequence of neutropenia. Many patients did reject their graft and the leukemia returned. Even worse, the few patients with successful engraftment without leukemia died from a unique and novel syndrome soon after return of hematopoiesis (engraftment). They developed a generalized rash, became icteric, and suffered from most severe diarrhea. Similar observations were made in mice. Most animals with a successful BMT did indeed survive the radiation-induced bone marrow aplasia (primary disease) but died 2 weeks later from a syndrome of wasting, rash, diarrhea and icterus named as 'secondary disease'. It did take time to understand this process known today as graft-versus-host disease (GVHD) [2, 3].

The Dawn of Graft-versus-Host Disease

Clinical and experimental animal BMT was performed simultaneously at many institutions in those early days. Experience stimulated research in a mutual way, sometimes obscuring findings as well. BMT development paralleled the early days of solid organ transplantation. Hence, organ graft rejection was a well-known obstacle to successful organ grafting, GVHD was not. It was Simonson, who brought up the concept of a graft-derived immune reaction. He observed pyroninophilic cells as early as 6 days after renal transplantation in the renal cortex. He postulated that graft-derived cells reacted against circulating host antigens. His interpretation was wrong, his observation correct; it was the beginning of a rejection episode. Still, his idea of a GVHD reaction was revolutionary at that time, novel but highly controversial. He finally could prove his model. He injected lymphocytes into newborn mice or chicken embryos. Both were unable to reject these cells and died from an immune reaction. Suddenly, many 'strange' experimental phenomena obtained a unifying explanation. 40 years earlier, Murphy observed lymphoid infiltrates in the spleen of chicken embryos, when he injected the allantois with chicken bone marrow cells, but not when he used goose cells. Chicken embryos could reject xenogeneic goose cells but not chicken cells. It could be explained by a GVHD reaction. Similarly, the secondary disease after total body irradiation and BMT called also the acute killing effect, homologous disease, runting disease, parent versus hybrid effect, embryo disease or parabiosis intoxication had all the same immunological basis. Billingham brought the puzzle together with his postulate of three requirements for GVHD: (a) immunocompetent transplanted cells, (b) antigens in the host which can be recognized by the transplanted cells but lack in the donor, and (c) sufficient time of complete engraftment to mount

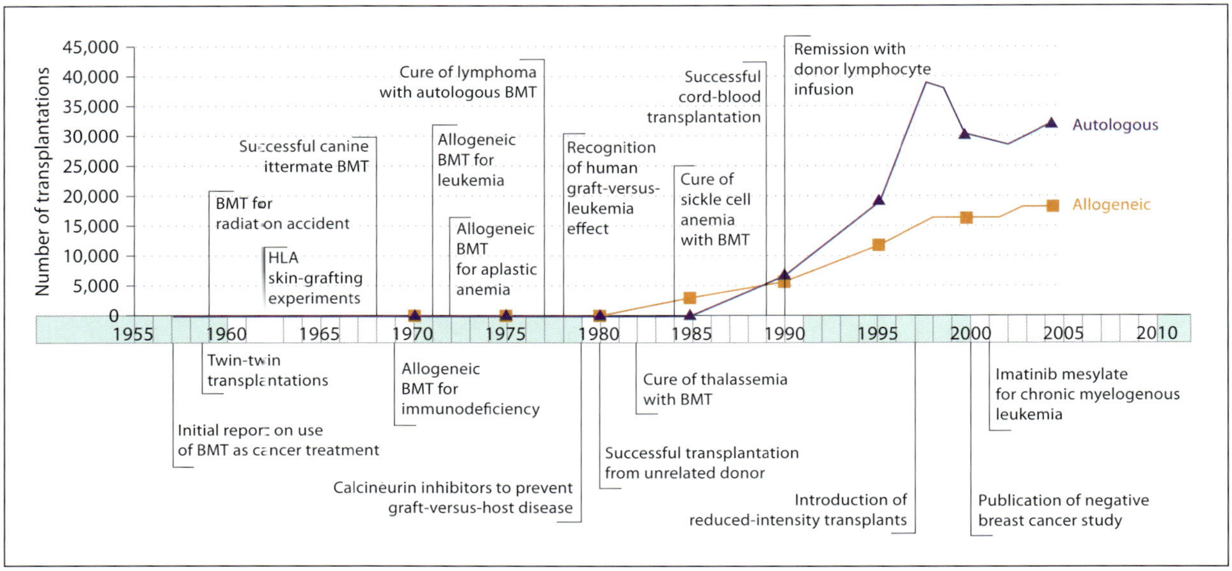

Fig. 1. Historical evolution of HSCT. Reprinted with permission from [13].

an immune response (security of tenure). These basic requirements remain valid today [6].

The Second Phase

Successful canine littermate BMT, the recognition of the major histocompatibility complex and the human leukocyte antigens as key targets of graft rejection and GVHD induced a second phase of human BMT trials (see fig. 1). They were initiated in 1968 by the parallel publication of three successful BMTs from human leukocyte antigen identical sibling donors for patients with congenital immune deficiency disorders. They were accompanied by massive basic and applied research into the mechanisms involved during this long process. Knowledge in supportive care, red blood cell and platelet transfusions as well as gnotobiotic measures supported by novel antibiotics and antifungal agents prepared the way to reduce the complications of pancytopenia after total body irradiation. Methotrexate proved successful to reduce the early impact of GVHD. Chronic GVHD and its close similarities to autoimmune disorders became recognized as well as the counterpart, the graft versus leukemia (GvL). Leukemia was not solely controlled by the toxic effects of the conditioning but also by the effects of the donor immune system against malignant host cells. E. Donnall Thomas from the Seattle Team [6] was awarded the Nobel Prize for medicine in 1990 for these pioneering contributions.

The Breakthrough

The modern era of BMT was initiated in the 1980s by two closely linked but independent moves, similar to the development in solid organ transplantations. The introduction of cyclosporine as a novel and potent immunosuppressive agent did provide a powerful tool to control GVHD. More important probably was the step to move BMT as a treatment plan to an earlier period for patients. Specifically, BMT was used for patients with acute leukemia in first complete remission, for patients with chronic leukemia in first chronic phase, for patients with aplastic anemia as soon in the disease process as a donor was identified. BMT was no longer a desperate measure for patients with refractory end-stage disease, but a planned undertaking. Survival dramatically improved. Moreover, results gave proof of principle that a hitherto incurable disease, chronic myeloid leukemia could be eradicated. Chronic myeloid leukemia became soon the most frequent indication for an allogeneic BMT. Improvement in the 1980s amplified in the 1990s, where, using registry and networking, recognition of risk factors for outcome led to better definition in indication for HSCT. Furthermore, important discoveries of GVHD pathophysiology were described: among them the cellular basis of GVHD by isolating the minor histocompatibility antigens and the importance of cytokines (cytokine storm).

In parallel, autologous BMT was investigated with success as an instrument to apply intensive therapy to patients with chemo- or radiotherapy-sensitive malignancies. It did permit dose intensifications up to the limits of extramedullary toxicity of the conditioning. The concept proved to be successful in prospective randomized studies for patients with lymphoid malignancies and some childhood tumors such as neuroblastoma; it failed to show a benefit in others, such as breast cancer. Discovery of stem cells in the blood and improvement of mobilization procedures significantly improved and facilitated not only autologous but later on also allogeneic BMT. Today, more than 90% of autologous and more than 50% of allogeneic transplants are performed with peripheral blood stem cells. Therefore, the definition BMT was replaced by HSCT.

Nevertheless, the clear documented advantage of HSCT, allogeneic in some, autologous in other indications, induced an expansion of indications, to the development of novel techniques and to a propagation of HSCT to many transplant teams worldwide. Today, it is an established procedure for many patients with congenital or acquired disorders of the hematopoietic system or with radio-, chemo- or immune sensitive malignancies. Indications include autoimmune disorders or single enzyme deficiencies where bone marrow-derived cells can restore the lacking enzyme (see fig. 2 for indications on HSCT in Europe). HSCT includes today bone marrow, peripheral blood or cord blood as stem cell source. For autologous transplantation, cells from the patients are used; otherwise cells can be taken from family members, from one of the more than 16 million typed volunteer donors

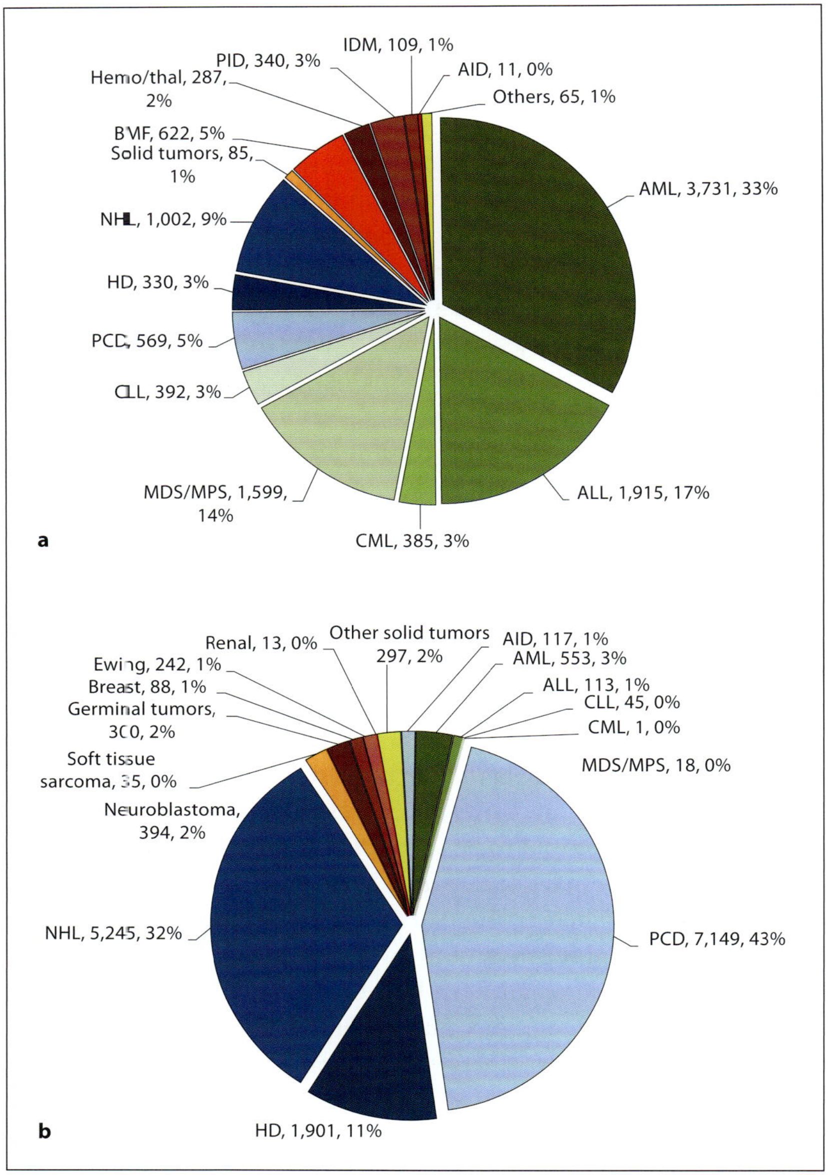

Fig. 2. Indications for HSCT. **a** Main indications for allogeneic HSCT. Based on EBMT data 2009. Reprinted with permission. **b** Main indications for autologous HSCT. Based on EBMT data 2009. Reprinted with permission from Baldomero et al. [12].

worldwide or from one of the more than half a million stored cord blood units. These hematopoietic stem cells are supplemented by additional cell donations, such as donor lymphocyte infusions, NK cells or mesenchymal stromal cells in order to facilitate engraftment, restore split chimerism, control acute GVHD or revert impending relapse.

Similarly, transplantation techniques have evolved. Complete or partial T cell depletion by negative or positive selection techniques is used to avoid GVHD but maintain, if possible, GvL. In patients without a donor, haploidentical HSCT from family members are increasingly used for curing patients for hematological malignancies using T cell depletion. Conditioning has been fine tuned for specific indications or adapted to the individual risk. Reduced intensity conditioning has been introduced for patients with advanced age or suffering from comorbidities. Its effect in disease control relies more on the immune-mediated GvL reaction than on cytoreduction. As a consequence, more than 60,000 such HSCT procedures are currently carried out worldwide; about two thirds are autologous and one third allogeneic HSCTs [7, 8]. The HSCT community today involves a global endeavor of physicians, of voluntary donors, of societies, of regulatory bodies, of global donor registries and of surveys unique in medicine. In this system, which not surprisingly is one of the most cost-intensive medical procedures, accreditation and excellence play an increasingly important role.

Macroeconomic Aspects of Hematopoietic Stem Cell Transplantation

Despite its success, HSCT remains associated with significant morbidity and mortality, and is considered as one of the most cost intensive medical procedures. As such, HSCT during its evolution was long restricted to a few affluent research-oriented countries. This has changed during the last decade. HSCT is no longer limited to high-income countries but has become a global undertaking (fig. 3). At the same time, studies on the evolution of HSCT have yielded novel insight into the macroeconomic aspects of medical technology use by itself [7, 9]. Not surprisingly, HSCT is mostly used in countries with higher gross national income per capita: a minimum of available resources is required. Furthermore, Governmental Health Care expenditures and team density (number of transplant teams per number of inhabitants) are associated with transplant rates (number of HSCT per number of inhabitants) in a given country. In summary, availability of resources, governmental support and access to the procedure determine the use.

The marked changes in HSCT utilization, e.g. the change from bone marrow to peripheral blood as stem cell source, the rise and fall of allogeneic HSCT for chronic myeloid leukemia or of autologous HSCT for breast cancer have permitted insight into the process of diffusion of a complex expensive medical technology. Economics of a country as expressed by gross national income per capita, evidence for an advantage of the novel procedure, external regulations and expectation of the transplant teams (4 'E') have been identified in the field of HSCT. It is highly likely that the same factors are decisive for any process of diffusion. As such, HSCT can serve as a model not only in regenerative medicine or transplantation immunology but in a broader field of medicine in general.

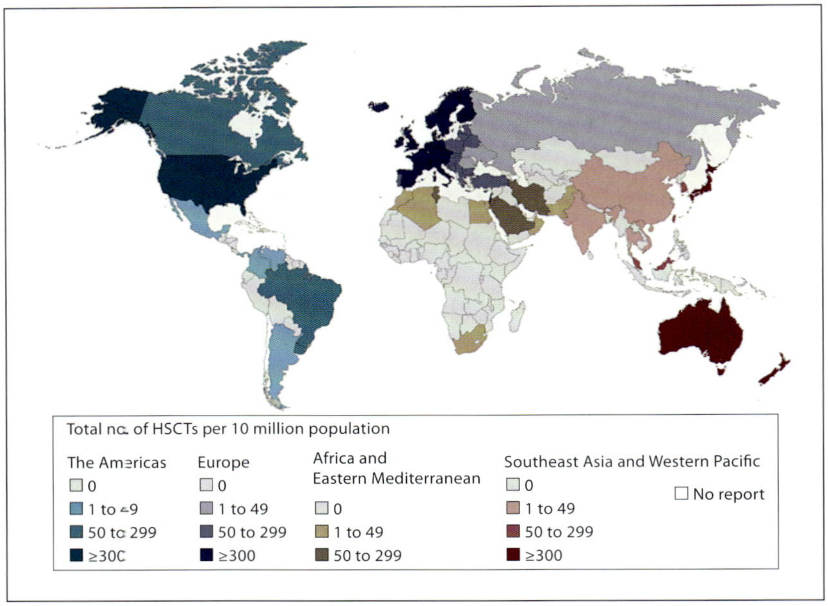

Fig. 3. HSCT rates worldwide in 2006 by WHO regions. Reprinted with permission (http://www.who.int/transplantation/hsctx/en/index.html).

The Changing Concepts of Chronic Graft-versus-Host Disease

The simultaneous appearance of different phenomenological disease characteristics mimicking autoimmune disorders, such as Sjögrens' syndrome, systemic sclerosis or biliary cirrhosis in recipients of allogeneic HSCT surviving the early phase of the procedure and of acute GVHD made it relatively easy to classify the syndrome as chronic GVHD and to explain its pathophysiology as an autoaggressive process. This model was supported by the close association of chronic GVHD with reduced relapse risk, hence a GvL reaction. Due to its antileukemic efficacy, mild chronic GVHD was even considered as beneficial. These concepts are again changing. There are no data so far that the beneficial effects of GvL outweigh the detrimental effects of GVHD in the long-term. There is increasing awareness that chronic GVHD might differ substantially in its pathophysiology from acute GVHD and is not just a chronic autoimmune process. It is of interest to note in this context that many aspects of chronic GVHD of the sclerosing type differ significantly from those in systemic sclerosis. It is more likely that chronic GVHD expresses a status of altered immunity and might be linked at least in part to premature ageing [10].

It will be of great interest to follow the evolution of patients with primary immune disorders who were treated with HSCT for their autoimmune disease. Incidental reports and several phase II studies indicate that primary autoimmune disease signs and symptoms can regress after autologous or allogeneic HSCT. Prospective randomized studies are currently underway and will give answer on the value of HSCT in this disease setting.

Outlook to Non-Hematopoietic Stem Cell Transplantation

The success of HSCT has stimulated many fields of regenerative medicine to use stem cell therapy in order to replace failed organs or failed organ function. Expectations were based in part on the potential of stem cells in their plasticity, expressed briefly in the slogan 'turn blood to brain'. So far, no other field of medicine has documented proof of efficacy, but many studies are ongoing. Hematopoietic stem cells are applied for non-hematopoietic use for cardiac, neurological or musculoskeletal repair. Non-hematopoietic stem cells are investigated for their potential to restore skin, musculoskeletal or neurological function. Autologous and allogeneic cells are used for these investigations from cord blood, bone marrow, the adipose tissue or from embryonic cell lines. More than a thousand such investigative procedures were reported in Europe in 2009 alone. Their numbers are rapidly increasing [11].

No results can yet be given, but a few predictions can be made based on the experience in HSCT. It took almost 50 years from the first clinical attempts of BMT to general clinical application of HSCT. It is likely that at least one or two decades of basic research will be required in non-hematopoietic stem cell transplantation. It is also easy to predict that the key impediments to HSCT will remain the same for non-hematopoietic stem cell transplantation: graft rejection, graft versus host reactions after successful engraftment and relapse of the basic disease despite successful initial therapy. At the same time, it can be predicted that one day replacement of failed organ function by stem cell therapy will become standard of care for many patients with failed organs.

References

1 Hochedlinger K, Jaenisch R: Nuclear transplantation, embryonic stem cells, and the potential for cell therapy. N Engl J Med 2003;349:275–286.

2 Copelan EA: Hematopoietic stem-cell transplantation. N Engl J Med 2006;27:1813–1826.

3 Thomas ED: A history of allogeneic hematopoietic cell transplantation; in Appelbaum FR, Forman S, Negrin RS, Blume KG (eds): Thomas' Hematopoietic Cell Transplantation, ed 4. Oxford, Wiley Blackwell, 2009, pp 3–7.

4 Armitage JO: The history of autologous hematopoietic cell transplantation; in Appelbaum FR, Forman S, Negrin RS, Blume KG (eds): Thomas' Hematopoietic Cell Transplantation, ed 4. Oxford, Wiley Blackwell, 2009, pp 8–14.

5 Gratwohl A: Historical aspects of cGvHD; in Vogelsang GB, Pavletic SZ (eds): Chronic Graft versus Host Disease. Cambridge, Cambridge University Press, 2009, pp 3–7.

6 Thomas ED, Storb R, Clift RA, et al: Bone marrow transplantation. II. N Engl J Med 1975;292:895–902.

7 Gratwohl A, Baldomero H, Aljurf M, et al: Hematopoietic stem cell transplantation: a global perspective. JAMA 2010;303:1617–1624.

8 Ljungman P, Bregni M, Brune M, et al: Allogeneic and autologous transplantation for haematological diseases, solid tumours and immune disorders: current practice in Europe 2009. Bone Marrow Transplant 2010;45:219–234.

9 Gratwohl A, Schwendener A, Baldomero H, Gratwohl M, Apperley J, Niederwieser D, Frauendorfer K: Changes in use of hematopoietic stem cell transplantation; a model for diffusion of medical technology. Haematologica 2010;95:637–643.
10 Filipovich AH, Weisdorf D, Pavletic S, Socie G, et al: National Institutes of Health consensus development project on criteria for clinical trials in chronic graft-versus-host disease. I. Diagnosis and staging working group report. Biol Blood Marrow Transplant 2005;11:945–956.
11 Martin I, Baldomero H, Bocelli-Tyndall C, Slaper-Cortenbach I, Passweg J, Tyndall A: The survey on cellular and engineered tissue therapies in Europe in 2009. Tissue Eng Part A 2011;17–18:2221–2230.
12 Baldomero H, Gratwohl M, Gratwohl A, Tichelli A, Niederwieser D, Madrigal A, Frauendorfer K, European Group for Blood and Marrow Transplantation EBMT: The EBMT activity survey 2009: trends over the past 5 years. Bone Marrow Transplant 2011;46:485–501.
13 Appelbaum FR: Hematopoietic-cell transplantation at 50. N Engl J Med 2007;357:1472–1475.

Prof. Dr. Alois Gratwohl, emeritus
Hematology, University Hospital Basel
Petersgraben 4
CH-4031 Basel (Switzerland)
Tel. +41 061 265 42 77, E-Mail alois.gratwohl@unibas.ch

Häusermann P, Steiger J, Passweg J (eds): Transplantation Dermatology.
Curr Probl Dermatol. Basel, Karger, 2012, vol 43, pp 91–100

Acute and Chronic Skin Graft-versus-Host Disease – Pathophysiological Aspects

Gerard Socié[a–c] · Regis Peffault de Latour[a] · Jean David Bouziz[b,d] · Michel Rybojad[d]

[a]AP-HP, Hematology Transplantation, Saint Louis Hospital, [b]Université Paris Diderot, Sorbonne Paris Cité, [c]INSERM U728, Hematology Institute, [d]AP-HP, Dermatology, Saint Louis Hospital, Paris, France

Abstract

Despite impressive advances in the field of allogeneic hematopoietic transplantation, graft-versus-host disease (GVHD) remains a significant obstacle to overcome. Whereas our understanding of the pathophysiology of acute GVHD has greatly improved, so has our knowledge of the complexities of the immune system. Much of the immunobiology of GVHD has been gleaned from preclinical models and far less from clinical observations or biological studies in human. In this chapter, we summarize some of the major advances in GVHD pathophysiology, and the potent translation of these from the bench to the bedside.

Graft-versus-host disease (GVHD) is a complex disease resulting from donor T cell recognition of a genetically disparate recipient that is unable to reject donor cells following allogeneic HSCT. From a clinical point of view, it has been classical to consider acute and chronic GVHD (cGVHD) separately. Acute GVHD usually develops early after transplant and mainly affects the skin, gut and liver. cGVHD is a frequent but highly polymorphic complication of allogeneic stem cell transplantation. Its clinical presentation varies from few lichenoid skin lesions to a highly aggressive disease with multi-organ involvement mimicking autoimmune disease such as scleroderma. Although cGVHD usually manifests itself more than 100 days after transplant, earlier disease onset could occur. More importantly, clinical syndromes with features of typical acute GVHD are increasingly recognized beyond 100 days after hematopoietic stem cell transplant, especially in recent years with the development of the reduced-intensity conditioning regimen. In addition, patients with acute GVHD may progress to cGVHD with symptoms of both acute GVHD and cGVHD. Thus, although we will still stick with the classical acute versus chronic aspects of the pathophysiology of the disease, we would like to stress the continuum of the immune process.

The classical scheme of GVHD development includes six basic steps.

- Step 1: Priming of the immune response. Cytoreductive conditioning induces tissue damage and the release of a storm of proinflammatory cytokines that promote the activation and maturation of antigen-presenting cells (APCs) and the rapid amplification of donor T cells [1–3].
- Step 2: T cell activation and costimulation. Activation occurs as the result of the recognition and interaction of the T cell receptor and costimulatory molecules with their cognate ligands expressed on the surface of the APC.
- Step 3: Alloreactive T cell expansion and differentiation.
- Step 4: Activated T cell trafficking. Activated T cell migration to GVHD target tissues is followed by the recruitment of other effector leukocytes.
- Step 5: Immune attack of the target tissues by effector T cells. Destruction occurs via exposure to cell surface and release of soluble immune effector molecules. Tissue damage then leads to increased inflammatory signals, perpetuating and augmenting the disease process by contributing to the cytokine storm that fuels GVHD.
- Step 6: Unregulated immune dysfunction and chronic inflammatory changes and fibrosis leading to cGVHD.

Previous reviews [1, 4–9] have detailed these phases of GVHD initiation and tissue destruction. We will focus on recent advances focusing on the pathophysiology of skin GVHD. The primary target cells in the skin have long been assigned to basal cells at rete tips. Murine data suggest that these cells are cytokeratin 15 positive and express an antiapoptotic phenotype during GVHD [10].

Priming of the Immune Response

The earliest phase of acute GVHD is set into motion by the damage caused by the underlying disease and exacerbated by conditioning regimens. Damaged skin secrete proinflammatory cytokines, such as TNF-α and IL-1, which contribute to the 'cytokine storm' increasing the expression of adhesion molecules, costimulatory molecules, MHC antigens, and chemokine gradients that alert the residual host and the infused donor immune cells. These 'danger signals' activate host tissue cells including APCs.

T Cell Activation and Costimulation

The core of the graft-versus-host immune reaction lies within the second step, in which donor T cells proliferate and differentiate in response to host APCs [11, 12].

Recent advances have indicated the presence of a subset of postmitotic, self-renewing CD44 (lo)/CD62L (hi)/CD8+ T cells that can generate and sustain all allogeneic T cell subsets in GVHD reactions, including central memory, effector memory and effector CD8+ T cells [13]. The danger signals generated in the first phase augment this activation, at least in part, by increasing expression of costimulatory molecules. In mouse models, in which genetic differences between donor and recipient strains can be tightly controlled, CD4+ T cells induce acute GVHD to MHC class II differences, and CD8+ T cells induce acute disease to MHC class I differences [11, 14–21]. Murine studies with minor histocompatibility antigen (MiHA)-disparate models have demonstrated that GVHD initiation requires donor T cell recognition of host antigen in the context of host APCs [11, 14–21]. Depletion of host Langerhans cells before experimental transplantation of donor alloreactive T cells prevents skin GVHD [22]. Donor-derived APCs then are able to augment CD8+ T cell-mediated GVHD by acquiring and presenting host antigens [21]. In humans, the incidence of acute GVHD is directly related to the degree of mismatch between HLA determinants. However, recipients of HLA-identical grafts still can develop systemic acute GVHD due to genetic differences that lie outside the MHC loci and that encode proteins referred to as MiHA. Thus, there is strong evidence for MiHA mismatch-mediated GVHD in humans [23–25]. In the skin, the in vitro skin explant model provided the first in situ evidence of direct involvement of MiHA targeting antigen-specific antigens [26]. Although individual human MiHA antigens associated with GVHD have been identified, the relative contribution of diverse MiHA and the existence (if any) of single, dominant MiHA in humans [such as B6dom and H60 that have been well characterized in rodents; 27, 28] is unknown. With respect to the donor versus host origin of APCs initiating GVHD in humans little data are available. However, recent studies on the fate of human Langerhans cells, dermal dendritic cell and macrophages in patients suggest that host-derived APCs at least participate in the early stage of the disease [29–31]. The fate of human Langerhans cells after allogeneic HSCT in human was studied by Collin et al. [31]. Recovery of Langerhans cells occurs rapidly within a month in the absence of acute GVHD but is markedly delayed (beyond 3 months) if GVHD is active.

A major role for GVHD initiation has been ascribed to CD28/CTLA-4 (CD152):B7 interactions which consists of both a positive (CD28/B7) and an inhibitory (CTLA-4:B7) pathway. Another B7 supergene family member, ICOS (CD278), binds the ligand B7h (CD275) expressed on host APCs, and thereby promotes T effector responses. Blockade or absence of ICOS on donor T cells diminishes gut and liver but not skin GVHD [32, 33]. In response to tissue injury and activated T cells, inhibitory pathways are upregulated in an attempt to protect the host against injury. CTLA-4 and programmed death-1 (PD-1; CD279) are upregulated on donor T cells during acute GVHD and serve to dampen the immune response. Both also are primarily expressed in the cytoplasm of activated T cells and CD4+CD25+Treg cells [for review see 5]. In rodents, selective blockade of CTLA-4:B7 interactions accelerated acute GVHD lethality. Blockade or absence of PD-1 on donor cells accelerates GVHD and is associated with increased IFN-γ production [34].

Acute GVHD and T Cell Subpopulations

Naïve T Cells

T cells can undergo a massive and much earlier than previously thought expansion in lymph nodes and Peyer patches [35]. In mice, naive CD44(lo)CD62L(hi) CD8+ T cells generate and sustain allogeneic CD8+ T cells in GVHD reactions [36, 37]. Murine memory T cells isolated from non-allosensitized donors fail to induce GVHD in experimental models [36]. In contrast, alloantigen-sensitized effector memory CD44(hi)CD62L(lo) as well as naive phenotype CD44(lo)CD62L(hi), but not central memory CD44(hi)CD62L(hi) CD8+ T cells, cause GVHD following adoptive transfer into secondary recipients [13].

Regulatory T Cells

CD4+CD25+Foxp3+ regulatory T cells (Tregs) have potent suppressor activity both in vitro and in vivo. Donor Treg cell infusion blocks acute GVHD. Murine L-selectin (CD62L) expressing Treg cells preferentially home to secondary lymphoid organs, and in particular lymph nodes, resulting in GVHD prevention [38]. Conversely, depletion of CD25+ T cells from the donor graft or in the recipient immediately following allogeneic HSCT promotes acute and cGVHD in various mouse models while still maintaining a graft-vs.-hematopoietic cell malignancy response in most but not all studies [39–43]. Experimental data both in mice and humans have demonstrated the extraordinary potential of T helper cell subsets (Th1, Th2, and Th17) and of Tregs to exhibit plasticity, shifting from one phenotype to another [reviewed in 44, 45].

Th17 Cells

Th17 cells [46] have recently emerged as a new player in GVHD. Although the role of this new T cell subset has been dissected in certain experimental models including inflammatory bowel disease, lung and skin GVHD, the study of its role in experimental GVHD has led to seemingly discordant GVHD lethality results that may be ascribed to different experimental conditions [47–49]. Our data indicate that Th17 cells in human GVHD Th17 cells are not as numerous as in Crohn's disease, but that the ratio of Th17 to Treg is associated with human pathology [50].

T Cell Trafficking

How T cells are recruited into tissues could be pivotal for understanding the stereotypical involvement of skin GVHD. During a GVHD reaction, donor T cells initially migrate to the spleen and peripheral lymphoid tissues within hours [51]. Naive donor T cells traffic to lymphoid tissues, where the subset of alloreactive T cells receive activation signals by APCs, and then subsequent migration to specific GVHD target organ sites, essential for the induction and pathogenesis of acute GVHD [52]. Almost all tissues express transplantation antigens; however, acute GVHD pathology is primarily limited to only a few locations – gut, skin, liver, lung, secondary lymphoid organs, and thymus. The ability of alloreactive donor T cells to home to specific organs is regulated by a unique combination of signals that bind to corresponding receptors on host tissues and counter-receptors expressed on donor T cells, including members of the chemokine family. MIP1a and other chemokines (such as CCL2–CCL5, CXCL2, CXCL9, CXCL10, CXCL11, CCL17, and CCL27) are overexpressed during GVHD generation and enhance the homing of cellular effectors to GVHD target organs [9, 53, 54]. CCR6+ donor CD4+ T cells target cells to the gut and skin in murine GVHD models [55], and activated effector T cells express CCR5 in human skin GVHD. Another study provided evidence of skin infiltration by CD4+ CCR10+ cells which correlates with enhanced epidermal expression of CCL27, the ligand of CCR10 [56]. The CLA is overexpressed on activated T cells almost a week before the onset of clinical signs of acute skin GHVD [57].

Effector Stage: T Cells and Others

After migration of alloreactive effector T cells to the target tissues of GVHD, these cells can mediate tissue destruction through both direct cytotoxic activity and the recruitment of other leukocytes. Targeting these effector pathways has been studied as a strategy to prevent or reduce GVHD severity. Researchers have considered acute GVHD to be a Th1/T cytotoxic type (IL-12, IL-2, and IFN-γ) disease on the basis of the predominance of cytotoxic T cell-mediated pathology and of increased production of Th1 type cytokines, including IFN-γ [58], which is detectable in the serum or donor T cells during acute GVHD. However, several recent studies have suggested that the influence of Th1 and Th2 cytokines in acute and cGVHD is not so simply explained [reviewed in 5]. The production of high levels of IFN-γ by both CD4+ and CD8+ donor T cells early after transplantation can limit the severity of acute GVHD in recipient mice after myeloablative conditioning due to the induction of T cell apoptosis [59]. Likewise, the proinflammatory cytokine IL-18, which promotes IFN-γ production, can inhibit CD4+-dependent GVHD. The use of donor T cells from mice lacking STAT4 or STAT6, transcription factors required for development to Th1 or Th2 phenotypes, respectively, or the ablation of either IL-2-producing

(Th1-type) or IL-4-producing (Th2-type) donor T cells following the onset of clinical symptoms of GVHD demonstrate that both Th1 and Th2 type donor T cells can induce acute GVHD [58, 60–65].

The concentration and timing of cytokine release into the circulation and relevant target organs appear to be critical for GVHD. For example, IL-10 promotes Th2 and type 1 regulatory T cell responses, which can be important in the induction of tolerance to allografts [reviewed in 5]. Higher production of IL-10, as demonstrated in human recipients with IL-10 production polymorphism is associated with reduced occurrence and severity of GVHD [66].

T cells mediate the final effector pathway in GVHD by multiple pathways [13, 67, 68]. The expression of both Fas and FasL is increased on CD8+ and CD4+ donor T cells during acute GVHD in patients and mice, and serum levels of soluble FasL and Fas were found to correlate with GVHD severity or the response to GVHD therapy. Several studies in experimental mouse models have analyzed the role of the Fas-FasL and perforin-granzyme pathways in the development of GVHD by using mice that are deficient for FasL, perforin or granzyme B as donors, or by the in vivo administration of neutralizing anti-FasL antibodies. Although these differences in experimental design affect the opportunity to draw a uniform conclusion, most studies have shown a role for the Fas-FasL pathway in GVHD mortality. With respect to the perforin-granzyme pathway, approximately two-thirds of studies demonstrated the importance of this pathway in GVHD pathogenesis [reviewed in 69].

However, cellular types other than T cells do participate in the effector phase of GVHD including macrophages, neutrophils and eosinophils. Nishiwaki et al. [70] reported that in the skin infiltrating macrophages were predictive of steroid-refractory GVHD. We also reported that degranulated eosinophils and the density of neutrophil infiltrate correlated with disease severity [71, 72].

Biology of Chronic Graft-versus-Host Disease

The biologic mechanisms leading to cGVHD are not as well understood as those leading to acute GVHD. Although acute GVHD has been recognized as a risk factor for cGVHD, not all cases of acute GVHD evolve into cGVHD, and cGVHD can develop in the absence of prior overt acute GVHD. In the skin, the initial phase of cGVHD is characterized by an intense mononuclear inflammatory infiltrate with destructive changes at the dermal-epidermal junction, accompanied by irregular acanthosis, hyperkeratosis, or atrophy, progressing to dermal fibrosis and sclerosis. Other hallmarks include destruction of tubuloalveolar glands and ducts in the skin, salivary, and lacrimal glands and respiratory epithelium, and destruction of bile ducts in the liver. Furthermore, damage of the endothelium by the conditioning regimen provides the initiation stimulus for recruitment of donor-derived endothelial cells and their progenitors. During the early inflammatory phase of GVHD, there is considerable neovascularization facilitating migration of inflammatory cells to target organs. In the course of GVHD, however, the vasculature itself becomes a target of alloreactive donor T cells. As a consequence, later stages of GVHD are characterized by fibrosis and rarefaction of blood vessels [reviewed in 4, 73].

One of the major challenges in studying the pathophysiology of cGVHD has been the lack of really good suitable experimental models [reviewed in 74]. In addition to the general mechanisms summarized for acute GVHD, cGVHD is characterized by 2 features: immune-mediated fibrosis and an acquired combined immune deficiency. Dysregulation of post-thymic T cells and thymic-dependent T cells, donor and recipient APCs, alloimmunity and autoimmunity, cellular and humoral immunity, explain complex and protean clinical manifestations of cGVHD. Additionally, differences in target antigen distribution and polymorphisms in the regulatory regions of genes that determine the nature of immune responses might also explain the diversity of clinical presentation among patients with cGVHD. Special attention has been paid to a specific and complex defect in B and Treg in cGVHD [reviewed in 4]. The fibrotic aspect of GVHD lesion appears to be immune mediated and active (at least early) rather than a consequence of end-stage healing process. Recent lines of evidence suggest the antibody against the platelet-derived growth factor receptor (PDGFR). Stimulatory antibodies to the PDGFR were first found in patients with scleroderma. The antibodies recognized native PDGFR, inducing tyrosine phosphorylation and ROS accumulation [75]. Subsequently, authors found similar antibodies in patients with cGVHD [76].

References

1 Hill GR, Ferrara JL: The primacy of the gastrointestinal tract as a target organ of acute graft-versus-host disease: rationale for the use of cytokine shields in allogeneic bone marrow transplantation. Blood 2000;95:2754–2759.

2 Nestel FP, Price KS, Seemayer TA, Lapp WS: Macrophage priming and lipopolysaccharide-triggered release of tumor necrosis factor alpha during graft-versus-host disease. J Exp Med 1992;175: 405–413.

3 Piguet PF, Grau GE, Allet B, Vassalli P: Tumor necrosis factor/cachectin is an effector of skin and gut lesions of the acute phase of graft-vs.-host disease. J Exp Med 1987;166:1280–1289.

4 Socie G, Blazar BR: Acute graft-versus-host disease: from the bench to the bedside. Blood 2009;114:4327–4336.

5 Welniak LA, Blazar BR, Murphy WJ: Immunobiology of allogeneic hematopoietic stem cell transplantation. Annu Rev Immunol 2007;25:139–170.

6 Ferrara JL, Levine JE, Reddy P, Holler E: Graft-versus-host disease. Lancet 2009;373:1550–1561.

7 Antin JH: Acute graft-versus-host disease: inflammation run amok? J Clin Invest 2001;107:1497–1498.

8 Ferrara JL, Reddy P: Pathophysiology of graft-versus-host disease. Semin Hematol 2006;43:3–10.

9 Wysocki CA, Panoskaltsis-Mortari A, Blazar BR, Serody JS: Leukocyte migration and graft-versus-host disease. Blood 2005;105:4191–4199.

10 Zhan Q, Signoretti S, Whitaker-Menezes D, Friedman TM, Korngold R, Murphy GF: Cytokeratin15-positive basal epithelial cells targeted in graft-versus-host disease express a constitutive antiapoptotic phenotype. J Invest Dermatol 2007; 127:106–115.

11 Teshima T, Ordemann R, Reddy P, Gagin S, Liu C, Cooke KR, et al: Acute graft-versus-host disease does not require alloantigen expression on host epithelium. Nat Med 2002;8:575–581.

12 Chakraverty R, Sykes M: The role of antigen-presenting cells in triggering graft-versus-host disease and graft-versus-leukemia. Blood 2007;110:9–17.

13 Zhang Y, Joe G, Hexner E, Zhu J, Emerson SG: Host-reactive CD8+ memory stem cells in graft-versus-host disease. Nat Med 2005;11:1299–1305.

14 Hadeiba H, Sato T, Habtezion A, Oderup C, Pan J, Butcher EC: CCR9 expression defines tolerogenic plasmacytoid dendritic cells able to suppress acute graft-versus-host disease. Nat Immunol 2008;9: 1253–1260.

15 Ferrara J: Location, location, location. Nat Immunol 2003;4:103–104.

16 Murai M, Yoneyama H, Ezaki T, Suematsu M, Terashima Y, Harada A, et al: Peyer's patch is the essential site in initiating murine acute and lethal graft-versus-host reaction. Nat Immunol 2003;4: 154–160.

17 Shlomchik WD, Couzens MS, Tang CB, McNiff J, Robert ME, Liu J, et al: Prevention of graft versus host disease by inactivation of host antigen-presenting cells. Science 1999;285:412–415.

18 Jones SC, Murphy GF, Friedman TM, Korngold R: Importance of minor histocompatibility antigen expression by nonhematopoietic tissues in a CD4+ T cell-mediated graft-versus-host disease model. J Clin Invest 2003;112:1880–1886.

19 Zhang Y, Louboutin JP, Zhu J, Rivera AJ, Emerson SG: Preterminal host dendritic cells in irradiated mice prime CD8+ T cell-mediated acute graft-versus-host disease. J Clin Invest 2002;109:1335–1344.

20 Ordemann R, Hutchinson R, Friedman J, Burakoff SJ, Reddy P, Duffner U, et al: Enhanced allostimulatory activity of host antigen-presenting cells in old mice intensifies acute graft-versus-host disease. J Clin Invest 2002;109:1249–1256.

21 Matte CC, Liu J, Cormier J, Anderson BE, Athanasiadis I, Jain D, et al: Donor APCs are required for maximal GVHD but not for GVL. Nat Med 2004;10:987–992.

22 Merad M, Hoffmann P, Ranheim E, Slaymaker S, Manz MG, Lira SA, et al: Depletion of host Langerhans cells before transplantation of donor alloreactive T cells prevents skin graft-versus-host disease. Nat Med 2004;10:510–517.

23 Mutis T, Gillespie G, Schrama E, Falkenburg JH, Moss P, Goulmy E: Tetrameric HLA class I-minor histocompatibility antigen peptide complexes demonstrate minor histocompatibility antigen-specific cytotoxic T lymphocytes in patients with graft-versus-host disease. Nat Med 1999;5:839–842.

24 Goulmy E, Gratama JW, Blokland E, Zwaan FE, van Rood JJ: A minor transplantation antigen detected by MHC-restricted cytotoxic T lymphocytes during graft-versus-host disease. Nature 1983;302:159–161.

25 Kamei M, Nannya Y, Torikai H, Kawase T, Taura K, Inamoto Y, et al: HapMap scanning of novel human minor histocompatibility antigens. Blood 2009;113: 5041–5048.

26 Dickinson AM, Wang XN, Sviland L, Vyth-Dreese FA, Jackson GH, Schumacher TN, et al: In situ dissection of the graft-versus-host activities of cytotoxic T cells specific for minor histocompatibility antigens. Nat Med 2002;8:410–414.

27 Fontaine P, Roy-Proulx G, Knafo L, Baron C, Roy DC, Perreault C: Adoptive transfer of minor histocompatibility antigen-specific T lymphocytes eradicates leukemia cells without causing graft-versus- host disease. Nat Med 2001;7:789–794.

28 Choi EY, Christianson GJ, Yoshimura Y, Sproule TJ, Jung N, Joyce S, et al: Immunodominance of H60 is caused by an abnormally high precursor T cell pool directed against its unique minor histocompatibility antigen peptide. Immunity 2002;17:593–603.

29 Haniffa M, Ginhoux F, Wang XN, Bigley V, Abel M, Dimmick I, et al: Differential rates of replacement of human dermal dendritic cells and macrophages during hematopoietic stem cell transplantation. J Exp Med 2009;206:371–385.

30 Ginhoux F, Collin MP, Bogunovic M, Abel M, Leboeuf M, Helft J, et al: Blood-derived dermal langerin+ dendritic cells survey the skin in the steady state. J Exp Med 2007;204:3133–146.

31 Collin MP, Hart DN, Jackson GH, Cook G, Cavet J, Mackinnon S, et al: The fate of human Langerhans cells in hematopoietic stem cell transplantation. J Exp Med 2006;203:27–33.

32 Hubbard VM, Eng JM, Ramirez-Montagut T, Tjoe KH, Muriglan SJ, Kochman AA, et al: Absence of inducible costimulator on alloreactive T cells reduces graft versus host disease and induces Th2 deviation. Blood 2005;106:3285–3292.

33 Taylor PA, Panoskaltsis-Mortari A, Freeman GJ, Sharpe AH, Noelle RJ, Rudensky AY, et al: Targeting of inducible costimulator (ICOS) expressed on alloreactive T cells down-regulates graft-versus-host disease (GVHD) and facilitates engraftment of allogeneic bone marrow (BM). Blood 2005;105:3372–3380.

34 Blazar BR, Carreno BM, Panoskaltsis-Mortari A, Carter L, Iwai Y, Yagita H, et al: Blockade of programmed death-1 engagement accelerates graft-versus-host disease lethality by an IFN-gamma-dependent mechanism. J Immunol 2003;171: 1272–1277.

35 Beilhack A, Schulz S, Baker J, Beilhack GF, Wieland CB, Herman EI, et al: In vivo analyses of early events in acute graft-versus-host disease reveal sequential infiltration of T-cell subsets. Blood 2005;106:1113–1122.

36 Anderson BE, McNiff J, Yan J, Doyle H, Mamula M, Shlomchik MJ, et al: Memory CD4+ T cells do not induce graft-versus-host disease. J Clin Invest 2003; 112:101–108.

37 Anderson BE, McNiff JM, Matte C, Athanasiadis I, Shlomchik WD, Shlomchik MJ: Recipient CD4+ T cells that survive irradiation regulate chronic graft-versus-host disease. Blood 2004;104:1565–1573.

38 Ermann J, Hoffmann P, Edinger M, Dutt S, Blankenberg FG, Higgins JP, et al: Only the CD62L+ subpopulation of CD4+CD25+ regulatory T cells protects from lethal acute GVHD. Blood 2005;105: 2220–2226.

39 Muriglan SJ, Ramirez-Montagut T, Alpdogan O, Van Huystee TW, Eng JM, Hubbard VM, et al: GITR activation induces an opposite effect on alloreactive CD4+ and CD8+ T cells in graft-versus-host disease. J Exp Med 2004;200:149–157.

40 Hoffmann P, Ermann J, Edinger M, Fathman CG, Strober S: Donor-type CD4+CD25+ regulatory T cells suppress lethal acute graft-versus-host disease after allogeneic bone marrow transplantation. J Exp Med 2002;196:389–399.

41 Cohen JL, Trenado A, Vasey D, Klatzmann D, Salomon BL: CD4+CD25+ immunoregulatory T cells: new therapeutics for graft-versus-host disease. J Exp Med 2002;196:401–406.

42 Edinger M, Hoffmann P, Ermann J, Drago K, Fathman CG, Strober S, et al: CD4+CD25+ regulatory T cells preserve graft-versus-tumor activity while inhibiting graft-versus-host disease after bone marrow transplantation. Nat Med 2003;9:1144–1150.

43 Taylor PA, Noelle RJ, Blazar BR: CD4+CD25+ immune regulatory cells are required for induction of tolerance to alloantigen via costimulatory blockade. J Exp Med 2001;193:1311–1318.

44 Annunziato F, Romagnani S: Do studies in humans better depict Th17 cells? Blood 2009;114:2213–2219.

45 Rowell E, Wilson CB: Programming perpetual T helper cell plasticity. Immunity 2009;30:7–9.

46 Dong C: TH17 cells in development: an updated view of their molecular identity and genetic programming. Nat Rev Immunol 2008;8:337–348.

47 Kappel LW, Goldberg GL, King CG, Suh DY, Smith OM, Ligh C, et al: IL-17 contributes to CD4-mediated graft-versus-host disease. Blood 2009;113: 945–952.

48 Yi T, Zhao D, Lin CL, Zhang C, Chen Y, Todorov I, et al: Absence of donor Th17 leads to augmented Th1 differentiation and exacerbated acute graft-versus-host disease. Blood 2008;112:2101–2110.

49 Carlson MJ, West ML, Coghill JM, Panoskaltsis-Mortari A, Blazar BR, Serody JS: In vitro-differentiated TH17 cells mediate lethal acute graft-versus-host disease with severe cutaneous and pulmonary pathologic manifestations. Blood 2009;113:1365–1374.

50 Ratajczak P, Janin A, Peffault de Latour R, Leboeuf C, Desveaux A, Keyvanfar K, et al: Th17/Treg ratio in human graft-versus-host disease. Blood 2011;116: 1165–1171.

51 Panoskaltsis-Mortari A, Price A, Hermanson JR, Taras E, Lees C, Serody JS, et al: In vivo imaging of graft-versus-host-disease in mice. Blood 2004;103: 3590–3598.

52 Chakraverty R, Cote D, Buchli J, Cotter P, Hsu R, Zhao G, et al: An inflammatory checkpoint regulates recruitment of graft-versus-host reactive T cells to peripheral tissues. J Exp Med 2006;203: 2021–2031.

53 Murai M, Yoneyama H, Harada A, Yi Z, Vestergaard C, Guo B, et al: Active participation of CCR5+CD8+ T lymphocytes in the pathogenesis of liver injury in graft-versus-host disease. J Clin Invest 1999;104: 49–57.

54 Wysocki CA, Jiang Q, Panoskaltsis-Mortari A, Taylor PA, McKinnon KP, Su L, et al: Critical role for CCR5 in the function of donor CD4+CD25+ regulatory T cells during acute graft-versus-host disease. Blood 2005;106:3300–3307.

55 Varona R, Cadenas V, Gomez L, Martinez AC, Marquez G: CCR6 regulates CD4+ T-cell-mediated acute graft-versus-host disease responses. Blood 2005;106:18–26.

56 Faaij CM, Lankester AC, Spierings E, Hoogeboom M, Bowman EP, Bierings M, et al: A possible role for CCL27/CTACK-CCR10 interaction in recruiting CD4 T cells to skin in human graft-versus-host disease. Br J Haematol 2006;133:538–549.

57 Tsuchiyama J, Yoshino T, Saito T, Furukawa T, Ito K, Fuse I, et al: Cutaneous lymphocyte antigen-positive T cells may predict the development of acute GVHD: alterations and differences of CLA+ T- and NK-cell fractions. Bone Marrow Transplant 2009; 43:863–873.

58 Nikolic B, Lee S, Bronson RT, Grusby MJ, Sykes M: Th1 and Th2 mediate acute graft-versus-host disease, each with distinct end-organ targets. J Clin Invest 2000;105:1289–1298.

59 Murphy WJ, Welniak LA, Taub DD, Wiltrout RH, Taylor PA, Vallera DA, et al: Differential effects of the absence of interferon-gamma and IL-4 in acute graft-versus-host disease after allogeneic bone marrow transplantation in mice. J Clin Invest 1998;102: 1742–1748.

60 Min CK, Maeda Y, Lowler K, Liu C, Clouthier S, Lofthus D, et al: Paradoxical effects of interleukin-18 on the severity of acute graft-versus-host disease mediated by CD4+ and CD8+ T-cell subsets after experimental allogeneic bone marrow transplantation. Blood 2004;104:3393–3399.
61 Reddy P, Teshima T, Hildebrandt G, Williams DL, Liu C, Cooke KR, et al: Pretreatment of donors with interleukin-18 attenuates acute graft-versus-host disease via STAT6 and preserves graft-versus-leukemia effects. Blood 2003;101:2877–2885.
62 Reddy P, Teshima T, Hildebrandt G, Duffner U, Maeda Y, Cooke KR, et al: Interleukin 18 preserves a perforin-dependent graft-versus-leukemia effect after allogeneic bone marrow transplantation. Blood 2002;100:3429–3431.
63 Reddy P, Teshima T, Kukuruga M, Ordemann R, Liu C, Lowler K, et al: Interleukin-18 regulates acute graft-versus-host disease by enhancing Fas-mediated donor T cell apoptosis. J Exp Med 2001; 194:1433–1440.
64 Itoi H, Fujimori Y, Tsutsui H, Matsui K, Futatsugi S, Okamura H, et al: Fas ligand-induced caspase-1-dependent accumulation of interleukin-18 in mice with acute graft-versus-host disease. Blood 2001;98: 235–237.
65 Okamoto I, Kohno K, Tanimoto T, Iwaki K, Ishihara T, Akamatsu S, et al: IL-18 prevents the development of chronic graft-versus-host disease in mice. J Immunol 2000;164:6067–6074.
66 Lin MT, Storer B, Martin PJ, Tseng LH, Gooley T, Chen PJ, et al: Relation of an interleukin-10 promoter polymorphism to graft-versus-host disease and survival after hematopoietic-cell transplantation. N Engl J Med 2003;349:2201–2210.
67 Braun MY, Lowin B, French L, Acha-Orbea H, Tschopp J: Cytotoxic T cells deficient in both functional fas ligand and perforin show residual cytolytic activity yet lose their capacity to induce lethal acute graft-versus-host disease. J Exp Med 1996;183:657–661.
68 Baker MB, Altman NH, Podack ER, Levy RB: The role of cell-mediated cytotoxicity in acute GVHD after MHC-matched allogeneic bone marrow transplantation in mice. J Exp Med 1996;183:2645–2656.
69 van den Brink MR, Burakoff SJ: Cytolytic pathways in haematopoietic stem-cell transplantation. Nat Rev Immunol 2002;2:273–281.
70 Nishiwaki S, Terakura S, Ito M, Goto T, Seto A, Watanabe K, et al: Impact of macrophage infiltration of skin lesions on survival after allogeneic stem cell transplantation: a clue to refractory graft-versus-host disease. Blood 2009;114:3113–3116.
71 Socie G, Mary JY, Lemann M, Daneshpouy M, Guardiola P, Meignin V, et al: Prognostic value of apoptotic cells and infiltrating neutrophils in graft-versus-host disease of the gastrointestinal tract in humans: TNF and Fas expression. Blood 2004;103: 50–57.
72 Daneshpouy M, Socie G, Lemann M, Rivet J, Gluckman E, Janin A: Activated eosinophils in upper gastrointestinal tract of patients with graft-versus-host disease. Blood 2002;99:3033–3040.
73 Penack O, Socie G, van den Brink MR: The importance of neovascularization and its inhibition for allogeneic hematopoietic stem cell transplantation. Blood 2011;117:4181–4189.
74 Chu YW, Gress RE: Murine models of chronic graft-versus-host disease: insights and unresolved issues. Biol Blood Marrow Transplant 2008;14:365–378.
75 Baroni SS, Santillo M, Bevilacqua F, Luchetti M, Spadoni T, Mancini M, et al: Stimulatory autoantibodies to the PDGF receptor in systemic sclerosis. N Engl J Med 2006;354:2667–2676.
76 Svegliati S, Olivieri A, Campelli N, Luchetti M, Poloni A, Trappolini S, et al: Stimulatory autoantibodies to PDGF receptor in patients with extensive chronic graft-versus-host disease. Blood 2007;110: 237–241.

Prof. Gerard Socié
Hematology/Transplantation
Hospital Saint Louis
1 Avenue Claude Vellefaux
F-75475 Paris CEDEX 10 (France)
Tel. +33 1 42 49 98 24, E-Mail gerard.socie@sls.aphp.fr

Häusermann P, Steiger J, Passweg J (eds): Transplantation Dermatology.
Curr Probl Dermatol. Basel, Karger, 2012, vol 43, pp 101–115

Cutaneous Graft-versus-Host Disease – Clinical Considerations and Management

Peggy A. Wu[a] · Edward W. Cowen[b]

[a]Department of Dermatology, Beth Israel Deaconess Medical Center, Boston, Mass.; [b]Dermatology Branch, Center for Cancer Research, National Cancer Institute, National Institutes of Health, Bethesda, Md., USA

Abstract

Graft-versus-host disease (GVHD) is the primary cause of non-relapse-related morbidity and mortality in patients who undergo hematopoietic stem cell transplantation. Dermatologic manifestations are common in both acute and chronic GVHD. In the acute setting, skin involvement often provides the first indication of GVHD and may progress to erythroderma and even skin necrolysis. In the chronic phase, skin involvement is extraordinarily polymorphic, potentially involves all layers of the skin and subcutaneous tissue, and presents in sclerotic and nonsclerotic forms. Management of cutaneous disease is challenging and ideally employs a multi-disciplinary approach and an understanding of the multiple medical issues facing patients with GVHD. The dermatologist plays a key role in caring for the patient with GVHD by providing an accurate diagnosis, determination of disease activity and response to treatment, and appropriate consideration of all available treatment modalities, including topical, systemic, and physical interventions (e.g. phototherapy, extracorporeal photopheresis). This chapter describes the cutaneous manifestations of acute and chronic GVHD and provides an evidence-based review of current treatment interventions for patients with GVHD skin disease.

Graft-versus-host disease (GVHD) affects approximately 50% of patients who undergo allogeneic hematopoietic stem cell transplantation (HSCT) and is the leading cause of non-relapse-related mortality. GVHD has been traditionally divided into acute and chronic manifestations based on clinical presentation and time of disease onset (i.e. before or after 100 days after transplant); however, evolving HSCT regimens, including non-myeloablative conditioning and donor lymphocyte infusion (DLI), the transfer of additional hematopoietic cells after transplant, have altered the timing of classic acute and chronic disease manifestations. Careful clinical classification is now the predominant factor in disease staging [1].

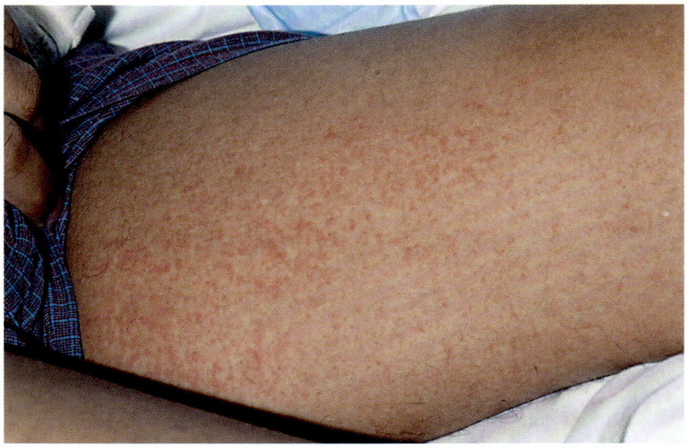

Fig. 1. aGVHD. Morbilliform eruption on the medial thigh.

Acute Graft-versus-Host Disease

Acute GVHD (aGVHD) occurs in approximately 40% of patients who undergo allogeneic HSCT [2, 3], typically 2–4 weeks after transplant. Late-onset aGVHD (after 100 days) may also occur following reduced intensity or nonmyeloablative preparatory regimens and following DLI. aGVHD primarily affects the skin, gastrointestinal tract, and liver. Frequently, skin involvement is the first sign of aGVHD, and most commonly presents as a rapid-onset, symmetric, morbilliform exanthem (fig. 1) or folliculocentric erythematous papules [4]. Initially, aGVHD may be most prominent on the acral surfaces, particularly the palms, and then extend over the upper trunk and lateral neck, face, and ears. Eruption of lymphocyte recovery and toxic erythema of chemotherapy may also occur in the first several weeks following HSCT, and can be difficult to distinguish from aGVHD. Rarely, aGVHD may progress to erythroderma, bullae formation, or necrolysis, resembling Stevens-Johnson syndrome/toxic epidermal necrolysis.

The characteristic histologic finding of aGVHD of the skin is an interface dermatitis with vacuolar change, particularly at the tips of the rete ridges. Similar changes may be present at the upper portions of eccrine and follicular structures. Histologic differentiation of aGVHD from viral exanthem and eruption of lymphocyte recovery can be challenging. In histologic grade I aGVHD, subtle vacuolization of the basal layer is seen. Grade II aGVHD is distinguished by keratinocyte apoptosis and satellitosis. Grades III and IV are characterized by subepidermal clefting and dermal-epidermal separation, respectively [3].

Clinical correlation is integral to the rapid and accurate diagnosis of aGVHD (table 1). Voluminous, watery diarrhea is suggestive of acute gastrointestinal involvement. Associated symptoms include abdominal pain, vomiting, or anorexia. Elevated total bilirubin is a marker of hepatic involvement, but may be difficult to

Table 1. Clinical manifestations of aGVHD

Skin	Erythema of palms, soles, ears Perifollicular erythema Generalized exanthem Bullae/necrolysis
Liver	Endothelialitis Pericholangitis Cholestasis (elevation of total bilirubin ≥2 mg/dl) Lymphocytic infiltration of portal system
Gastrointestinal tract	Upper: mucositis, vomiting, abdominal pain, anorexia Lower: secretory diarrhea (≥500 ml)

differentiate from other causes of liver dysfunction, including drug hypersensitivity and viral infection. The prognosis for patients with aGVHD is determined by the overall severity of skin, hepatic, and gastrointestinal involvement. Acute skin GVHD is staged as follows: (1) <25% body surface area (BSA); (2) 25–50% BSA; (3) >50% BSA or erythroderma, and (4) erythroderma with bullae. Similar staging of hepatic and gastrointestinal aGVHD based on bilirubin elevation, quantity of diarrhea and presence of pain/ileus is used to determine an overall aGVHD grade. Grade III and IV aGVHD is associated with approximately 31% and 9% 5-year survival, respectively [3, 5].

Chronic Graft-versus-Host Disease

Chronic GVHD (cGVHD) develops in approximately 30–70% of patients who undergo allogeneic HSCT. The median onset is 4–6 months following HSCT and symptoms usually present within 3 years of transplantation [1, 6]. cGVHD may evolve from aGVHD (progressive), occur following resolution of aGVHD (quiescent), or arise de novo. Similar to aGVHD, chronic disease may result in significant morbidity and mortality [6]. Unlike aGVHD, however, the pathophysiology behind cGHVD is less well understood. Patients often demonstrate features of autoimmunity with symptoms similar to well-characterized autoimmune diseases such as scleroderma and Sjögren's syndrome. Recently reported autoantibodies found in cGVHD patients provide further evidence for dysfunctional humoral immunity [7, 8]. Risk factors associated with cGVHD include history of aGVHD, older age at time of HSCT, HLA-antigen mismatch, female donor and male recipient, DLIs, and peripheral blood as the stem cell source [9].

Nearly any organ system may be affected by cGVHD, and 50% of patients will have involvement of three or more organ systems [6]. The skin is the most common target for cGVHD, but it varies markedly in clinical presentation. A National Institutes of Health consensus effort led to a set of proposed cGVHD disease definitions [1]. Diagnostic manifestations are those that are sufficiently unique to cGVHD to render the diagnosis, whereas distinctive manifestations require additional histologic or laboratory confirmation (table 2). According to the National Institutes of Health criteria, diagnosis of cGVHD requires: (1) at least one diagnostic sign of cGVHD, or the presence of at least 1 distinctive manifestation confirmed by biopsy or relevant tests, and (2) exclusion of other diagnoses, including aGVHD.

Chronic Graft-versus-Host Disease Skin and Mucosal Manifestations

Diagnostic skin manifestations of cGVHD include poikiloderma, lichen planus-like, lichen-sclerosus-like, morphea-like eruptions, as well as scleroderma-like disease and subcutaneous fibrosis/fasciitis (fig. 2b–f). Approximately 10% of patients with cGVHD develop sclerotic skin involvement [10]. Sclerotic changes in the skin may occur at any level from the upper dermis to the muscle fascia. Involvement of the upper dermis results in well-circumscribed hyperpigmented plaques of superficial morphea or gray-white atrophic plaques of lichen sclerosus. Diffuse sclerotic involvement resembles scleroderma [10]. Fibrosis of the subcutaneous fat and/or fascia causes skin, particularly of the medial arms or thighs, to 'ripple' and 'dimple,' resembling eosinophilic fasciitis. Fascial disease can also manifest as a 'groove sign' – linear depressions between muscle groups or along the course of superficial blood vessels. New-onset limb edema may portend sclerotic skin involvement, or fascial involvement may occur insidiously, leading to range of motion deficits and joint contractures without skin changes. If sclerotic changes are suspected, evaluation of joint range of motion in the affected area is recommended to follow progression of disease. Magnetic resonance imaging may aid in the diagnosis of fascial involvement [11].

Other less specific cGVHD skin changes include pruritus, decreased sweating, erythema and maculopapular rash. Nail changes include longitudinal ridging, splitting, brittle features, pterygium and partial or complete nail loss (fig. 2a). In the setting of non-diagnostic cutaneous signs or symptoms after HSCT, alternative dermatologic diagnoses should be considered. Drug eruptions and viral exanthems may mimic cGVHD, or may also induce a flare of cutaneous cGVHD. Phototoxicity from voriconazole, an antifungal agent commonly employed in the HSCT setting, should also be considered in the differential diagnosis of a cGVHD flare [12]. Dermatologic exam should also include evaluation for genital and oral mucosal cGVHD. In a prospective study, 49% of women manifested vulvo-vaginal involvement 2 years after transplant [13]. Women may describe dryness, vulvodynia,

Table 2. Common clinical manifestations of cGVHD

Organ/system	Sign/symptom
Skin	**Poikiloderma** **Lichen planus-like disease** **Lichen sclerosus-like disease** **Superficial morphea-like disease** **Scleroderma-like disease** **Subcutaneous fibrosis/fasciitis** Erythema Hypo-/hyperpigmentation Ichthyosis Keratosis pilaris-like eruption Maculopapular rash Pruritus Sweat impairment
Scalp and body hair	Alopecia (scarring or nonscarring)
Nails	Pterygium unguis Splitting, ridging, brittle nails Onycholysis
Eyes	Dry eyes Cicatricial conjunctivitis
Oral	Xerostomia **White reticulated plaques** **Restriction of mouth opening** Ulceration
Genitalia	**Lichen planus-like disease** **Vaginal sclerosis** Erosions
Lung	**Bronchiolitis obliterans**
Gastrointestinal	Dysphagia **Esophageal webbing** **Esophageal stenosis or strictures, upper to mid-third**
Liver	Elevated total bilirubin, alkaline phosphatase, ALT, AST
Musculoskeletal	**Fasciitis** **Joint stiffness, contractures** Edema
Hematologic	Thrombocytopenia Venous thromboembolism

Diagnostic criteria (sufficient to establish diagnosis of cGVHD) in **bold**. Adapted from Filipovich et al. [1].

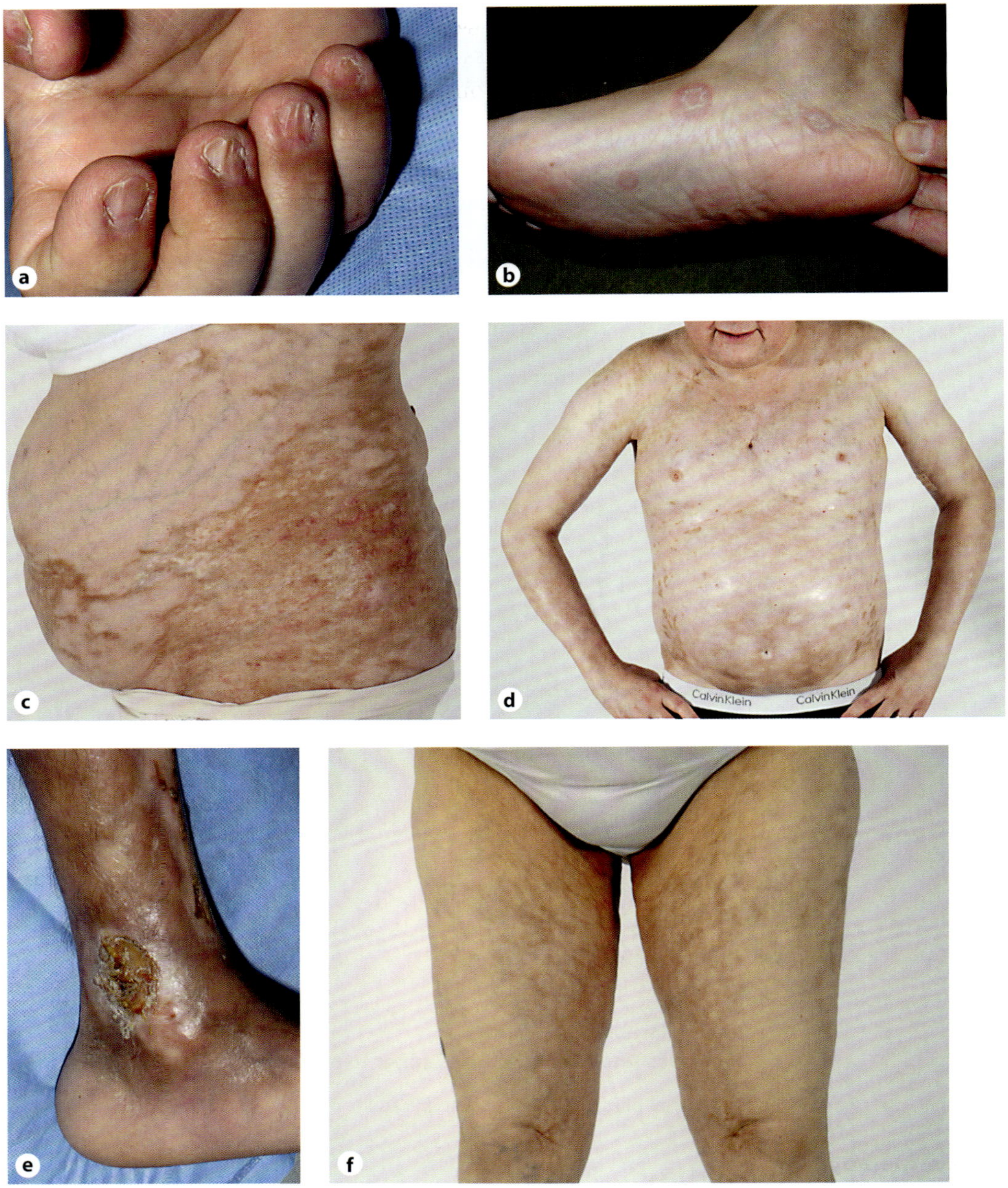

Fig. 2. The spectrum of chronic cutaneous GVHD. **a** Nail thinning, ridging and micronychia. **b** Lichen planus-like plaques. **c** Morphea-like sclerotic changes on the abdomen and flank. **d** Extensive sclerosis of the chest and abdomen with dyspigmentation. **e** Scleroderma-like skin fibrosis of the distal ankle with ulceration. **f** Subcutaneous/fascial cGVHD, rippling of the skin of the medial thighs with overlying hyperpigmentation.

pruritus, or dyspareunia. Diagnostic findings include vaginal scarring/stenosis and lichen planus-like features. Erosions, fissures and ulcers are also common. Involvement of the oral cavity is also common in cGVHD and manifests as erythema, lichenoid changes, xerostomia, ulcers and/or mucoceles [14]. Oral cGVHD may resemble oral lichen planus with lacy white reticular plaques. Perioral sclerosis may result in a restricted ability to open the mouth. Candidiasis may result from salivary gland dysfunction.

Histologic findings of cGVHD reflect the variable clinical presentation of the disease. Lichen planus-like cGVHD displays satellitosis and vacuolization of the epidermal basal layer, reminiscent of aGVHD [15]. Lichen sclerosus-like GVHD, morphea-like cGVHD, and cGVHD fascial involvement are reflected by thickening, homogenization and compaction of collagen in the papillary dermis, reticular dermis, or fascial tissue, respectively.

Weight loss, diarrhea, dyspnea, ocular sicca, and fatigue are other features suggestive of active cGVHD. Nausea, vomiting, anorexia, or dysphagia, from esophageal webbing and strictures may indicate cGVHD gastrointestinal disease. In the lungs, cGVHD can manifest as bronchiolitis obliterans syndrome, with dry cough, wheezing, and dyspnea. Hematologic abnormalities include lymphopenia, eosinophilia, and hyper- or hypogammaglobulinemia.

Therapy

The following section provides an overview of therapies for GVHD that might be utilized under a dermatologist's care. Phototherapy and extracorporeal photopheresis will be reviewed separately in the chapter by Greinix and Tanew [this vol., pp. 116–131]. Treatment for cGVHD of the skin can be divided into skin-directed (including phototherapy) and systemic interventions. Systemic intervention may be chosen based on the severity of skin involvement, multiple organ involvement, or lack of response to skin-directed therapy. Other important considerations are risk of malignancy relapse, risk of infection, and rate of cGVHD disease progression.

Topical Therapy

Topical corticosteroids are first-line therapy for limited chronic cutaneous, oral and mucosal cGVHD, and may also be useful for symptomatic relief of mild cutaneous aGVHD. Medium-high potency topical corticosteroids provide relief for superficial skin changes such as a lichen planus-like rash or pruritus symptoms and avoid interference with graft-versus-malignancy effects. Unfortunately, topical corticosteroids may provide only short-term relief, and may lead to poor wound healing, skin atrophy, striae formation, and increased risk of local infection. Therefore it is recommended that topical medications only be used for short periods and withdrawn or tapered following symptom relief [16].

The nonsteroidal topical immunomodulators, tacrolimus and pimicrolimus are particularly beneficial for sites at risk of skin atrophy with topical steroids. Choi and Nghiem [17] described a cGVHD response to tacrolimus 0.01% in 13/18 (72%) patients. Topical tacrolimus has also been used to treat ocular and oral GVHD symptoms [18–23]. Pimecrolimus has similarly been reported in several case reports [23, 24]. Topical calcineurin inhibitor therapy is generally well tolerated; however, systemic absorption has been reported in GVHD patients following use on mucosal surfaces and in the pediatric setting [21].

Systemic Therapy

Corticosteroids

Corticosteroids are first-line therapy for both aGVHD and cGVHD. Prednisone 1 mg/kg/day is commonly used for aGVHD [25]. Higher-dose steroid regimens (e.g. 2 mg/kg/day) were not found to provide additional benefit in grade I–II aGVHD [26]. Doses less than 1 mg/kg/day are sometimes used in practice, but evidence is lacking in clinical trials [25]. Corticosteroids are effective for approximately 50% of patients with aGVHD, particularly those with skin-limited disease [27]. For cGVHD, a common regimen is 1 mg/kg/day for 2 weeks, followed by reducing dosage over a period of 6–8 weeks [25]. Most patients who will respond to steroid therapy will do so within 3 months [28]. Alternate day steroid dosing is commonly employed to minimize steroid-induced adverse effects; however, there have been no randomized studies comparing daily versus alternate day dosing. Side effects of systemic corticosteroids in the transplant setting include bone density loss, avascular necrosis of bone, and diabetes mellitus. Because prolonged treatment is often required for control of GVHD, steroid-sparing agents are commonly employed. However, there is no single steroid alternative therapy that has demonstrated proven superiority.

Tacrolimus and Cyclosporine

The systemic calcineurin inhibitors tacrolimus and cyclosporine are used for GVHD prophylaxis as well as for active aGVHD [27]. Although they are frequently employed with systemic steroids for cGVHD, the evidence supporting their additive benefit in this setting is limited [25]. In a nonrandomized trial, complete response and 4-year survival rates of 33 and 51%, respectively, were observed in the CsA/prednisone group, compared to 16 and 26% with prednisone alone [29]. In contrast, a randomized trial of 287 patients found no difference in overall survival [30]. However, treatment-related mortality, recurrent malignancy, need for secondary therapy and/or immunosuppression, avascular necrosis, and disease-free survival were significantly improved in the CsA/prednisone cohort. Important complications of calcineurin inhibitor treatment include renal insufficiency, hypertension and infection.

Mycophenolate Mofetil

Mycophenolate mofetil (MMF) is an inhibitor of purine synthesis via the inosine monophosphate dehydrogenase enzyme, and preferentially suppresses proliferation of B and T cells. It is associated with dose-dependent cytopenias and gastrointestinal adverse effects such as upper and lower enteritis. Small retrospective trials for aGVHD and cGVHD have demonstrated partial or complete response in the majority of patients [31–34]. However, in a multicenter, double-blind, trial comparing MMF to standard immunosuppressive therapy for initial treatment of cGVHD, no difference was found in treatment success ($p = 0.22$) between the two arms, and in fact, the cumulative incidence of treatment failure appeared to be higher in the MMF group ($p = 0.03$) [35].

Sirolimus

Sirolimus, or rapamycin, is a bacterial macrolide antibiotic with immunosuppressive properties and antiproliferative effects on fibroblasts and smooth muscle cells. It inhibits the mammalian target of rapamycin, which leads to downregulation of DNA transcription, translation and protein synthesis [36]. Sirolimus may also decrease the risk of cutaneous malignancy [37, 38]. In a prospective randomized controlled trial of sirolimus versus standard immunosuppressive therapy in the renal allograft setting, 12/17 patients in the standard treatment group had progression of actinic keratoses or verruca vulgaris at 12 months, whereas no patients (0/16) in the sirolimus group had progression of skin lesions [39]. In a retrospective review of sirolimus for steroid-refractory aGVHD, improvement was seen in 20/22 patients [36]. Response rates for cGVHD range between 56 and 81% [16]. Jedlickova et al. [40] reported a 76% response in a series of 34 patients with scleroderma-like GVHD. Adverse effects include cytopenias, impaired wound healing and transplant-associated microangiopathy, which is increased with concomitant calcineurin inhibitor therapy.

Hydroxychloroquine

Hydroxychloroquine (HCQ), a 4-aminoquinolone antimalarial drug, has also been employed in cGVHD with variable success. HCQ reduces proinflammatory cytokines such as IL-1, IL-6 and tumor necrosis factor-α, and has also been shown to interfere with antigen processing and presentation and to work synergistically with the calcineurin inhibitors to suppress proliferative T-cell responses in vitro [41, 42]. In a multi-institutional phase II study, 50% of patients with cGVHD treated with HCQ 800 mg daily in addition to their existing immunosuppressive therapy experienced improvement [41]. Responses were observed most commonly in skin, oral, and liver GVHD, and platelet count. Three cases of HCQ-related neuropathy or myopathy were reported. Other common side effects are gastrointestinal symptoms and retinopathy. More recently, a double-blind, placebo-controlled trial of 800 mg daily HCQ in newly diagnosed cGVHD (18 HCQ, 24 placebo) failed to demonstrate a difference between treatment groups [43].

Rituximab

Rituximab is a chimeric mouse/human anti-CD20 antibody, which has been used for the treatment of B-cell malignancies and autoimmune disease. Recent studies have implicated B cells in the pathogenesis of cGVHD [7, 8], and rituximab is thought to modulate both the Th2 and humoral components of the disease. Therapeutic response rates of 43–86% (median 67%) have been reported for steroid-refractory cGVHD [16, 44]. Responses have been reported most frequently for skin involvement, followed by oral mucosa, liver, and lung [45].

Imatinib Mesylate

Imatinib mesylate is a multikinase inhibitor originally used for treatment of BCR-ABL-positive malignancies such as chronic myelogenous leukemia. It inhibits c-Abl, a downstream signaling molecule of transforming growth factor-β (TGFβ), as well as PDGF receptors [46]. TGFβ and PDGF have been implicated in fibroblast activation, leading to accumulation of extracellular matrix characteristic of sclerotic disease [47]. Patients with extensive cGVHD were found to produce stimulatory antibodies to the PDGF receptor in one study [48]. In preclinical murine studies, imatinib prevented fibrosis induced by bleomycin and in the TSK-1 model of scleroderma [49, 50]. Successful treatment of sclerotic-type cGVHD with imatinib 100 mg/day in the clinical setting was first reported in 2008 [51]. Olivieri et al. [52] subsequently reported 19 treatment-refractory cGVHD patients with sclerotic features treated with imatinib 50–200 mg/day. At median follow-up of 17 months, the overall response rate was 63%. In a second series, 14 patients with refractory sclerotic cGVHD treated with imatinib 400 mg/day (adults) or 100 mg/day (children) demonstrated an overall response rate of 50% [53]. Side effects of imatinib include fluid retention, muscle cramps, diarrhea, and bone marrow toxicity.

Thalidomide

Although its mechanisms of action are not completely understood, thalidomide is thought to inhibit expression of adhesion molecules, angiogenesis, NFκB activity, and cytokines, including tumor necrosis factor-α. It has shown some modest success in lichen planus-like cGVHD, but does not have efficacy in sclerotic disease [54, 55]. Vogelsang et al. [56] reported responses in 26/44 (59%) patients with refractory or high-risk cGVHD. In contrast, high-dose thalidomide at 200–800 mg/day resulted in an 11% response rate in a second study [55]. Another group found that thalidomide did not improve clinical response when added to a regimen of prednisone and cyclosporine [57], and use as cGVHD prophylaxis has been reported to increase risk of cGVHD [58]. Side effects of thalidomide include teratogenicity, sensory neuropathy, sedation, constipation, and granulocytopenia [27, 59].

Systemic Retinoids

Retinoids are vitamin A derivatives that induce normal differentiation of epithelial tissue, promote induction of T regulatory cells, block Th17 cell induction, and inhibit fibroblast proliferation as well as collagen production [16]. They have been used in various dermatologic contexts, including systemic sclerosis [60], but experience with GVHD is limited. A study of etretinate for sclerotic cGHVD in patients who had not responded to systemic steroids and/or cyclosporine described responses in 20/27 patients by 3 months [61]. However, ulceration of the skin and skin breakdown caused 6 patients to stop treatment. Other well-recognized side effects such as nail cracking, xerosis, hypercholesterolemia, eye irritation, chelitis, pruritus, and scaling were also common.

Mesenchymal Stem Cells

Mesenchymal stem cells (MSC) are multipotent progenitor cells found in the bone marrow and adipose tissue which are distinct from hematopoietic cells. They have generated considerable interest for their immunomodulating effects, which have been demonstrated in vivo and in vitro [62–64]. MSCs are thought to modulate T cell alloreactivity through a variety of mechanisms. Interestingly, the immunomodulatory effects of MSCs are similar regardless of whether the cells are derived from HLA-identical, partially matched or completely mismatched donors [65]. In a series of 55 patients with grade II–IV aGVHD treated with MSC, 30 (55%) had a complete response and 9 (16%) demonstrated a partial response [66]. Similarly, Weng et al. [67] demonstrated an overall skin response rate of 78% in patients with refractory cGVHD. More recently, Zhou et al. [68] demonstrated >70% improvement in

Rodnan skin score, decreased symptoms, healing of ulcers and increased skin mobility in 4 patients with scleroderma-like cGVHD. To date, significant adverse events related to MSC infusion have not been reported. However, additional clinical data are needed to characterize optimal dosage, number of infusions and time intervals, MSC growth medium, origin of MSC cells (adipose versus bone marrow) and the value of HLA matching.

Supportive Care Measures

Comprehensive management of the skin issues in the post-HSCT setting requires attention to the other risks intrinsic to this population, including drug exposures, infection and skin cancer. Ultraviolet radiation, drug eruptions and systemic infections all may induce a flare of GVHD. Sun protection with chemical and/or physical blockers should be emphasized, particularly in patients taking photosensitizing antimicrobial agents, including voriconazole, which has also been associated with increased risk of squamous cell carcinoma in the immunocompromised setting [12, 69]. Patients should be educated regarding skin cancer risk and require regular surveillance for skin cancer. In addition, prompt evaluation of new areas of skin breakdown and other possible areas of skin infection are warranted.

References

1 Filipovich AH, Weisdorf D, Pavletic S, Socie G, Wingard JR, Lee SJ, et al: National Institutes of Health consensus development project on criteria for clinical trials in chronic graft-versus-host disease. I. Diagnosis and staging working group report. Biol Blood Marrow Transplant 2005;11:945–956.

2 Hari P, Carreras J, Zhang MJ, Gale RP, Bolwell BJ, Bredeson CN, et al: Allogeneic transplants in follicular lymphoma: higher risk of disease progression after reduced-intensity compared to myeloablative conditioning. Biol Blood Marrow Transplant 2008; 14:236–245.

3 Ferrara JL, Levine JE, Reddy P, Holler E: Graft-versus-host disease. Lancet 2009;373:1550–1561.

4 Hausermann P, Walter RB, Halter J, Biedermann BC, Tichelli A, Itin P, et al: Cutaneous graft-versus-host disease: a guide for the dermatologist. Dermatology 2008;216:287–304.

5 Gratwohl A, Hermans J, Apperley J, Arcese W, Bacigalupo A, Bandini G, et al: Acute graft-versus-host disease: grade and outcome in patients with chronic myelogenous leukemia. Working Party Chronic Leukemia of the European Group for Blood and Marrow Transplantation. Blood 1995;86:813–818.

6 Lee SJ: Have we made progress in the management of chronic graft-vs-host disease? Best Pract Res Clin Haematol 2010;23:529–535.

7 Miklos DB, Kim HT, Miller KH, Guo L, Zorn E, Lee SJ, et al: Antibody responses to H-Y minor histocompatibility antigens correlate with chronic graft-versus-host disease and disease remission. Blood 2005;105:2973–2978.

8 Miklos DB, Kim HT, Zorn E, Hochberg EP, Guo L, Mattes-Ritz A, et al: Antibody response to DBY minor histocompatibility antigen is induced after allogeneic stem cell transplantation and in healthy female donors. Blood 2004;103:353–359.

9 Flowers ME, Inamoto Y, Carpenter PA, Lee SJ, Kiem HP, Petersdorf EW, et al: Comparative analysis of risk factors for acute graft-versus-host disease and for chronic graft-versus-host disease according to National Institutes of Health consensus criteria. Blood 2011;117:3214–3219.
10 Kroft EB, Berkhof NJ, van de Kerkhof PC, Gerritsen RM, de Jong EM: Ultraviolet A phototherapy for sclerotic skin diseases: a systematic review. J Am Acad Dermatol 2008;59:1017–1030.
11 Clark J, Yao L, Pavletic SZ, Krumlauf M, Mitchell S, Turner ML, et al: Magnetic resonance imaging in sclerotic-type chronic graft-vs-host disease. Arch Dermatol 2009;145:918–922.
12 Patel AR, Turner ML, Baird K, Gea-Banacloche J, Mitchell S, Pavletic SZ, et al: Voriconazole-induced phototoxicity masquerading as chronic graft-versus-host disease of the skin in allogeneic hematopoietic cell transplant recipients. Biol Blood Marrow Transplant 2009;15:370–376.
13 Zantomio D, Grigg AP, MacGregor L, Panek-Hudson Y, Szer J, Ayton R: Female genital tract graft-versus-host disease: incidence, risk factors and recommendations for management. Bone Marrow Transplant 2006;38:567–572.
14 Carpenter PA: How I conduct a comprehensive chronic graft-versus host disease assessment. Blood 2011;118:2679–2687.
15 Shulman HM, Kleiner D, Lee SJ, Morton T, Pavletic SZ, Farmer E, et al: Histopathologic diagnosis of chronic graft-versus-host disease: National Institutes of Health Consensus Development Project on Criteria for Clinical Trials in Chronic Graft-versus-Host Disease. II. Pathology Working Group Report. Biol Blood Marrow Transplant 2006;12:31–47.
16 Wolff D, Schleuning M, von Harsdorf S, Bacher U, Gerbitz A, Stadler M, et al: Consensus conference on clinical practice in chronic GVHD: second-line treatment of chronic graft-versus-host disease. Biol Blood Marrow Transplant 2011;17:1–17.
17 Choi CJ, Nghiem P: Tacrolimus ointment in the treatment of chronic cutaneous graft-vs-host disease: a case series of 18 patients. Arch Dermatol 2001;137:1202–1206.
18 Riemens A, te Boome L, Imhof S, Kuball J, Rothova A: Current insights into ocular graft-versus-host disease. Curr Opin Ophthalmol 2010;21:485–494.
19 Mawardi H, Stevenson K, Gokani B, Soiffer R, Treister N: Combined topical dexamethasone/tacrolimus therapy for management of oral chronic GVHD. Bone Marrow Transplant 2010;45:1062–1067.
20 Tam PM, Young AL, Cheng LL, Lam PT: Topical 0.03% tacrolimus ointment in the management of ocular surface inflammation in chronic GVHD. Bone Marrow Transplant 2010;45:957–958.
21 Prot-Labarthe S, Therrien R, Champagne MA, Duval M, Joubert C: Toxic serum levels of tacrolimus after topical administration in an infant with severe cutaneous graft-versus-host disease. Bone Marrow Transplant 2007;40:295–296.
22 Administration FaD: Protopic (tacrolimus) ointment 0.03% Ointment 0.1%. http://www.accessdata.fda.gov/scripts/cder/drugsatfda/index.cfm?fuseaction=Search.Label_ApprovalHistory#apphist.
23 Ziemer M, Gruhn B, Thiele JJ, Elsner P: Treatment of extensive chronic cutaneous graft-versus-host disease in an infant with topical pimecrolimus. J Am Acad Dermatol 2004;50:946–948.
24 Schmook T, Kraft J, Benninghoff B, Nindl I, Roewert J, Ulrich C, et al: Treatment of cutaneous chronic graft-versus-host disease with topical pimecrolimus. Bone Marrow Transplant 2005;36:87–88.
25 Wolff D, Gerbitz A, Ayuk F, Kiani A, Hildebrandt GC, Vogelsang GB, et al: Consensus conference on clinical practice in chronic graft-versus-host disease (GVHD): first-line and topical treatment of chronic GVHD. Biol Blood Marrow Transplant 2010;16: 1611–1628.
26 Mielcarek M, Storer BE, Boeckh M, Carpenter PA, McDonald GB, Deeg HJ, et al: Initial therapy of acute graft-versus-host disease with low-dose prednisone does not compromise patient outcomes. Blood 2009;113:2888–2894.
27 Penas PF, Fernandez-Herrera J, Garcia-Diez A: Dermatologic treatment of cutaneous graft versus host disease. Am J Clin Dermatol 2004;5:403–416.
28 Vogelsang GB: How I treat chronic graft-versus-host disease. Blood 2001;97:1196–1201.
29 Sullivan KM, Witherspoon RP, Storb R, Deeg HJ, Dahlberg S, Sanders JE, et al: Alternating-day cyclosporine and prednisone for treatment of high-risk chronic graft-v-host disease. Blood 1988;72: 555–561.
30 Koc S, Leisenring W, Flowers ME, Anasetti C, Deeg HJ, Nash RA, et al: Therapy for chronic graft-versus-host disease: a randomized trial comparing cyclosporine plus prednisone versus prednisone alone. Blood 2002;100:48–51.
31 Vogelsang GB, Arai S: Mycophenolate mofetil for the prevention and treatment of graft-versus-host disease following stem cell transplantation: preliminary findings. Bone Marrow Transplant 2001;27: 1255–1262.

32 Krejci M, Doubek M, Buchler T, Brychtova Y, Vorlicek J, Mayer J: Mycophenolate mofetil for the treatment of acute and chronic steroid-refractory graft-versus-host disease. Ann Hematol 2005;84: 681–685.

33 Takami A, Mochizuki K, Okumura H, Ito S, Suga Y, Yamazaki H, et al: Mycophenolate mofetil is effective and well tolerated in the treatment of refractory acute and chronic graft-versus-host disease. Int J Hematol 2006;83:80–85.

34 Onishi C, Ohashi K, Sawada T, Nakano M, Kobayashi T, Yamashita T, et al: A high risk of life-threatening infectious complications in mycophenolate mofetil treatment for acute or chronic graft-versus-host disease. Int J Hematol 2010;91: 464–470.

35 Martin PJ, Storer BE, Rowley SD, Flowers ME, Lee SJ, Carpenter PA, et al: Evaluation of mycophenolate mofetil for initial treatment of chronic graft-versus-host disease. Blood 2009;113:5074–5082.

36 Ghez D, Rubio MT, Maillard N, Suarez F, Chandesris MO, Delarue R, et al: Rapamycin for refractory acute graft-versus-host disease. Transplantation 2009;88:1081–1087.

37 Alberu J, Pascoe MD, Campistol JM, Schena FP, Rial MD, Polinsky M, et al: Lower malignancy rates in renal allograft recipients converted to sirolimus-based, calcineurin inhibitor-free immunotherapy: 24-month results from the CONVERT trial. Transplantation 2011;92:303–310.

38 Mathew T, Kreis H, Friend P: Two-year incidence of malignancy in sirolimus-treated renal transplant recipients: results from five multicenter studies. Clin Transplant 2004;18:446–449.

39 Salgo R, Gossmann J, Schofer H, Kachel HG, Kuck J, Geiger H, et al: Switch to a sirolimus-based immunosuppression in long-term renal transplant recipients: reduced rate of (pre-)malignancies and nonmelanoma skin cancer in a prospective, randomized, assessor-blinded, controlled clinical trial. Am J Transplant 2010;10:1385–1393.

40 Jedlickova Z, Burlakova I, Bug G, Baurmann H, Schwerdtfeger R, Schleuning M: Therapy of sclerodermatous chronic graft-versus-host disease with mammalian target of rapamycin inhibitors. Biol Blood Marrow Transplant 2010;17:657–663.

41 Gilman AL, Chan KW, Mogul A, Morris C, Goldman FD, Boyer M, et al: Hydroxychloroquine for the treatment of chronic graft-versus-host disease. Biol Blood Marrow Transplant 2000;6:327–334.

42 Ziegler HK, Unanue ER: Decrease in macrophage antigen catabolism caused by ammonia and chloroquine is associated with inhibition of antigen presentation to T cells. Proc Natl Acad Sci USA 1982;79:175–178.

43 Gilman AL, Schultz KR, Goldman FD, Sale GE, Krailo MD, Chen Z, et al: Randomized trial of hydroxychloroquine for newly diagnosed chronic graft-versus-host disease in children: A Children's Oncology Group Study. Biol Blood Marrow Transplant 2011, Epub ahead of print.

44 Cutler C, Miklos D, Kim HT, Treister N, Woo SB, Bienfang D, et al: Rituximab for steroid-refractory chronic graft-versus-host disease. Blood 2006;108: 756–762.

45 Kharfan-Dabaja MA, Mhaskar AR, Djulbegovic B, Cutler C, Mohty M, Kumar A: Efficacy of rituximab in the setting of steroid-refractory chronic graft-versus-host disease: a systematic review and meta-analysis. Biol Blood Marrow Transplant 2009;15: 1005–1013.

46 Daniels CE, Wilkes MC, Edens M, Kottom TJ, Murphy SJ, Limper AH, et al: Imatinib mesylate inhibits the profibrogenic activity of TGF-beta and prevents bleomycin-mediated lung fibrosis. J Clin Invest 2004;114:1308–1316.

47 Varga J, Abraham D: Systemic sclerosis: a prototypic multisystem fibrotic disorder. J Clin Invest 2007;117: 557–567.

48 Svegliati S, Olivieri A, Campelli N, Luchetti M, Poloni A, Trappolini S, et al: Stimulatory autoantibodies to PDGF receptor in patients with extensive chronic graft-versus-host disease. Blood 2007;110: 237–241.

49 Akhmetshina A, Venalis P, Dees C, Busch N, Zwerina J, Schett G, et al: Treatment with imatinib prevents fibrosis in different preclinical models of systemic sclerosis and induces regression of established fibrosis. Arthritis Rheum 2009;60:219–224.

50 Distler JH, Jungel A, Huber LC, Schulze-Horsel U, Zwerina J, Gay RE, et al: Imatinib mesylate reduces production of extracellular matrix and prevents development of experimental dermal fibrosis. Arthritis Rheum 2007;56:311–322.

51 Moreno-Romero JA, Fernandez-Aviles F, Carreras E, Rovira M, Martinez C, Mascaro JM Jr: Imatinib as a potential treatment for sclerodermatous chronic graft-vs-host disease. Arch Dermatol 2008;144: 1106–1109.

52 Olivieri A, Locatelli F, Zecca M, Sanna A, Cimminiello M, Raimondi R, et al: Imatinib for refractory chronic graft-versus-host disease with fibrotic features. Blood 2009;114:709–718.

53 Magro L, Mohty M, Catteau B, Coiteux V, Chevallier P, Terriou L, et al: Imatinib mesylate as salvage therapy for refractory sclerotic chronic graft-versus-host disease. Blood 2009;114:719–722.
54 Penas PF, Jones-Caballero M, Aragues M, Fernandez-Herrera J, Fraga J, Garcia-Diez A: Sclerodermatous graft-vs-host disease: clinical and pathological study of 17 patients. Arch Dermatol 2002;138:924–934.
55 Parker PM, Chao N, Nademanee A, O'Donnell MR, Schmidt GM, Snyder DS, et al: Thalidomide as salvage therapy for chronic graft-versus-host disease. Blood 1995;86:3604–3609.
56 Vogelsang GB, Farmer ER, Hess AD, Altamonte V, Beschorner WE, Jabs DA, et al: Thalidomide for the treatment of chronic graft-versus-host disease. N Engl J Med 1992;326:1055–1058.
57 Arora M, Wagner JE, Davies SM, Blazar BR, Defor T, Enright H, et al: Randomized clinical trial of thalidomide, cyclosporine, and prednisone versus cyclosporine and prednisone as initial therapy for chronic graft-versus-host disease. Biol Blood Marrow Transplant 2001;7:265–273.
58 Chao NJ, Parker PM, Niland JC, Wong RM, Dagis A, Long GD, et al: Paradoxical effect of thalidomide prophylaxis on chronic graft-vs-host disease. Biol Blood Marrow Transplant 1996;2:86–92.
59 Koc S, Leisenring W, Flowers ME, Anasetti C, Deeg HJ, Nash RA, et al: Thalidomide for treatment of patients with chronic graft-versus-host disease. Blood 2000;96:3995–3996.
60 Maurice PD, Bunker CB, Dowd PM: Isotretinoin in the treatment of systemic sclerosis. Br J Dermatol 1989;121:367–374.
61 Marcellus DC, Altomonte VL, Farmer ER, Horn TD, Freemer CS, Grant J, et al: Etretinate therapy for refractory sclerodermatous chronic graft-versus-host disease. Blood 1999;93:66–70.
62 Bartholomew A, Sturgeon C, Siatskas M, Ferrer K, McIntosh K, Patil S, et al: Mesenchymal stem cells suppress lymphocyte proliferation in vitro and prolong skin graft survival in vivo. Exp Hematol 2002; 30:42–48.
63 Le Blanc K, Tammik L, Sundberg B, Haynesworth SE, Ringden O: Mesenchymal stem cells inhibit and stimulate mixed lymphocyte cultures and mitogenic responses independently of the major histocompatibility complex. Scand J Immunol 2003;57:11–20.
64 Tse WT, Pendleton JD, Beyer WM, Egalka MC, Guinan EC: Suppression of allogeneic T-cell proliferation by human marrow stromal cells: implications in transplantation. Transplantation 2003;75: 389–397.
65 Ringden O, Le Blanc K: Mesenchymal stem cells for treatment of acute and chronic graft-versus-host disease, tissue toxicity and hemorrhages. Best Pract Res Clin Haematol 2011;24:65–72.
66 Le Blanc K, Frassoni F, Ball L, Locatelli F, Roelofs H, Lewis I, et al: Mesenchymal stem cells for treatment of steroid-resistant, severe, acute graft-versus-host disease: a phase II study. Lancet 2008;371:1579–1586.
67 Weng JY, Du X, Geng SX, Peng YW, Wang Z, Lu ZS, et al: Mesenchymal stem cell as salvage treatment for refractory chronic GVHD. Bone Marrow Transplant 2010;45:1732–1740.
68 Zhou H, Guo M, Bian C, Sun Z, Yang Z, Zeng Y, et al: Efficacy of bone marrow-derived mesenchymal stem cells in the treatment of sclerodermatous chronic graft-versus-host disease: clinical report. Biol Blood Marrow Transplant 2010;16:403–412.
69 Cowen EW, Nguyen JC, Miller DD, McShane D, Arron ST, Prose NS, et al: Chronic phototoxicity and aggressive squamous cell carcinoma of the skin in children and adults during treatment with voriconazole. J Am Acad Dermatol 2010;62:31–37.

Edward W. Cowen, MD, MHSc
Dermatology Branch
Center for Cancer Research
National Cancer Institute
10 Center Dr., MSC 1908
Bethesda, MD 20892 (USA)
Tel. +1 301 496 4299, E-Mail cowene@mail.nih.gov

Häusermann P, Steiger J, Passweg J (eds): Transplantation Dermatology.
Curr Probl Dermatol. Basel, Karger, 2012, vol 43, pp 116–131

UV Treatment of Chronic Skin Graft-versus-Host Disease – Focus on UVA1 and Extracorporeal Photopheresis

Hildegard T. Greinix[a] · Adrian Tanew[b]

[a]Bone Marrow Transplantation, Department of Internal Medicine I, and [b]Department of Dermatology, Medical University of Vienna, Vienna, Austria

Abstract

Chronic graft-versus-host disease (GVHD) is a serious and life-threatening complication after allogeneic hematopoietic stem cell transplantation. Cutaneous manifestations such as lichenoid or sclerotic-type skin changes have been frequently observed in these patients. UVA1 phototherapy appears as a very effective treatment option for treatment-refractory lichenoid and sclerodermatous GVHD. Substantial improvements can often be achieved within 8–12 weeks of treatment allowing for subsequent reduction or withdrawal of immunosuppressive medications. UVA1 treatment acts via a local effect and is therefore only indicated for cutaneous manifestations of GVHD. In patients with multiorgan involvement by chronic GVHD, extracorporeal photopheresis is an efficacious and safe second-line therapy for steroid-refractory disease in both pediatric as well as adult patients. Besides high response rates in cutaneous and extracutaneous manifestations of chronic GVHD, a substantial corticosteroid-sparing effect and improved survival rates have been reported in patients given extracorporeal photopheresis treatment.

Chronic graft-versus-host disease (GVHD) remains a severe and clinically challenging complication after allogeneic hematopoietic stem cell transplantation (HCT) with a significant negative impact on quality of life and patient survival. It is a multisystem disorder with a variety of clinical phenotypes resembling autoimmune disorders such as scleroderma, systemic lupus erythematosus, Sjögren syndrome and rheumatoid arthritis. The most frequent organ manifestations of chronic GVHD are skin in up to 90% of patients, oral mucosa in 60%, eyes in 60% and liver in 60%, respectively [1]. Lichenoid-type changes represent the early form of cutaneous manifestations of chronic GVHD, whereas late ones may lead to superficial and deep sclerosis of the skin resulting in severe impairment of patients' activities and quality of life.

In general, patients with mild chronic GVHD defined as 1 or 2 organ involvement except lung without clinically significant functional impairment [2] may receive topical immunosuppressive therapy either alone or in combination with systemic immunosuppressive medication. In moderate and severe chronic GVHD, topical immunosuppression may be applied as an adjunct to increase local response rates and to spare patients of long-lasting corticosteroid medications and its toxicity. Topical immunosuppression may also be an important therapeutic modality in patients with chronic GVHD and high risk of relapse since no negative impact on the beneficial graft-versus-leukemia/tumor effect is to be expected. Close follow-up of patients under topical therapy alone is warranted to avoid progression of chronic GVHD to other organs. For treatment of cutaneous chronic GVHD, a number of effective topical therapeutic options are available including PUVA that denotes irradiation with UVA light irradiation after administration of the photosensitizer 8-methoxypsoralen (8-MOP), UVA1 irradiation, narrow-band and broad-band UVB irradiation. Since all these topical therapeutic modalities solely impact cutaneous manifestations of chronic GVHD, patients with extracutaneous involvements should receive systemic immunosuppressive medications and/or extracorporeal photopheresis (ECP). Response of chronic GVHD to topical and/or systemic immunosuppressive therapy should be assessed every 8–12 weeks [3]. If patients have progression of chronic GVHD after 4 weeks, a new therapeutic option should be initiated. Since patients with chronic GVHD are immunocompromised, they should receive infection prevention measures as previously published [4].

UVA1

Historical Background and Terminology

Phototherapy using short-wave ultraviolet light (UVB, 290–320 nm) has a long tradition in dermatology and has been successfully employed for a wide range of inflammatory skin diseases [5]. In contrast, the therapeutic use of long-wave ultraviolet light (UVA, 320–400 nm) has for a long time been hampered by the fact that photons in the UVA range are biologically much less effective than UVB wavelengths and that high-output irradiation units have not been available until the beginning of the 1980s [6]. In 1985, Thomas B. Fitzpatrick, an eminent photobiologist from Boston, proposed to further subdivide UVA into UVA 2 (far UVA, 320–340 nm) and UVA 1 (near UVA, 340–400 nm). This suggestion was based on the observation that wavelengths in the UVA 2 region produced pigmentary changes in the epidermis similar to those seen following UVB exposure and different from the pigmentation induced by near UVA [7]. In 1992, the principle of UVA1 phototherapy was introduced into dermatology by Krutmann and colleagues who were the first to report on the successful use of high-dose of UVA1 for patients with severe atopic dermatitis [8]. Since then, the effectiveness of UVA1 treatment was explored for a variety of other skin diseases such as urticaria pigmentosa, granuloma annulare, mycosis fungoides, polymorphic light eruption and localized as well as systemic scleroderma.

UVA1 Treatment of Chronic GVHD

In contrast to the large body of evidence demonstrating the high efficacy of UVA1 phototherapy for sclerosing skin conditions [9, 10], there is a paucity of data on its use in chronic GVHD [11]. This is due to the fact that the latter is often encountered in the setting of a multiorgan affection requiring a systemic rather than a locally acting treatment. Furthermore, UVA1 is not considered as a first-line treatment for chronic GVHD and is often used only when other treatments have failed. Finally, UVA1 irradiation units (that are substantially more expensive than conventional PUVA or UVB phototherapy units) are not widely available and essentially restricted to a few university-based phototherapeutic centers within Europe.

In 2000, Grundmann-Kollmann et al. [12] described a 42-year-old male patient with chronic myeloid leukemia who received allogeneic bone marrow transplantation from his HLA-identical brother. One year later, the patient developed chronic sclerodermatous GVHD not responding to a combination therapy of cyclosporine and corticosteroids and later mycophenolate mofetil plus corticosteroids. A combination therapy of mycophenolate mofetil and low-dose UVA1 therapy (single doses of 20 J/cm^2, 4 times per week over 6 weeks) resulted in striking clinical improvement of the sclerotic skin changes as early as after 12 treatments.

This first report on a beneficial effect of UVA1 radiation for cutaneous GVHD was subsequently corroborated by Ständer et al. [13] in a small case series of 6 patients with refractory chronic sclerodermatous GVHD. One of these patients, a 12-year-old boy with extremely severe sclerotic changes had been receiving systemic immunosuppressive therapy and ECP for 8 weeks. Since this regimen did not at all affect the sclerotic lesions, UVA1 therapy was also administered 5 times weekly with single exposure doses of 50 and 20 J/cm^2 (for the child), respectively. Within 4–6 weeks after initiation of UVAl therapy, a remarkable improvement was observed in all patients. The sclerotic changes became much softer, all erosive lesions healed and joint mobility improved.

In 2003, Calzavara Pinton et al. [14] published their experiences with UVA1 phototherapy for patients with both chronic lichenoid (4 patients) and sclerodermatous (5 patients) refractory GVHD. Treatment was administered 3 times weekly with fixed doses of 50 J/cm^2. After 12–21 UVA1 exposures, 2 of the 4 patients with generalized lichenoid GVHD showed complete remission (CR) while the other 2 patients responded partially (>50% decrease of skin affection). Out of the 5 patients with sclerodermatous GVHD, 3 experienced a CR (healing of erosions and resolution of induration) and 2 had a partial response after 15–33 UVA1 exposures. The improvement of the clinical findings was confirmed by histopathology showing a marked reduction of the lichenoid and sclerotic changes after treatment. Of note, areas inaccessible to UVA1 radiation such as the armpits, perineocrural region or intergluteal clefts did not improve during UVA1 phototherapy, thus ruling out spontaneous improvement and demonstrating that UVA1 acts via a local and not a systemic effect. Likewise, extracutaneous GVHD manifestations, when present, remained unchanged. All patients with lichenoid GVHD had an early relapse that required prolonged maintenance treatment. In contrast, the 3 complete responders with localized sclerodermatous GVHD remained in persistent remission after discontinuation of treatment.

The finding that debilitating chronic GVHD in children may also be well amenable to UVA1 treatment has been supported by an anecdotal report on 2 children with severe lichenoid and sclerodermatous lesions [15]. After 32 and 20 treatments with fixed UVA1 doses of 50 and 20 J/cm^2, respectively, a marked decrease in the sclerotic changes (objectified by 20 MHz ultrasound examination) and improved joint motility was observed. The condition remained stable after cessation of treatment and allowed for complete withdrawal of the systemic immunosuppressive therapy.

The most recent report summarized the therapeutic results for medium-dose (50–60 J/cm^2) UVA1 as an adjunct to systemic immunosuppressive treatment in 7 patients with chronic lichenoid and 3 patients with sclerodermatous GVHD. CR was achieved in 6 and partial remission in 1 of the patients with lichenoid GVHD after 13–36 irradiations. Relapses occurred in 2 patients. All 3 patients with sclerodermatous GVHD showed significant reduction in sclerosis but required a much longer treatment duration (29–91 exposures) [16].

It is also our experience that lichenoid GVHD has a more favorable prognosis and that sustained remissions can often be achieved (fig. 1). In contrast, complete resolution of long-standing sclerodermatous GVHD is an unrealistic expectation although a substantial decrease in skin thickening, and gain in joint motility can be induced by UVA1 treatment (fig. 2). Our empirical data in patients with sclerodermatous GVHD indicate that there is a negative correlation between disease duration and treatment response, as has been observed with ECP. Therefore, treatment should be initiated at the earliest signs of skin affection.

An interesting yet unexplored field of clinical research is the question whether the efficacy of UVA1 phototherapy can be enhanced by combination with other treatments for GVHD. There is preliminary evidence that the adjunctive administration of isotretinoin improves the response to bath PUVA in patients with sclerodermatous GVHD [17]. Likewise, as mentioned above, the addition of UVA1 treatment to ECP and immunosuppressive therapy has resulted in a favorable outcome in a child with severe sclerodermatous GVHD. Thus, the potential of combining UVA1 with other interventions requires further investigation and may be considered in unresponsive patients.

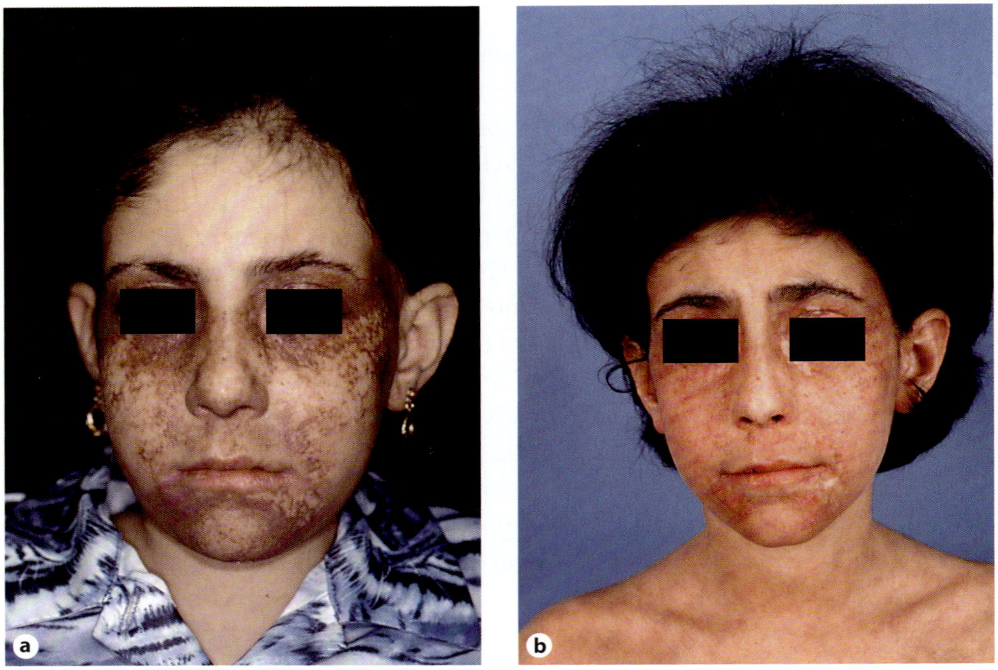

Fig. 1. **a** Chronic steroid-refractory lichenoid GVHD in a 12-year-old girl. **b** Almost complete resolution of the lichenoid skin changes after UVA1 phototherapy.

Mechanism of Action

UVA1 phototherapy has a profound effect on cutaneous inflammatory disorders by depleting activated skin-infiltrating T helper cells [18]. In vitro studies have shown that UVA1 radiation generates singlet oxygen which is followed by cellular membrane damage and subsequent immediate apoptosis of CD4+ cells [19]. In addition, UVA1 phototherapy exerts a direct effect on the connective tissue by inducing the synthesis of collagenase I, a member of the matrix metalloproteinase family, in dermal fibroblasts. The increased expression of this collagen-degrading enzyme and a decreased production of procollagen are major contributors to the high efficacy of UVA1 phototherapy for sclerodermatous GVHD and sclerosing skin diseases in general [10].

Side Effects

The most common acute side effect is painless UVA1 erythema occurring a few hours after irradiation and resolving within 24 h. Rarely, polymorphic light eruption can be elicited. UVA1-induced tanning can unmask a subclinical sclerodermic affection of

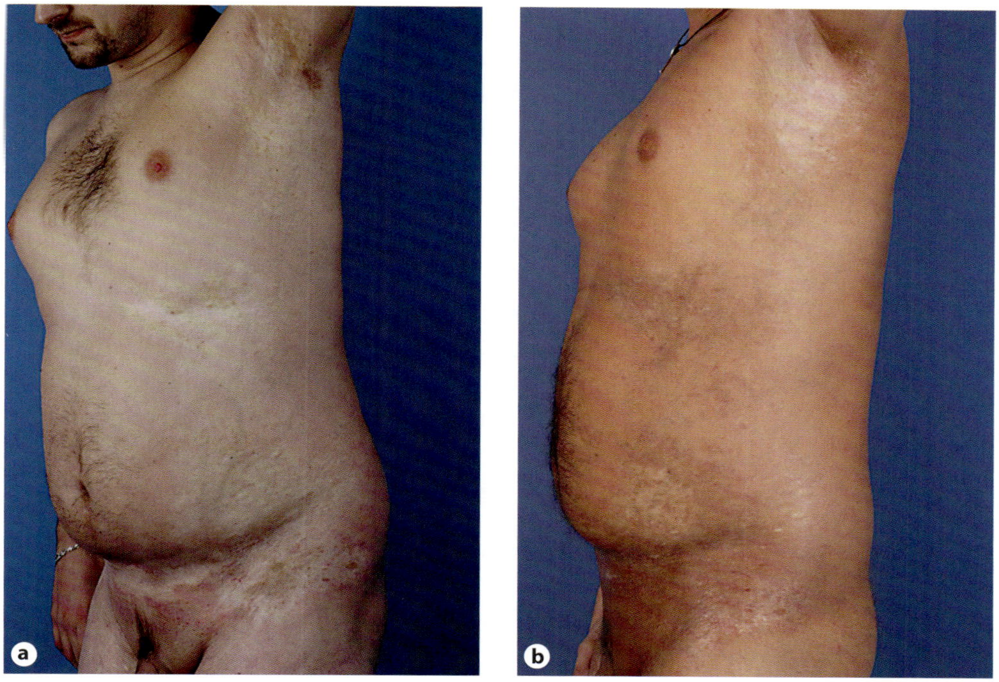

Fig. 2. **a** 26-year-old man at 5 months after the onset of rapidly progressing sclerodermatous GVHD. **b** Marked decrease in the sclerotic skin changes after 3 months of UVA1 phototherapy.

the skin during the early phase of treatment and give the false impression of a seeming progression of the disease.

The long-term risks of UVA1 phototherapy are unknown. UVA1 radiation is known to exert immunosuppressive effects [20] and to induce cyclobutane pyrimidine dimers in human skin in vivo [21]. It is, thus conceivable that UVA1 treatment might be associated with an increased risk for skin cancer when given over prolonged periods of time. However, the occurrence of skin cancer after UVA1 treatment has, so far, not been reported in the literature.

Practical Aspects

UVA1 phototherapy is basically easy to perform. Prior to treatment, a detailed dermatological history should be taken with particular emphasis on the presence of abnormal light sensitivity or the intake of photosensitizing medications. In positive or doubtful cases, a photodiagnostic evaluation including the determination of the minimal erythema dose for UVA1 might be required. It is also mandatory to examine the whole skin for the presence of atypical nevi or malignant skin tumors before starting UVA1 treatment.

In the average patient (Fitzpatrick skin types III–IV), one might start with an initial exposure dose of 30 J/cm^2. If this dose is well tolerated, treatment can be continued with fixed single exposure doses of 50 J/cm^2. In patients with a fair complexion (Fitzpatrick skin types I–II) or abnormal light sensitivity, an initial UVA1 dose below the minimal erythema dose should be chosen.

The optimum UVA1 exposure dose for the treatment of chronic GVHD remains to be determined. Whereas it has been shown in localized scleroderma that medium-dose UVA1 (50–70 J/cm^2) provides for better therapeutic results than low-dose (20 J/cm^2) UVA1 [22], it is as yet unknown whether this also applies for the treatment of chronic cutaneous GVHD.

Treatment can be given 3 or 5 times weekly until a satisfactory response is achieved. Maintenance therapy should be reserved for patients with early relapse after discontinuation of UVA1 phototherapy.

Summary

UVA1 phototherapy appears as a very effective treatment option for treatment-refractory lichenoid and sclerodermatous GVHD. It has a rapid onset of action, and substantial improvement can often be achieved within 8–12 weeks of treatment allowing for subsequent reduction or withdrawal of immunosuppressive medications. UVA1 treatment acts via a local effect, and is therefore only indicated for cutaneous manifestations of GVHD. In patients with multiorgan involvement, UVA1 treatment might be used as a valuable adjunctive treatment to systemic immunosuppressants or ECP.

Extracorporeal Photopheresis

ECP is a leukapheresis-based immunomodulatory therapy that has been approved for the palliative treatment of cutaneous T cell lymphoma [23]. It has also shown promising efficacy in a variety of T cell-mediated diseases including prevention and therapy of rejection after solid organ transplantation, Crohn's disease and systemic sclerosis [23]. During the last years, clinicians in numerous allogeneic HCT centers worldwide have been frequently using ECP for treatment of steroid-refractory or steroid-dependent chronic GVHD patients.

The exact mechanisms of action of ECP have been the focus of exciting and ongoing research projects leading to improved insights. Ex vivo-administered 8-MOP in the presence of UVA irradiation forms covalent bonds with DNA pyrimidine bases, intercalating into its structure and cross-linking the two DNA strands [23]. ECP induces apoptosis in all leukocyte subsets within 24–48 h. Circulating apoptotic cells are phagocytosed by antigen-presenting cells leading to inhibition of proinflammatory cytokines, production of anti-inflammatory cytokines and induction of regulatory T cells [24–26]. Furthermore, tolerogenic or immunomodulatory properties might be induced in antigen-presenting cells during ECP [27].

ECP has an excellent safety profile and does not cause general immunosuppression since T and B cell responses to novel or recall antigens remain unaltered [28], and thus no increases in infectious complications or relapse have been reported [24, 29, 30].

Technical Aspects

During ECP, up to 15% of the patient's total blood volume is removed with an antecubital angiocatheter and passed through the UVAR or CELLEX photopheresis system (Therakos, Raritan, N.J., USA) centrifuge. Then, collected white blood cells are incubated with liquid 8-MOP administered into the treatment bag and passed through a disposable plastic device, exposed to UVA and then reinfused into the patient.

To avoid catheter-related infectious complications, ECP treatments should be performed by peripheral venous access. Various schedules of ECP have been reported including weekly treatments on 2–4 days, biweekly therapy on 2 consecutive days and prolongation of ECP intervals to 4 weeks in responding patients. So far, no clear association between dose intensity of ECP and response has been observed in chronic GVHD patients [24, 31]. At the Medical University of Vienna, most patients with chronic GVHD receive ECP on 2 consecutive days every 2 weeks until partial response followed by ECP every 4 weeks [24, 29].

Cutaneous Responses in Adult Patients

In 1994, Owsianowski et al. [32] reported the first patient given ECP for steroid-refractory chronic extensive GVHD with severe sclerodermatous manifestations including joint contractures and liver involvement resulting in a partial resolution of cutaneous manifestations and CR of hepatic involvement. Of note, complete healing of cutaneous ulcerations occurred 24–30 weeks after start of ECP and joint mobility improved dramatically.

During the last years, around 430 adult patients with steroid-refractory chronic cutaneous GVHD given ECP therapy have been reported and all larger studies are summarized in table 1 [24, 29, 31–41]. Median reported overall response rate in cutaneous chronic GVHD is 70% with a range of 31–100% demonstrating the favorable response of skin involvement to ECP treatment. A substantial number of patients achieved CR of cutaneous manifestations mainly when ECP had been administered over prolonged periods of time [24, 29, 31, 33, 34]. Besides improvements in skin scores and cutaneous texture, healing of skin ulcerations during ECP treatment have been reported [31, 32, 35].

Table 1. ECP in chronic cutaneous GVHD – results in adult patients

First author	Patients	Response			Comments
		CR	PR	ORR, %	
Owsianowski [32]	1	0	1	100	healing of ulcerations, improved mobility
Greinix [29]	15	12	3	100	median of 18 (7–47) cycles of ECP within 4–31 months, 93% alive a median of 15 months after discontinuation of ECP
Smith [35]	10	2	2	40	healing of ulcers
Miller [35]	7	5[1]	71		
Sniecinski [35]	15	12[1]	80		
Child [36]	10	10[1]		100	median 48% (16.5–95%) reduction in skin score, steroid sparing
Seaton [37]	21	1	9	48	after 6 months skin score 50% lower in sclerodermoid and lichenoid
Apisarnthanarax [33]	32	8	11	59	median of 36 (12–98) ECP sessions over a median of 5 (1–28) months, no defined schedule, median of 6 ECP sessions per month, 59% alive
Foss [31]	25	0	16	64	median duration 9 (3–24) months, 6 patients had healing of ulcerations, 6 patients had softening of sclerodermatous changes, 60% alive
Rubegni [38]	27	14	8	81	
Couriel [39]	58	33[1]	0	57	2–4 ECP per week, 53% alive after 1 year
Greinix [24]	44	30	11	93	2 days every 2 weeks, then every 4 weeks; 89% alive
Flowers [40]	48	18[1]	0	40	randomized study, 40% ORR vs. 10% ($p < 0.0001$) in non-ECP arm at 12 weeks
Dignan [34]	62	7	50	92	2 days every 2 weeks, median of 15 (1.5–32) ECP cycles, steroid sparing, 3-year OS 69%
Greinix [41]	29	9[1]	0	31	steroid sparing, progressive improvement

CR = Complete resolution; PR = partial resolution; ORR = overall response rate; OS = overall survival.
[1] No distinction between CR and PR in publication.

In the first multicenter, prospective, randomized phase II study of ECP in steroid-refractory/dependent/intolerant chronic cutaneous GVHD, 95 patients were randomized to either standard immunosuppressive treatment with corticosteroids, calcineurin inhibitors and/or mycophenolate mofetil or standard immunosuppressive therapy combined with ECP [40]. Ninety-four percent of patients in both study arms had extensive chronic GVHD. Whereas median percent improvement in total skin score (TSS) per se was not significantly different between the study arms after 12 weeks (14.5% for the ECP arm and 8.5% for the control arm), a significant steroid-sparing effect of ECP defined as at least 50% reduction of corticosteroid dose together with an at least 25% reduction in the TSS were observed in the ECP arm (8.3% in the ECP arm at week 12 and 0% in the control arm, $p = 0.04$). Furthermore, 21% of patients in the ECP arm compared to 6% in the control arm had at least a 50% reduction of the corticosteroid dose and a final corticosteroid dose below 10 mg/day at the end of therapy. In addition, by week 12 significantly more patients in the ECP arm achieved a complete and partial resolution of cutaneous manifestations of chronic GVHD as assessed by the clinical investigator compared to the control arm (40 vs. 10%, $p < 0.001$). No significant differences in adverse events and serious adverse events between the study arms were observed.

In a prospective open-label crossover ECP study in 29 eligible patients randomized initially to the standard of care non-ECP (control) arm of the above mentioned randomized study, complete and partial skin responses at week 24 were observed in 9 patients (31%) [41]. The median percent of decrease in TSS from baseline to weeks 12 and 24 was –7.9 and –25.8, respectively. Thus, progressive improvement in skin involvement was observed during longer duration of ECP. By analyzing the trajectory of chronic cutaneous GVHD manifestations in patients initially treated prospectively with standard therapy and then crossed over to receive ECP treatment, significantly higher responses in skin (26 vs. 8%, $p = 0.04$) were observed at 12 weeks after crossing over to ECP treatment compared to the same previous period under standard therapy. Despite longer duration of chronic GVHD, responses observed in ECP were comparable to previously reported ones [31].

ECP in Sclerotic-Type Chronic GVHD

Sclerotic-type chronic GVHD of the skin encompasses several cutaneous presentations characterized by inflammation and progressive fibrosis of the dermis and subcutaneous tissues resembling morphea, systemic sclerosis, or eosinophilic fasciitis. Sclerotic-type cutaneous manifestations occur late in the course of chronic GVHD and may lead to significant functional disability and morbidity due to skin ulceration and poor wound healing. Sclerotic-type chronic GVHD responds poorly to topical interventions and often is recalcitrant to systemic immunosuppressive treatment [42].

Promising results on the use of ECP in sclerotic-type chronic GVHD have been reported as shown in table 2 [29, 32, 33, 39, 43, 44]. Complete and partial resolution

Table 2. ECP in chronic cutaneous GVHD – results in sclerotic-type manifestations

First author	Patients	Response			Schedule of ECP	Comments
		CR	PR	ORR, %		
Owsianowski [32]	1	0	1	100	2 days every 4 weeks	healing of ulcers after 24–30 weeks
Dall'Amico [43]	3	0	2	67	2 days every 3 weeks for 6 months, then every 4 weeks	histologic confirmation of improvement
Greinix [29]	12	9	3	100	2 days every 2 weeks, after PR every 4 weeks	median duration of ECP 12 (4–31) months, same ORR as in lichenoid
Apisarnthanarax [33]	17	2	7	53	not defined	same ORR as in lichenoid
Bisaccia [44]	12	1	4	42	3 days every week	median time to response 6 (2–15) months, 5-year OS 77%
Couriel [39]	21		14[1]	67	2–4 every week	higher ORR than in lichenoid

[1] No distinction between CR and PR in publication

of cutaneous manifestations has been observed in 42–100% of patients with the best results obtained in studies investigating ECP over prolonged periods of time. Thus, not treatment intensity defined by number of ECP treatments per week but treatment duration seem to be of importance especially in patients with longstanding skin involvement and sclerotic-type features. Whereas some investigators reported similar response rates in sclerotic-type compared to lichenoid chronic GVHD [29, 33], Couriel et al. [39] observed higher response rates in sclerotic-type cutaneous chronic GVHD manifestations.

Cutaneous Responses in Pediatric Patients

As shown in table 3, around 140 pediatric patients given ECP for treatment of chronic steroid-refractory cutaneous GVHD have been reported in the literature. Complete and partial resolution of skin involvement was achieved in a median of 78% of pediatric patients with a range from 43 to 100% [30, 43, 45–53].

Table 3. ECP in chronic cutaneous GVHD – results in pediatric patients

First author	Patients	Response		Side effects	Comments
		CR + PR	ORR, %		
Rossetti [51]	7	3	43		2 ECP every 3 weeks, duration of ECP 3–30 months
Dall'Amico [43]	3	2	67		improvement of skin score >70%
Salvaneschi [46]	12	10	83	decrease in Hb >2 g/dl in 93% of patients	5 CR, maximal improvement after a median of 6 (3–26) months, 79% alive
Perseghin [52]	8	7	87.5		duration of ECP 2–28 months
Messina [30]	36	20	55.5	1 pulmonary hemorrhage in thrombocytopenic patient	2 days per week, 77% alive
Halle [53]	8	7	87.5		duration of ECP 2–20 months
Kanold [47]	12	9	75	9% adverse events 6.5% RBC transfusions	67% alive after median 52 (6–108) months after end of ECP
Perseghin [48]	25	22	88		response after a median of 19 (8–38) treatments, median treatment duration 177 (28–454) days, 19 (76%) alive a median of 24 (0.6–81) months after end of ECP
Gonzales-Vicent [49]	3	3	100		all patients alive
Perotti [50]	23	22	95.6		steroid sparing, 83% survival at 5 years

Messina et al. [30] reported the so far largest pediatric patient population treated with ECP for steroid-refractory chronic GVHD. Besides high response rates in cutaneous (56%) and hepatic (60%) manifestations of chronic GVHD, ECP responders had a significantly longer overall survival at 5 years (96 vs. 58%, $p = 0.04$) and an improved quality of life with Karnofsky performance scores rising from 50 to 60% prior to ECP to ≥90% after completion of ECP. Furthermore, a clinical response was more frequently (64%) observed in pediatric patients who started ECP earlier (before the median time of 8.9 months) after diagnosis of chronic GVHD. Age, gender, diagnosis, type of donor and source of stem cells did not influence the outcome in univariate analysis.

Besides excellent response rates comparable to adult patients, ECP was in general tolerated well by pediatric patients. Side effects observed in children during ECP were generally mild consisting mainly of decreases in hemoglobin levels, the need for central venous catheters and the psychological impact of repeated apheresis procedures [30, 46, 47]. Of note, children weighing less than 25 kg were not more susceptible to side effects [47].

Influence of Extracorporeal Photopheresis on Patient Outcome after Hematopoietic Stem Cell Transplantation

Besides improvement of cutaneous manifestations, a steroid-sparing effect was observed in ECP-responding patients with chronic GVHD [24, 29, 31, 36, 39, 40, 41, 46]. Of note, Foss et al. [31] reported a reduction in dosage or discontinuation of corticosteroids or other immunosuppressive medications in 80% of patients during ECP.

In a prospective, randomized study on steroid-refractory/dependent/intolerant cutaneous chronic GVHD, a targeted symptom assessment evaluating the symptom burden and suffering of patients revealed a median improvement of 19% in the ECP arm compared with 2.5% improvement in the control arm [40], thus confirming the beneficial effects of ECP on patients' quality of life that has also been observed by others [29, 30].

Messina et al. [30] observed a significantly longer survival in ECP responders of 96% compared with 58% in nonresponders at 5 years. Couriel et al. [39] reported a significantly reduced nonrelapse mortality in ECP responders compared with nonresponders.

Conclusions

Results of retrospective and prospective studies demonstrate high response rates of steroid-refractory cutaneous chronic GVHD to ECP including sclerotic-type features. Due to ECP's steroid-sparing capacity and excellent safety profile, its use for treatment of chronic GVHD has been recommended by independent study groups such as the German/Austrian/Swiss consensus conference on clinical practice in chronic GVHD [3]. The latter recommended ECP for second-line therapy of chronic GVHD and suggested ECP as reasonable first choice in certain clinical scenarios. This is in agreement with Kanold et al. [47] who recommended ECP as second-line therapy of chronic GVHD in pediatric patients in clinical practice guidelines.

References

1 Kuzmina Z, Eder S, Böhm A, Pernicka E, Vormittag L, Kalhs P, Petkov V, Stary G, Nepp J, Knobler R, Just U, Krenn K, Worel N, Greinix HT: Significantly worse survival of patients with NIH-defined chronic graft-versus-host disease and thrombocytopenia or progressive onset type: results of a prospective study. Leukemia, DOI:10.1038/leu.2011.257.

2 Filipovich AH, Weisdorf D, Pavletic S, Socie G, et al: National Institutes of Health consensus development project on criteria for clinical trials in chronic graft-versus-host disease. I. Diagnosis and staging working group report. Biol Blood Marrow Transplant 2005;11:945–955.

3 Wolff D, Schleuning M, von Harsdorf S, Bacher U, Gerbitz A, Stadler M, Ayuk F, Kiani A, Schwerdtfeger R, Vogelsang GB, Kobbe G, Gramatzki M, Lawitschka A, Mohty M, Pavletic SZ, Greinix H, Holler E: Consensus conference on clinical practice in chronic GVHD: second-line treatment of chronic graft-versus-host disease. Biol Blood Marrow Transplant 2011;17:1–17.

4 Tomblyn M, Chiller T, Einsele H, Gress R, Sepkowitz K, Storek J: Guidelines for preventing infectious complications among hematopoietic cell transplant recipients: a global perspective. Biol Blood Marrow Transplant 2009;15:1143–1238.

5 Hönigsmann H, Szeimies R, Knobler R: Photochemotherapy and Photodynamic Therapy; in Wolff K, Goldsmith LA, Katz SI, Gilchrest BA, Paller AS, Leffell DJ (eds): Fitzpatrick's Dermatology in General Medicine, ed 7. New York, McGraw-Hill, 2008, pp 2249–2262.

6 Mutzhas MF, Hölzle E, Hofmann C, Plewig G: A new apparatus with high radiation energy between 320–460 nm: physical description and dermatological applications. J Invest Dermatol 1981;76:42–47.

7 Fitzpatrick TB: Ultraviolet-induced pigmentary changes: benefits and hazards; in Hönigsmann H, Stingl G (eds): Therapeutic Photomedicine. Curr Probl Derm. Basel, Karger, 1986, vol 15, pp 25–38.

8 Krutmann J, Czech W, Diepgen T, Niedner R, Kapp A, Schöpf E: High-dose UVA1 therapy in the treatment of patients with atopic dermatitis. J Am Acad Dermatol 1992;26:225–230.

9 Kroft EBM, Berkhof NJG, van de Kerkhof PCM, Gerritsen RMJP, de Jong EMGJ: Ultraviolet A phototherapy for sclerotic skin diseases: a systematic review. J Am Acad Dermatol 2008;59:1017–1030.

10 Vasquez R, Jacobe H: Phototherapy for sclerosing skin conditions. Exp Rev Dermatol 2011;6:595–612.

11 Marks C, Stadler M, Häusermann P, Wolff D, Buchholz S, Stary G, Lee S, Lawitschka A, Bertz H: German-Austrian-Swiss consensus conference on clinical practice in chronic graft-versus-host disease (GVHD): guidance for supportive therapy of chronic cutaneous and musculoskeletal GVHD. Br J Dermatol 2011;165:18–29.

12 Grundmann-Kollmann M, Behrens S, Gruss C, Gottlöber P, Peter RU, Kerscher M: Chronic sclerodermic graft-versus-host disease refractory to immunosuppressive treatment responds to UVA_1 phototherapy. J Am Acad Dermatol 2000;42:134–136.

13 Ständer H, Schiller M, Schwarz T: UVA1 therapy for sclerodermic graft-versus-host disease of the skin. J Am Acad Dermatol 2002;46:799–800.

14 Calzavara Pinton P, Porta F, Izzi T, Venturini M, Capezzera R, Zane C, Notarangelo LD: Prospects for ultraviolet A1 phototherapy as a treatment for chronic cutaneous graft-versus-host disease. Haematologica 2003;88:1169–1175.

15 Ziemer M, Thiele JJ, Gruhn B, Elsner P: Chronic cutaneous graft-versus-host disease in two children responds to UVA1 therapy: improvement of skin lesions, joint mobility, and quality of life. J Am Acad Dermatol 2004;51:318–319.

16 Wetzig T, Sticherling M, Simon JC, Hegenbart U, Niederwieser D, Al-Ali HK: Medium dose long-wavelength ultraviolet A (UVA1) phototherapy for the treatment of acute and chronic graft-versus-host disease of the skin. Bone Marrow Transplant 2005; 35:515–519.

17 Ghoreschi K, Thomas P, Penovici M, Ullmann J, Sander CA, Ledderose G, Plewig G, Kolb HJ, Röcken M: PUVA-bath photochemotherapy and isotretinoin in sclerodermatous graft-versus-host disease. Eur J Dermatol 2008;18:667–670.

18 Grundmann SA, Beissert S: Regulation of cellular immunity by photo(chemo)therapy. Front Biosci 2009;14:4326–4336.

19 Morita A, Werfel T, Stege H, Ahrens C, Karmann K, Grewe M, Grether-Beck S, Ruzicka T, Kapp A, Klotz LO, Sies H, Krutmann J: Evidence that singlet oxygen-induced human T helper cell apoptosis is the basic mechanism of ultraviolet-A radiation phototherapy. J Exp Med 1997;186:1763–1768.

20 Damian DL, Matthews YJ, Phan TA, Halliday GM: An action spectrum for ultraviolet radiation-induced immunosuppression in humans. Br J Dermatol 2011;164:657–659.

21 Tewari A, Sarkany RP, Young AR: UVA1 induces cyclobutane pyrimidine dimers but not 6–4 photoproducts in human skin in vivo. J Invest Dermatol, DOI: 10.1038/jid.2011.283.

22 Sator PG, Radakovic S, Schulmeister K, Hönigsmann H, Tanew A: Medium-dose is more effective than low-dose ultraviolet A1 phototherapy for localized scleroderma as shown by 20-MHz ultrasound assessment. J Am Acad Dermatol 2009;60:786–791.
23 Knobler R, Barr ML, Couriel DR, Ferrara JLM, French LE, Jaksch P, Reinisch W, Rook AH, Schwarz T, Greinix H: Extracorporeal photopheresis: past, present and future. J Am Acad Dermatol 2009;61: 652–665.
24 Greinix HT, Socie G, Bacigalupo A, Holler E, Edinger MG, Apperley JF, Schwarz T, Ullrich SE, Albert ML, Knobler RM, Peritt D, Ferrara JLM: Assessing the potential role of photopheresis in hematopoietic stem cell transplant. Bone Marrow Transplant 2006;38:265–273.
25 Gatza E, Rogers CE, Clouthier SG, Lowler KP, Tawara I, Liu C, Reddy P, Ferrara JLM: Extracorporeal photopheresis reverses experimental graft-versus-host disease through regulatory T cells. Blood 2008;112:1515–1521.
26 Di Biaso I, Di Maio L, Bugarin C, Gaipa G, Dander E, Balduzzi A, Parma M, D'Amico G, Perseghin P, Biondi A, Biagi E: Regulatory T cells and extracorporeal photochemotherapy: correlation with clinical response and decreased frequency of proinflammatory cells. Transplant 2009;87:1422–1425.
27 Holtick U, Marshall SR, Wang XN, Hilkens CM, Dickinson AM: Impact of psoralen/UVA-treatment on survival, activation and immunostimulatory capacity of monocyte-derived dendritic cells. Transplant 2008;85:757–766.
28 Suchin KR, Cassin M, Washko R, Nahass G, Berkson M, Stouch B, Vowels BR, Rook AH: Extracorporeal photochemotherapy does not suppress T- or B-cell responses to novel or recall antigens. J Am Acad Dermatol 1999;41:980–986.
29 Greinix HT, Volc-Platzer B, Rabitsch W, Gmeinhart B, Guevara-Pineda C, Kalhs P, Krutmann J, Hönigsmann H, Ciovica M, Knobler RM: Successful use of extracorporeal photochemotherapy in the treatment of severe acute and chronic graft-versus-host disease. Blood 1998;92:3098–3104.
30 Messina C, Locatelli F, Lanino E, Uderzo C, et al: Extracorporeal photochemotherapy for paediatric patients with graft-versus-host disease after haematopoietic stem cell transplantation. Br J Haematol 203;122:118–127.
31 Foss FM, DiVenuti GM, Chin K, Sprague K, Grodman H, Klein A, Chan G, Stiffler K, Miller KB: Prospective study of extracorporeal photopheresis in steroid-refractory or steroid-resistant extensive chronic graft-versus-host disease: analysis of response and survival incorporating prognostic factors. Bone Marrow Transplant 2005;35:1187–1193.
32 Owsianowski M, Gollnick H, Siegert W, Schwerdtfeger R, Orfanos CE: Successful treatment of chronic graft-versus-host disease with extracorporeal photopheresis. Bone Marrow Transplant 1994;14:845–848.
33 Apisarnthanarax N, Donato M, Korbling M, Couriel D, Gajewski J, Giralt S, Khouri I, Hosing C, Champlin R, Duvic M, Anderlini P: Extracorporeal photopheresis therapy in the management of steroid-refractory or steroid-dependent cutaneous chronic graft-versus-host disease after allogeneic stem cell transplantation: feasibility and results. Bone Marrow Transplant 2003;31:459–465.
34 Dignan FL, Greenblatt D, Cox M, Cavenagh J, Oakervee H, Apperley JF, Fielding AK, Pagliuca A, Mufti G, Raj K, Marks DI, Amrolia P, Peniket A, Medd P, Potter MN, Shaw BE, Scarisbrick JJ: Efficacy of bimonthly extracorporeal photopheresis in refractory chronic mucocutaneous GVHD. Bone Marrow Transplant, DOI:10.1038/bmt.2011.186.
35 Dall'Amico R, Messina C: Extracorporeal photochemotherapy for the treatment of graft-versus-host disease. Ther Apheresis 2002;6:296–304.
36 Child FJ, Ratnavel R, Watkins P, Samson D, Apperley J, Ball J, Taylor P, Russell-Jones R: Extracorporeal photopheresis (ECP) in the treatment of chronic graft-versus-host disease (GVHD). Bone Marrow Transplant 1999;23:881–887.
37 Seaton ED, Szydlo RM, Kanfer E, Apperley JF, Russell-Jones R: Influence of extracorporeal photopheresis on clinical and laboratory parameters in chronic graft-versus-host disease and analysis of predictors of response. Blood 2003;102:1217–1223.
38 Rubegni P, Cuccia A, Sbano P, Cevenini G, Calcagni MR, D'Ascenzo G, De Aloe G, Guidi S, Guglielmetti P, Marotta G, Lauria F, Bosi A, Fimiani M: Role of extracorporeal photochemotherapy in patients with refractory chronic graft-versus-host disease. Br J Haematol 2005;130:271–275.
39 Couriel DR, Hosing C, Saliba R, Shpall EJ, Anderlini P, Rhodes B, Smith V, Khouri I, Giralt S, De Lima M, Hsu Y, Ghosh S, Neumann J, Andersson B, Qazibash M, Hymes S, Kim S, Champlin R, Donato M: Extracorporeal photochemotherapy for the treatment of steroid-resistant chronic GVHD. Blood 2006;107:3074–3080.
40 Flowers ME, Apperley JF, van Besien K, Elmaagacli A, Grigg A, Reddy V, Bacigalupo A, Kolb HJ, Bouzas L, Michallet M, Prince HM, Knobler R, Parenti D, Gallo J, Greinix HT: A multicenter prospective phase 2 randomized study of extracorporeal photopheresis for treatment of chronic graft-versus-host disease. Blood 2008;112:2667–2674.

41 Greinix HT, van Besien K, Elmaagacli AH, Hillen U, Grigg A, Knobler R, Parenti D, Reddy V, Theunissen K, Michallet M, Flowers MED: Progressive improvement in cutaneous and extracutaneous chronic graft-versus-host disease after a 24-week course of extracorporeal photopheresis – results of a crossover randomized study. Biol Blood Marrow Transplant 2011;17:1775–1782.
42 Couriel D, Carpenter PA, Cutler C, Bolanos-Meade J, et al: Ancillary therapy and supportive care of chronic graft-versus-host disease: National Institutes of Health consensus development project on criteria for clinical trials in chronic graft-versus-host disease. V. Ancillary therapy and supportive care working group report. Biol Blood Marrow Transplant 2006;12:375–396.
43 Dall'Amico R, Rossetti F, Zulian F, Montini G, Murer L, Andreetta B, Messina C, Baraldi E, Montesco MC, Dini G, Locatelli F, Argiolu F, Zacchello G: Photopheresis in paediatric patients with drug-resistant chronic graft-versus-host disease. Br J Haematol 1997;97:848–854.
44 Bisaccia E, Palangio M, Ganzalez J, Adler KR, Scarborough R, Goldberg SL, Rowley SD: Treatment of extensive chronic graft-versus-host disease with extracorporeal photochemotherapy. J Clin Apher 2006;21:181–187.
45 Kanold J, Paillard C, Halle P, D'Incan M, Bordigoni P, Demeocq F: Extracorporeal photochemotherapy for graft versus host disease in pediatric patients. Transfus Apheres Sci 2003;28:71–80.
46 Salvaneschi L, Perotti C, Zecca M, Bernuzzi S, Viarengo G, Georgiani G, Del Fante C, Bergamaschi P, Maccario R, Pession A, Locatelli F: Extracorporeal photochemotherapy for treatment of acute and chronic GVHD in childhood. Transfusion 2001;41: 1299–1305.
47 Kanold J, Merlin E, Halle P, Paillard C, Marabelle A, Rapatel C, Evrard B, Berger C, Stephan JL, Galambrun C, Piguet C, D'Incan M, Bordigoni P, Demeocq F: Photopheresis in pediatric graft-versus-host disease after allogeneic marrow transplantation: clinical practice guidelines based on field experience and review of the literature. Transfusion 2007;47:2276–2289.
48 Perseghin P, Galimberti S, Balduzzi A, Bonanomi S, Baldini V, Rovelli A, Dassi M, Rambaldi A, Castagna L, Corti P, Pogliani EM, Uderzo C: Extracorporeal photochemotherapy for the treatment of chronic graft-versus-host disease: trend for a possible cell dose-related effect? Therap Aph Dial 2007;11:85–93.
49 Gonzalez-Vicent M, Ramirez M, Perez A, Lassaletta A, Sevilla J, Diaz MA: Extracorporeal photochemotherapy for steroid-refractory graft-versus-host disease in low-weight pediatric patients. Haematol 2008;93:1278–1280.
50 Perotti C, Del Fante C, Tinelli C, Viarengo G, Scudeller L, Zecca M, Locatelli F, Salvaneschi L: Extracorporeal photochemotherapy in graft-versus-host disease: a longitudinal study on factors influencing the response and survival in pediatric patients. Transfusion 2010;50:1359–1369.
51 Rossetti F, Zulian F, Dall'Amico R, et al: Extracorporeal photochemotherapy as single therapy for extensive, cutaneous, chronic graft-versus-host disease. Transplantation 1995;59:149–151.
52 Perseghin P, Dassi M, Balduzzi A, Rovelli A, Bonanomi S, Uderzo C: Mononuclear cell collection in patients undergoing extracorporeal photochemotherapy for acute and chronic graft vs host disease: comparison between Cobe pectra version 4.7 and 6.0. J Clin Apher 2002;17:65–71.
53 Halle P, Paillard C, D'Incan M, et al: Successful extracorporeal photochemotherapy for chronic graft-versus-host disease in pediatric patients. J Hematother Stem Cell Res 2002;11:501–512.

Prof. Dr. Hildegard T. Greinix
Klinik für Innere Medizin I
Währinger Gürtel 18–20
AT–1090 Vienna (Austria)
Tel. +43 1 40400 4457, E-Mail hildegard.greinix@meduniwien.ac.at

Häusermann P, Steiger J, Passweg J (eds): Transplantation Dermatology.
Curr Probl Dermatol. Basel, Karger, 2012, vol 43, pp 132–149

Late Effects after Hematopoietic Stem Cell Transplantation – Critical Issues

André Tichelli[a] · Alicia Rovó[a] · Gérard Socié[b]

[a]Hematology, University Hospital, Basel, Switzerland; [b]Service d'Hématologie-Greffe, Hôpital Saint-Louis, Paris, France

Abstract

Today, long-term prognosis after hematopoietic stem cell transplantation (HSCT) has greatly improved. Nevertheless, there are still a number of malignant and nonmalignant late effects that can cause substantial morbidity, with considerable impact on the health status and quality of life in the long-term survivors. Transplant-preparative regimen and graft-versus-host disease are considered the main risk factors after allogeneic HSCT. The continuous changes in the transplantation practice and in the type of patients selected are responsible that the pattern of the late effects after HSCT is changing over time. Relevant recent changes concern the avoidance of total body irradiation conditioning whenever possible, the higher age of the patients transplanted, the increasing use of unrelated donors as well as the introduction of reduced intensity conditioning. The detection of an increasing number of late effects should not be considered as a drawback of HSCT. The experience gathered during the past decades has become the main source of information on which the current management of the long-term survivors is based. A broad expertise is mandatory to manage long-term survivors. Aftercare of long-term survivors includes a standardized screening, counseling of the patients as well as prevention and treatment of late effects. Counseling should include self-examination for early cancer detection, and advice for healthy lifestyle behavior. Beyond immediate survival, allogeneic HSCT is a lifelong commitment between long-term survivors and the transplant team, involving the recipient's family and the general health care providers. Proper information on 'life after HSCT' should also be provided to the whole community, which plays a key role in the social reinsertion of the long-term survivors.

With the growing number of transplants performed yearly and improvement in outcome, long-term survivorship becomes of increasing interest to patients treated with hematopoietic stem cell transplantation (HSCT). The principal aim of the HSCT is to cure the primary disease. However, long-term survivors additionally wish to regain complete health status, with satisfying physical and psychological functioning, restore social integration in the family and at work, and achieve a subjective well-being. Despite the improvement in the results of HSCT, outcome of patients surviving

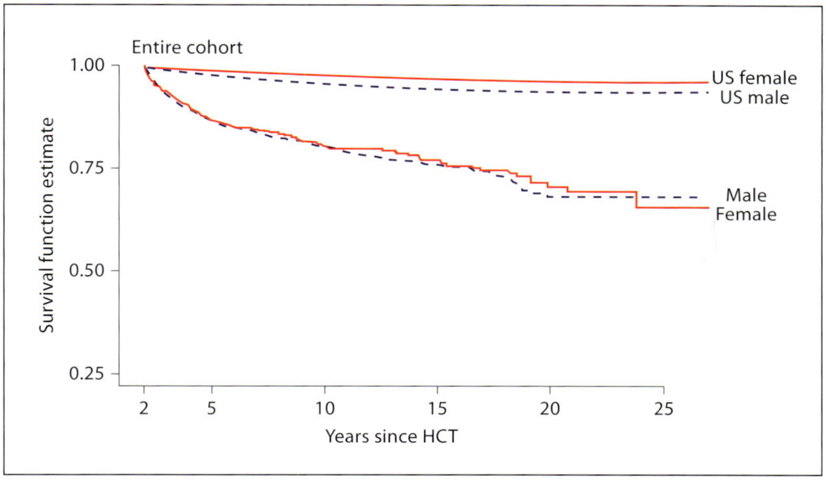

Fig. 1. All-cause mortality in a cohort of 1,479 long-term survivors after allogeneic HSCT. From Bhatia et al. [1].

at least 2 years after HSCT is still decreased when compared to a matched general population; after allogeneic HSCT, death rate is higher than expected, even more than 20 years after transplantation (fig. 1). Increased late death rates are necessarily associated with excess of morbidity [1].

Long-term survivorship and health status of the patients treated with allogeneic HSCT depends on the patient characteristics (age, gender, comorbidity before HSCT), the primary disease, its risk category and remission status before transplantation, the treatment used before transplantation, the type of conditioning regimen, the cell source, as well as the onset of graft-versus-host disease (GVHD) and the drugs used for its treatment.

A list of the most relevant late events is shown in table 1. In this chapter, we will not describe systematically all possible late effects. There are excellent reviews on it [2–4]. We will focus on general considerations of long-term survivorship and late effects after HSCT, and illustrate the arguments with typical examples of late effects. Cutaneous late effects and the particular aspects of late effects related to chronic GVHD will be outlined in different chapters of this book.

Late Effects of Stem Cell Transplantation

Late effects after HSCT are complications with relevant long-term consequences in recipients. Some of the complications can appear within the first year after transplant, while other events become apparent only years or even decades after HSCT [5]. Late events after HSCT are usually divided into malignant and nonmalignant complications. The major risk factors for late effects after allogeneic HSCT are chronic GVHD and/or its

Table 1. List of the most important late effects after HSCT, with risk factors, screening, patient counseling, prevention and treatment

Late effect	Main risk factor	Screening	Counseling	Prevention	Treatment
GVHD – infections	HLA disparity, donor source	clinical assessment, blood count, lymphocyte subsets, immunoglobulin levels, CMV monitoring	vaccination schedule, consider functional asplenia	antibiotic prophylaxis, PCP prophylaxis	always indicated if a pathogen has been identified
Thyroid dysfunction	local irradiation, TBI	TSH, fT3		fractionation of TBI if irradiation is indicated	substitution with L-thyroxin in overt hypothyroidism
Growth failure	cranial irradiation, TBI	monitor growth velocity (particular pubertal growth), growth hormone (repetitive if abnormal growth)	during childhood and adolescence regular controls are mandatory	timing of puberty induction	growth hormone treatment if indicated according to endocrinologist
Fertility and gonadal failure	TBI, older age	FSH, LH testosterone in males, seminal fluid analysis, post-HSCT in males	high likelihood of post-HSCT infertility, contraception if indicated	cryopreservation of sperms, embryo or oocyte banking	hormonal substitution if indicated
Respiratory tract complications	chronic GVHD TBI	clinical assessment, pulmonary function tests, radiographic evaluation if indicated	avoiding smoking, vaccination schedule	avoiding risk of a viral infection (influenza, RSV, etc.)	steroids, bronchiodilatators, treatment of GVHD, treatment of infections
Cardiac complications	anthracyclines	check blood pressure, cardiac rhythm, cardiac function			pace maker, surgical intervention if indicated, transplantation (?)
Vascular complications	TBI, GVHD, dyslipidemia, diabetes, chronic kidney disease, hypertension, smoking, physical inactivity	check blood pressure, weight (BMI), lipidogram, glucose tolerance	healthy heart lifestyle, regular exercise, compliance with the treatment/ prevention, cardiovascular risk factors	early treatment of cardiovascular risk factors	surgical intervention if indicated

Table 1. Continued

Late effect	Main risk factor	Screening	Counseling	Prevention	Treatment
Renal complications	calcineurin inhibitors, chronic GVHD	check blood pressure, serum creatinine and glomerular filtration rate, urine sediment, check for proteinuria	suspend nephrotoxic drugs whenever possible	adapt dosage of calcineurin inhibitors, choose alternative	dialysis, renal transplantation
Liver complications	HCV infection, iron overload	liver function testing, HCV monitoring during treatment, ferritin, liver biopsy in patients at risk	importance of compliance of treatment (HCV infection)	phlebotomy or iron chelation	consider pegylated-IFN-α and ribavirin treatment in HCV infection
Avascular necrosis	TBI, prolonged steroid therapy, GVHD	MRI if necessary		avoidance of long-term treatment with corticosteroids	treatment of pain, orthopedic measures, surgical repair
Osteoporosis	TBI, prolonged steroid treatment, calcineurin inhibitors, inactivity, gonadal failure	bone density measurement	regular physical activity	sex hormone substitution, bisphosphonates, avoidance of long-term treatment with corticosteroids	treatment of bone fractures
Cataract formation	TBI, steroids	split lamp		fractionation of TBI if irradiation indicated	surgical repair
Kerato-conjunctivitis	GVHD irradiation infection	ophthalmologic assessment, Schirmer testing	instructions regarding sicca	artificial tears	local therapy with steroids and/or cyclosporine, systemic therapy of GVHD
Oral complication	GVHD, irradiation, poor oral hygiene	clinical assessment, dental assessment	instruction regarding sicca, importance of oral hygiene, regular dental assessment, avoidance of sugar-containing drinks	teeth brushing with fluoride-containing toothpaste, remineralization solutions	treatment of GVHD

Table 1. Continued

Late effect	Main risk factor	Screening	Counseling	Prevention	Treatment
Genital tract complications	GVHD, peripheral blood stem cells	clinical assessment, cervical cytology	self-surveillance, instruction on early recognition of symptoms, on importance of genital hygiene, and on the use of vaginal dilatators	topical application of immunosuppressive agents, use of vaginal dilatator, systemic estrogen and progesterone replacement	treatment of local infections, surgical therapy if indicated
Complications of the skin and appendages	GVHD	clinical assessment	self-examination of the skin	skin inspection for cancer	topical treatment, treatment of GVHD
Central and peripheral system complications	TBI, cranial radiation therapy, intrathecal chemo-therapy, GVHD	clinical assessment, MRI, electromyography, CNS or nerve biopsy			treatment of infection, adapt dosage of calcineurin inhibitors, choose alternative in case of toxicity
Malignant hematological neoplasms	pretransplant chemotherapy and radiation therapy, TBI	blood counts and smears, chimerism analysis of normal/malignant cells			treatment of the malignant disease
Nonsquamous cell carcinoma: breast cancer, thyroid cancer, colon cancer	TBI, fludarabine (?), pretransplant radiation therapy, younger age, longer follow-up	mammography in females, ultrasonography of the thyroid gland	self-examination of breast, skin, mucosa, regular clinical assessment		early treatment of the cancer
Squamous cell carcinoma of the oral cavity	GVHD	regular clinical controls	self-examination of oral mucosa, regular clinical assessment		early treatment of the cancer
Performance, quality of life, sexuality	GVHD, late effects	inquiries about general performance, social and familial life, depression, fatigue, sexual function	counseling by specialist of the recipient, involving partner and family	consider lifestyle, rapid reinsertion in professional life, consider non pharmaceutical measures	psychological support, pharmaceutical support

FSH = Follicle-stimulating hormone; LH = luteinizing hormone.

treatment, as well as total body irradiation (TBI) used for conditioning. Nonmalignant late effects are heterogeneous in nature and intensity. The type and severity of these late effects depend on the type, duration and intensity of the treatment applied. Patients treated with TBI are at particular risk for specific organ or tissue complications such as pulmonary late effects, liver and cardiac complications, ocular problems, bone and joint complications, endocrine dysfunctions and fertility abnormality. In theory, any organ can be the target of a late effect, and frequently multiple causes are involved (table 1).

Secondary malignancies are known complications of conventional chemotherapy and radiation therapy in cancer patients. They are increasingly recognized as a serious complication among HSCT recipients. The estimated risk is reported to be 3.5% at 10 years, increasing to 12.8% at 15 years among recipients of allogeneic HSCT. However, with longer follow-up, the cumulative incidence is continuously increasing. Secondary malignancies after HSCT include late hematological malignancies and solid cancers. Three types of late hematological malignancies may be observed in long-term survivors: late relapse of the primary malignant disease, therapy-related myelodysplastic syndrome/acute myeloid leukemia after autologous HSCT, and donor type leukemia after allogeneic HSCT.

Chronic GVHG is the main cause of transplant-related mortality and contributes directly or indirectly to many of the malignant and nonmalignant late effects. In a particular patient, GVHD may involve one or several organs, and almost all organ systems may be affected. In some patients, the manifestations of the GVHD have little impact on the daily activity and do not require any treatment. In other cases, GVHD greatly affects the general health status and the quality of life after HSCT. The profound immune deficiency related with chronic GVHD is responsible for most deaths attributable to infection [6].

Late effects, although often not life threatening, significantly impair the quality of life in long-term survivors. Even though quality of life is generally perceived as satisfactory to good in a majority of long-term survivors after HSCT, fatigue and sleeping disorders have been reported in up to 65% patients and may persist over years after transplantation [7, 8]. Problems with sexuality have been reported in approximately 25% of patients. Quality of life does not necessarily correlate with the patient's health status. Some patients with more advanced disease report better quality of life after transplantation than patients with early effects. This can be explained because quality of life is subjective and reflects the patient view, while health status corresponds to an objective assessment of the situation. Coping strategies of some patients with late effects may lead to lower self-perception of illness and therefore improve quality of life.

Changes of the Pattern of Late Effects over Time

The pattern of late effects after HSCT may change over time. The main reasons are changes in practice regarding the conditioning regimen and transplant procedure.

While TBI was universally used for more than two decades, today nonradiation protocols have become established. Therefore, cataract, which was an almost obligatory late complication after HSCT [9, 10] has been decreasing in frequency over the last decade. In a group of 620 patients transplanted between 1997 and 2007, only 8 patients presented with steroid-induced cataract [11]. However, although TBI may no longer form part of standard condition regimens, the knowledge of its late consequences is still mandatory, because patients who received TBI remain at risk of radiation-related complications. Indeed, some radiation-related late effects, such a secondary breast cancers [12] or therapy-related cardiovascular diseases (CVD) may appear more than 10 or even 20 years after HSCT [13], and will therefore continue increasing during the next decades. On the other hand, the increasing age of the patients receiving allogeneic HSCT as well as more frequent use of an alternative donor has led to an increased incidence of late effects related to chronic GVHD. Accordingly, the incidence of avascular necrosis of the bone and bronchiolitis obliterans syndrome may increase in near future. Finally, the increasing use of reduced intensity conditioning (RIC) will certainly change type and prevalence of late events. This will be discussed later in this review.

Late Effects as a Direct Consequence of the Transplant Procedure

Many of the late effects are the direct consequence of the transplant procedure and its conditioning regimen. Examples of a direct relationship between HSCT and late effects in long-term survivors are cataract formation, endocrine dysfunctions, secondary malignancies and infertility (see fig. 3a). They are all closely related to TBI conditioning. For instance, radiation therapy plays a key role in inducing late thyroid dysfunction [14]. The severity of the endocrine dysfunction depends on the dose and type of irradiation. The risk is 5–6 times higher when single dose instead of fractionated TBI is applied. After conditioning with busulfan and cyclophosphamide, the incidence and severity of thyroid dysfunction is lower. Recipients conditioned with TBI are also at significantly higher risk of secondary thyroid cancer than the general population, especially when HSCT is performed during childhood and adolescence [15].

Gonadal damage and loss of fertility after HSCT is dependent on age of the patient at transplantation and the conditioning regimen received for HSCT. Ovaries are more vulnerable than testes. In female patients, infertility and hypergonadotropic hypogonadism is almost the rule after TBI, with elevated serum follicle-stimulating hormone and luteinizing hormone [16–18]. Damage by radiation therapy is dependent on the dose and radiation schedule. Fractionation of the dose has a sparing effect on the ovaries. Busulfan, despite being one of the most gonadotoxic chemotherapeutic agents, induces less gonadal dysfunction and infertility than TBI. Conditioning with cyclophosphamide alone has the highest probability of recovery of gonadal function and

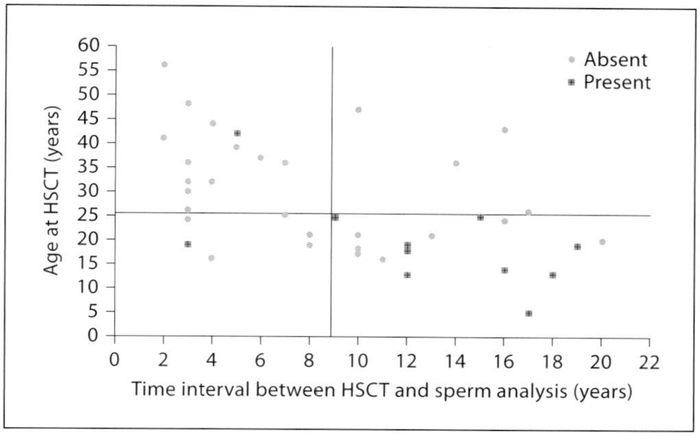

Fig. 2. Presence or absence of spermatozoa after HSCT (HSCT) as a function of age at transplantation and time interval from HSCT. From Rovó et al. [20].

fertility. The age at transplantation is of major significance: the younger the age, the better the chances for gonadal recovery. In a recent retrospective study from seven European centers, gonadal function of 138 female and 206 male patients treated with allogeneic HSCT as a child were evaluated. Two thirds of the long-term survivors showed signs of impaired fertility. Significant risk factors were TBI for males and the use of busulfan for females [19].

The absence of spermatozoa is a common long-term sequel in male recipients receiving chemotherapy and irradiation prior to HSCT and as pretransplantation conditioning. With TBI conditioning of at least 7.5 Gy, azoospermia is the rule. Azoospermia is less frequent in patients conditioned with busulfan and cyclophosphamide (50%), and uncommon when treated with cyclophosphamide alone (10%). However, even when conditioned with standard-dose TBI, male recipients surviving more than10 years, younger than 25 years at HSCT, and apparently without chronic GVHD have a reasonable likelihood of spermatogenesis [20] (fig. 2).

Infertility is a distinct late effect. Long-term survivors consider reproductive health issues, and the possibility to have a child of great importance. Therefore, even though infertility does not produce direct physical symptoms, this late effect is associated with significant psychological distress, with levels of depression twice that of the normal population. Infertility may directly affect quality of life of the patients and their respective partner wishing to conceive a child [21].

Late Effects Occurring as a Secondary and Tertiary Event

Some of the late effects are indirectly related to the transplant procedure, and emerge as a secondary or even a tertiary event of a primary late complication or its treatment. Typical examples of secondary occurring late effects are osteoporosis and dental

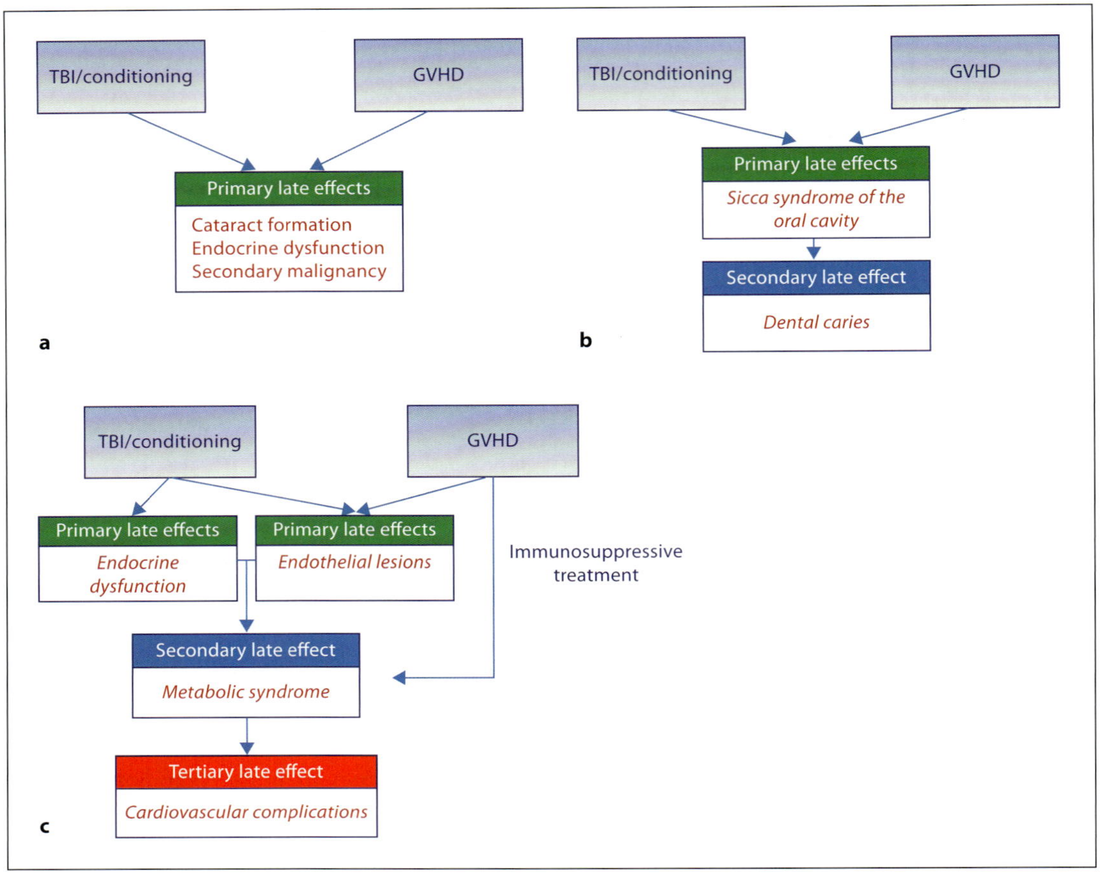

Fig. 3. **a** Primary late effects as a direct consequence of the transplant procedure. Conditioning with total body irradiation is directly responsible for cataract formation, endocrine dysfunction or secondary malignancies. **b** Secondary late effects as a consequence of a primary late effect from transplant procedure. As an example, sicca syndrome of the oral cavity is the primary late effect after TBI and/or the onset of chronic GVHD. Without any preventive intervention, this sicca syndrome will lead to severe dental caries, which are in this case the secondary late effects. **c** Tertiary late effects as a consequence of primary and secondary late effects from the transplant procedure. Vascular complications are an example of tertiary late-occurring effects after HSCT, as a consequence of a metabolic syndrome (secondary late effect), which in turn is secondary to endocrine dysfunction and endothelial damage (primary late effects).

caries (fig. 3b). Osteoporosis in long-term HSCT survivors may be multifactorial, and appears as a secondary event of post-transplant gonadal failure, of treatment with corticosteroids for chronic GVHD, and of prolonged immobility caused by the burden of morbidity and chronic health condition. Therapy-related dental caries are another example of a secondary occurring late effect. Rampant dental decay may occur in patients with abnormal decreased salivary flow due to conditioning with TBI and/or chronic GVHD. Therapy-related CVD after HSCT is even more complex, and will be discussed here in more detail as an example of a tertiary occurring late effect.

Cardiovascular complications have for a long time not been considered belonging to late effects of HSCT. CVD are common in the general population, and therefore any additional event occurring after HSCT could appear meaningless. Furthermore, CVD occurs usually very late after HSCT, and therefore a relationship between transplantation and the vascular complication is not obvious. Today, the increased risk of vascular events after allogeneic HSCT has been definitively established [5, 22]. In a retrospective study, the cumulative incidence of a CVD after HSCT was 22% at 25 years. Adjusted for age of the patients, recipients of allogeneic HSCT presented significantly more vascular events than patients treated with autologous HSCT [13]. In a recent publication on 1,491 long-term survivors, transplant recipients experienced higher cardiovascular deaths and showed increased cumulative incidence of ischemic heart disease, cardiomyopathy, heart failure, stroke and rhythm disorders, when compared to a matched control cohort [23].

A number of pre- and posttransplant factors may contribute to the accelerated atherosclerosis and lead to therapy-related CVD. In two retrospective studies, an unequivocal relationship between posttransplant cardiovascular risk factors and CVD in HSCT long-term survivors has been demonstrated [13, 24]. Hypertension, diabetes, and dyslipidemia appearing after HSCT, as well as physical inactivity and ongoing tobacco smoking were related to increased risk of late CVD. Patients presenting more than 50% of these risk factors after HSCT had a cumulative incidence of a CVD at 15 years of 17%, compared to 4% for patients with less risk factors present.

The risk factors for therapy-related CVD are in part those found in a general population. However, their incidence is higher after allogeneic HSCT when compared to patients treated with autologous HSCT, to sibling donors [25, 26] and to a general population [23]. In a large cohort of 1,089 HSCT patients, recipients who survived at least 2 years and were not taking immunosuppressants, the prevalence of diabetes and hypertension was increased. Patients treated with allogeneic HSCT have a 2.2-fold increased risk of a metabolic syndrome compared to an age- and sex-matched population. The causes of a metabolic-like syndrome appearing after allogeneic HSCT are probably multifactorial: therapy-related endocrine dysfunctions, such as hypothyroidism, gonadal dysfunction and growth hormone failure may be involved.

In addition to these well-established cardiovascular risk factors, radiation therapy may play a role. Cancer patients not treated with HSCT and receiving local radiation therapy have an increased risk of CVD, as demonstrated in patients with Hodgkin disease [27, 28], breast cancer [29, 30], and head and neck cancer [31]. In long-term survivors of HSCT, chest radiation before transplantation and the posttransplant development of multiple cardiovascular risk factors are primarily responsible for the excess of CVD. Pretransplant chest radiation exposure is associated with a 9.5-fold higher risk of CVD [32]. The influence of TBI on the development of cardiovascular risk factors is more controversial.

Therefore, therapy-related CVD can be considered as a typical example of a tertiary occurring late effect: the clinical manifestations of the vascular disease are the ultimate consequence of endocrine dysfunctions and endothelial damages initiated during the acute phase of the transplantation. These primary late effects favor the development of a metabolic-like syndrome, the secondary occurring late effect, which, if untreated will be directly involved in the development of therapy-related CVD (fig. 3c).

Does Graft-versus-Host Disease or Its Treatment Play the Major Role in Late Organ Dysfunction?

Chronic GVHD is the leading cause of nonrelapse mortality in patients surviving more than 2 years since transplantation. An extended review on chronic GVHD is published in this volume. We focus here on the respective influence of GVHD and its treatment on the development of late organ dysfunction. In some situations, the direct effect of GVHD is obvious. For instance, GVHD is strongly involved in the development of bronchiolitis obliterans syndrome, and plays an important role in the sicca syndrome of the eye, the mucosa and the skin. For some late effects, however, it is not possible to discern the influence of GVHD itself and the effect due to its treatment. Chronic kidney disease and avascular necrosis of the bone are two late effects demonstrating this inextricable relationship.

Chronic kidney disease is defined as a sustained decrease in glomerular filtration rate (GFR) below 60 ml/min/1.73 m^2. Patients treated with HSCT have a significant risk of chronic kidney disease. Severe kidney disease after HSCT, with GFR below 30 ml/min/1.73 m^2 has been reported in 3% of the patients; half of them are end-stage diseases requiring chronic dialysis. In a study on 148 patients who received allogeneic HSCT and were alive after 2 years without relapse, chronic kidney disease correlated with TBI and chronic GVHD [33]. Among 1,190 long-term adult patients who underwent HSCT and survived for at least 1 year, the estimated cumulative incidence of chronic kidney disease was 4.4% at 5 years, and 5.7% at 10 years after HSCT. The large majority of events occurred within the first 10 years [34]. Older age at transplantation, exposure to calcineurin inhibitors for GVHD prophylaxis or treatment, patients with multiple myeloma, and nephrotoxic drugs used before HSCT, during conditioning and in the early phase after transplant were the main risk factors. In another large cohort study of 1,635 patients treated with HSCT, a strong association was observed between acute and chronic GVHD and renal dysfunction [35]. However, it was not possible to distinguish the respective contribution of GVHD itself and of its treatment for the development of chronic kidney disease.

A similar condition is observed for avascular bone necrosis. The incidence after HSCT varies from 4 to over 10% in the largest series [36, 37]. The mean time from transplant to avascular bone necrosis is 18 months. Pain is usually the first sign. MRI

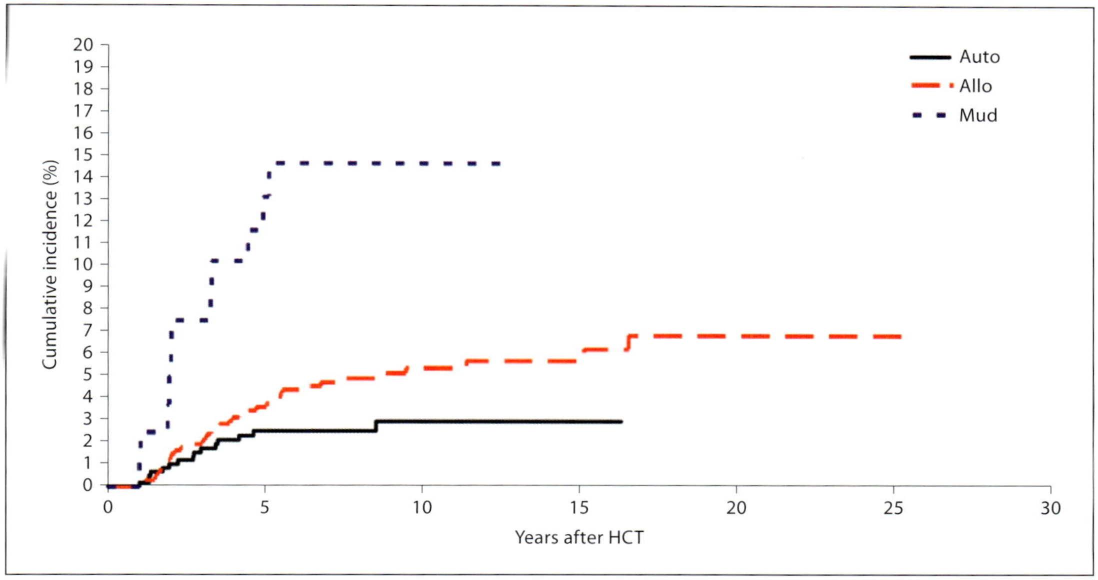

Fig. 4. Cumulative Incidence of avascular bone necrosis by type of hematopoietic cell transplant. From Campbell et al. [38].

is the investigational method of choice for early diagnosis. The hip is affected in over 80% of cases with bilateral involvement in 60% cases. Other locations include the knee, wrist and ankle. Studies evaluating risk factors for avascular bone necrosis have clearly identified total dose and duration corticosteroid therapy, and TBI, mainly with administration of single doses of 10 Gy or higher or >12 Gy in fractionated doses. In a recent series involving more than 1,300 patients at the City of Hope, the cumulative incidence of avascular bone necrosis at 10 years was 4% after autologous HSCT, 6% after allogeneic sibling donor HSCT, and 15% after unrelated donor HSCT [38]. Unrelated donor HSCT recipients were at increased risk of developing avascular necrosis compared with autologous HSCT patients (fig. 4). Among allogeneic HSCT recipients, the risk was increased in male patients, those diagnosed with chronic GVHD, or those exposed to at least three of the following drugs: cyclosporine, tacrolimus, prednisone and mycophenolate mofetil [7]. Again, because of the strong correlation between the use of systemic prednisone and the presence of chronic GVHD, it was not possible to attribute the risk of avascular necrosis to GVHD alone.

Does Reduced Intensity Conditioning Reduce the Risk of Late Effects?

It has become standard to offer RIC transplantation to patients older than 55 years, and in younger patients with comorbidity. The current available data suggest that RIC provides similar donor engraftment, increases the probability of relapse, decreases the transplant-related mortality, but does not affect overall survival [39]. So far, there have been nearly no data on late effects after conditioning with RIC. However, from the actual understanding of late effects, we can hypothesize about the type of late effects expected in long-term survivors treated with RIC. Indeed, most of the late effects of allogeneic HSCT are related either to the transplant immunobiology or to the transplant preparative regimen [40]. After RIC, we expect similar incidence of late effects due to GVHD and its treatment, but lower risks of late effects related to the preparative regimen. In addition to these hypothetical considerations, new factors of undetermined relevance in respect of late effects, such as older age, higher rates of comorbidity, or the use of new drugs used for conditioning, such as fludarabine, might generate completely new prerequisites.

Consequently, avascular bone necrosis, chronic kidney disease, or bronchiolitis obliterans syndrome, which are GVHD and GVHD treatment-related late effects should appear in similar frequency and severity than in patients treated with myeloablative conditioning. Likewise, second squamous cell cancers of the oral cavity are expected to occur in the same frequency as in patients treated with myeloablative conditioning. Indeed, squamous cell carcinomas of the oral cavity are significantly increased in patients with HSCT [41–43]. Multifocal oral cancer is found in 28% of cases, and localized recurrence is observed in 44% of cases. These cancers are strongly related to chronic GVHD of the oral cavity and male sex, but not to the transplant-preparative regimen. Furthermore, they show little variation in risk by age at HSCT and with longer follow-up time [44].

On the other hand, patients treated with RIC should be at lower risk of endocrine dysfunctions and loss of fertility, strongly related to the transplant preparative regimen [40]. Conditioning with cyclophosphamide alone for patients with severe aplastic anemia can be considered as an RIC. These patients have a higher probability of gonadal recovery. Fifty percent of adult female survivors from Seattle had return of menstruation and normal gonadotropin and estradiol levels, and half of them subsequently conceived a child. Likewise, 61% of male survivors had sperm recovery, and 26% fathered a child, compared to 6% of patient conditioned with busulfan and cyclophosphamide, and 1% of patients conditioned with TBI [17]. The risk of nonsquamous cell carcinoma is significantly increased in patients treated with myeloablative conditioning. For instance, breast and thyroid gland cancers are linked to radiation conditioning regimens received at a young age [44] (fig. 5). The cumulative incidence of nonsquamous cell cancers increases with longer follow-up since HSCT. As a result, we can assume that the frequency of nonsquamous cell carcinoma should be lower after RIC when compared to patients conditioned with TBI, provided that the patient did not have chest radiation therapy before HSCT.

The effect of RIC on health-related quality of life was prospectively compared in 115 adult patients with myeloid malignancies undergoing allogeneic HSCT and receiving either myeloablative or reduced intensity conditioning. Patients treated with

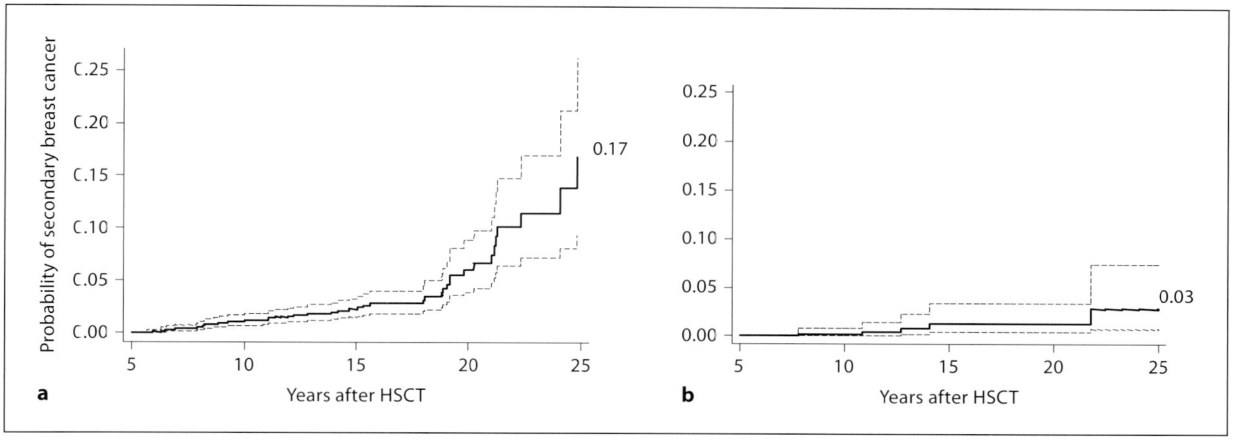

Fig. 5. Cumulative incidence of secondary breast cancer, a nonsquamous cell cancer after allogeneic HSCT, with (**a**) and without (**b**) TBI. From Friedman et al. [12].

RIC were significantly older at the time of HSCT. However, no significant difference was found for overall survival at one year, cumulative incidence of acute and chronic GVHD, nonrelapse mortality, relapse and quality of life outcomes [45].

Thus, although there are nearly no data for RIC-treated patients, we may assume that late effects will appear. But they will differ in some aspects from the late effects of patients treated with myeloablative conditioning. Some types of the late effects are predictable, while the consequence of other factors, such as patient selection, comorbidity, and new drugs used for conditioning cannot be anticipated yet. Particularly, secondary malignancies might be of importance in this elderly group of patients.

Relevance of Knowing about Late Effects after Hematopoietic Stem Cell Transplantation

Research on malignant and nonmalignant late complications after HSCT is sometimes considered as fouling one's own nest. There is criticism that efforts are undertaken in order to denigrate the acquisitions obtained over the last decades regarding HSCT and adoptive therapy. It is important to know about late effects first because, the patient, his family, as well as the health care providers have to be aware of all possible long-term complications that may occur, once the acute phase of the HSCT has ended. Secondly, the knowledge on late effects allows introducing appropriate screening and management to prevent or attenuate late effects after the HSCT.

Encouraging healthy lifestyle behaviors and counseling cancer screening practice should become integral part of the specialized long-term surveillance. In a questionnaire-based survey, 1,040 long-term survivors were less likely to report risky health behaviors such as smoking or excessive alcohol intake, and had similar or better cancer screening practices when compared with siblings. The vast majority of female survivors reported having a recent clinical breast examination or Papanicolaou smear performed. But younger survivors, those without health insurance and with lower education continued to engage in high-risk behaviors [46].

The knowledge on late effects should be used as a guidance to prevent clinical manifestations. Thus, knowledge on therapy-related CVD will focus the management on early treatment of the risk factors for CVD after HSCT, long time before the appearance of vascular complications. However, some of the cardiovascular risk factors are not modifiable: age, sex and hereditary factors. Furthermore, pretransplant factors, the conditioning regimen and the type of transplantation are usually determined by other considerations. Therefore, the main effort has to be devoted to the management of the modifiable cardiovascular risk factors. Mainly two complementary approaches can be considered: the treatment of the endocrine dysfunctions that may be responsible for the development of the cardiovascular risk factors, and the treatment of these cardiovascular risk factors themselves, which are hypertension, diabetes, obesity, and dyslipidemia. The counseling of healthy heart lifestyle is an integrated part of the preventive practices.

The approach of late gonadal dysfunction related to HSCT will be different. The impact of HSCT on fertility and symptoms due to gonadal failure has to be discussed with patients before HSCT and repeatedly throughout the treatment period after HSCT. Consideration should be given to sperm or embryo cryopreservation before HSCT. To represent an acceptable option, however, embryo cryopreservation requires prior to HSCT a delay of a minimum of 4–6 weeks to induce the ovarian hyperstimulation and perform egg collection. It also requires that the patient has a committed partner to provide sperms. An alternative possibility is the use of donor eggs. Paradoxically, despite the high probability of infertility, the potential spermatogenesis recovery also alerts about the need of counseling regarding birth control during post-transplantation follow-up.

Conclusions

The knowledge and experience on long-term survivorship and late effects have greatly improved. It has become evident that there is a substantial burden of morbidity with considerable impact on the health state and quality of life in the long-term survivors. This implies a great need for a standardized approach in screening, prevention and treatment of late effects. The large experience collected during the past decades has become the main source of information on which the current management of the long-term survivors is based. There are still obstacles to overcome. With the increasing follow-up time since HSCT, many of the long-term survivors will no longer receive direct care from their transplant center, but are regularly controlled by their hematologist or primary care physician. The broad expertise that is mandatory to correctly manage long-term survivors risks to get lost. Therefore, aftercare of long-term survivors does not only need recommendations for standardized screening, counseling of the patients as well as prevention and treatment of late effects. These recommendations have to be shared regularly with the general health providers. Furthermore, the type of late effects will continuously change according to the modifications brought in the transplant procedure. However, consequences of any change in the transplant protocol will be evaluable only years and decades later in long-term survivors. Finally, recommendations on screening and prevention exist, but they are mainly based on the experiences of the general population. So far, there have been nearly no data on the effects of these preventive measures in long-term survivors. The effort brought into new preventive measures and treatment of complications will become evident much later. For all these reasons, beyond immediate survival, allogeneic HSCT is a lifelong commitment between long-term survivors and the transplant team, involving the recipient's family and the general health care providers. Proper information on 'life after HSCT' should also be provided to the whole community, which plays a key role in the social reinsertion of the long-term survivors.

References

1 Bhatia S, Francisco L, Carter A, et al: Late mortality after allogeneic hematopoietic cell transplantation and functional status of long-term survivors: report from the Bone Marrow Transplant Survivor Study. Blood 2007;110:3784–3792.

2 Bhatia S: Long-term health impacts of hematopoietic stem cell transplantation inform recommendations for follow-up. Expert Rev Hematol 2011;4: 437–454.

3 Socie G, Salooja N, Cohen A, et al: Nonmalignant late effects after allogeneic stem cell transplantation. Blood 2003;101:3373–3385.

4 Tichelli A, Rovo A, Passweg J, et al: Late complications after hematopoietic stem cell transplantation. Expert Rev Hematol 2009;2:583–601.

5 Tichelli A, Bhatia S, Socie G: Cardiac and cardiovascular consequences after haematopoietic stem cell transplantation. Br J Haematol 2008;142:11–26.

6 Lee SJ, Vogelsang G, Flowers ME: Chronic graft-versus-host disease. Biol Blood Marrow Transplant 2003;9:215–233.

7 Carlson LE, Smith D, Russell J, Fibich C, Whittaker T: Individualized exercise program for the treatment of severe fatigue in patients after allogeneic hematopoietic stem-cell transplant: a pilot study. Bone Marrow Transplant 2006;37:945–954.

8 Hjermstad MJ, Knobel H, Brinch L, et al: A prospective study of health-related quality of life, fatigue, anxiety and depression 3–5 years after stem cell transplantation. Bone Marrow Transplant 2004;34: 257–266.

9 Belkacemi Y, Labopin M, Vernant JP, et al: Cataracts after total body irradiation and bone marrow transplantation in patients with acute leukemia in complete remission: a study of the European Group for Blood and Marrow Transplantation. Int J Radiat Oncol Biol Phys 1998;41:659–668.

10 Tichelli A, Gratwohl A, Egger T, et al: Cataract formation after bone marrow transplantation. Ann Intern Med 1993;119:1175–1180.

11 Tabbara KF, Al-Ghamdi A, Al-Mohareb F, et al: Ocular findings after allogeneic hematopoietic stem cell transplantation. Ophthalmology 2009;116: 1624–1629.

12 Friedman DL, Rovo A, Leisenring W, et al: Increased risk of breast cancer among survivors of allogeneic hematopoietic cell transplantation: a report from the FHCRC and the EBMT-Late Effect Working Party. Blood 2008;111:939–944.

13 Tichelli A, Bucher C, Rovo A, et al: Premature cardiovascular disease after allogeneic hematopoietic stem-cell transplantation. Blood 2007;110:3463–3471.

14 Cohen A, Bekassy AN, Gaiero A, et al: Endocrinological late complications after hematopoietic SCT in children. Bone Marrow Transplant 2008;41(suppl 2):S43–S48.
15 Cohen A, Rovelli A, Merlo DF, et al: Risk for secondary thyroid carcinoma after hematopoietic stem-cell transplantation: an EBMT Late Effects Working Party Study. J Clin Oncol 2007;25:2449–2454.
16 Salooja N, Szydlo RM, Socie G, et al: Pregnancy outcomes after peripheral blood or bone marrow transplantation: a retrospective survey. Lancet 2001;358: 271–276.
17 Sanders JE, Hawley J, Levy W, et al: Pregnancies following high-dose cyclophosphamide with or without high-dose busulfan or total-body irradiation and bone marrow transplantation. Blood 1996;87: 3045–3052.
18 Spinelli S, Chiodi S, Bacigalupo A, et al: Ovarian recovery after total body irradiation and allogeneic bone marrow transplantation: long-term follow up of 79 females. Bone Marrow Transplant 1994;14: 373–380.
19 Borgmann-Staudt A, Rendtorff R, Reinmuth S, et al: Fertility after allogeneic haematopoietic stem cell transplantation in childhood and adolescence. Bone Marrow Transplant, DOI:10.1038/bmt.2011.78.
20 Rovo A, Tichelli A, Passweg JR, et al: Spermatogenesis in long-term survivors after allogeneic hematopoietic stem cell transplantation is associated with age, time interval since transplantation, and apparently absence of chronic GvHD. Blood 2006;108:1100–1105.
21 Duffy C, Allen S: Medical and psychosocial aspects of fertility after cancer. Cancer J 2009;15:27–33.
22 Armenian SH, Bhatia S: Cardiovascular disease after hematopoietic cell transplantation – lessons learned. Haematologica 2008;93:1132–1136.
23 Chow EJ, Mueller BA, Baker KS, et al: Cardiovascular hospitalizations and mortality among recipients of hematopoietic stem cell transplantation. Ann Intern Med 2011;155:21–32.
24 Tichelli A, Passweg J, Wojcik D, et al: Late cardiovascular events after allogeneic hematopoietic stem cell transplantation: a retrospective multicenter study of the Late Effects Working Party of the European Group for Blood and Marrow Transplantation. Haematologica 2008;93:1203–1210.
25 Baker KS, Ness KK, Steinberger J, et al: Diabetes, hypertension, and cardiovascular events in survivors of hematopoietic cell transplantation: a report from the bone marrow transplantation survivor study. Blood 2007;109:1765–1772.
26 Rovo A, Daikeler T, Halter J, et al: Late altered organ function in very long-term survivors after allogeneic hematopoietic stem cell transplantation: a paired comparison with their HLA-identical sibling donor. Haematologica 2011;96:150–155.
27 Adams MJ, Lipsitz SR, Colan SD, et al: Cardiovascular status in long-term survivors of Hodgkin's disease treated with chest radiotherapy. J Clin Oncol 2004; 22:3139–3148.
28 Aleman BMP, van den Belt-Dusebout A, De Bruin ML, et al: Late cardiotoxicity after treatment for Hodgkin lymphoma. Blood 2007;109:1878–1886.
29 Bouillon K, Haddy N, Delaloge S, et al: Long-term cardiovascular mortality after radiotherapy for breast cancer. J Am Coll Cardiol 2011;57:445–452.
30 Nilsson G, Holmberg L, Garmo H, Terent A, Blomqvist C: Increased incidence of stroke in women with breast cancer. Eur J Cancer 2005;41: 423–429.
31 Dorresteijn LD, Kappelle AC, Boogerd W, et al: Increased risk of ischemic stroke after radiotherapy on the neck in patients younger than 60 years. J Clin Oncol 2002;20:282–288.
32 Armenian SH, Sun CL, Mills G, et al: Predictors of late cardiovascular complications in survivors of hematopoietic cell transplantation. Biol Blood Marrow Transplant 2010;16:1138–1144.
33 Abboud I, Porcher R, Robin M, et al: Chronic kidney dysfunction in patients alive without relapse 2 years after allogeneic hematopoietic stem cell transplantation. Biol Blood Marrow Transplant 2009;15:1251–1257.
34 Choi M, Sun CL, Kurian S, et al: Incidence and predictors of delayed chronic kidney disease in long-term survivors of hematopoietic cell transplantation. Cancer 2008;113:1580–1587.
35 Hingorani S, Guthrie KA, Schoch G, Weiss NS, McDonald GB: Chronic kidney disease in long-term survivors of hematopoietic cell transplant. Bone Marrow Transplant 2007;39:223–229.
36 Schulte CM, Beelen DW: Avascular osteonecrosis after allogeneic hematopoietic stem-cell transplantation: diagnosis and gender matter. Transplantation 2004;78:1055–1063.
37 Socie G, Cahn JY, Carmelo J, et al: Avascular necrosis of bone after allogeneic bone marrow transplantation: analysis of risk factors for 4388 patients by the Societe Francaise de Greffe de Moelle (SFGM). Br J Haematol 1997;97:865–870.
38 Campbell S, Sun CL, Kurian S, et al: Predictors of avascular necrosis of bone in long-term survivors of hematopoietic cell transplantation. Cancer 2009;115: 4127–4135.

39 Horwitz ME: Reduced intensity versus myeloablative allogeneic stem cell transplantation for the treatment of acute myeloid leukemia, myelodysplastic syndrome and acute lymphoid leukemia. Curr Opin Oncol 2011;23:197–202.
40 Dahllof G, Hingorani SR, Sanders JE: Late effects following hematopoietic cell transplantation for children. Biol Blood Marrow Transplant 2008;14:88–93.
41 Chen MH, Chang PM, Li WY, et al: High incidence of oral squamous cell carcinoma independent of HPV infection after allogeneic hematopoietic SCT in Taiwan. Bone Marrow Transplant 2011;46:567–572.
42 Curtis RE, Metayer C, Rizzo JD, et al: Impact of chronic GVHD therapy on the development of squamous-cell cancers after hematopoietic stem-cell transplantation: an international case-control study. Blood 2005;105:3802–3811.
43 Mawardi H, Elad S, Correa ME, et al: Oral epithelial dysplasia and squamous cell carcinoma following allogeneic hematopoietic stem cell transplantation: clinical presentation and treatment outcomes. Bone Marrow Transplant 2011;46:884–891.
44 Rizzo JD, Curtis RE, Socie G, et al: Solid cancers after allogeneic hematopoietic cell transplantation. Blood 2009;113:1175–1183.
45 Gupta V, Panzarella T, Li L, et al: A prospective study comparing the outcomes and health-related quality of life in adult patients with myeloid malignancies undergoing allogeneic transplantation using myeloablative or reduced-intensity conditioning. Biol Blood Marrow Transplant 2011, Epub ahead of print.
46 Armenian SH, Sun CL, Francisco L, et al: Health behaviors and cancer screening practices in long-term survivors of hematopoietic cell transplantation (HCT): a report from the BMT Survivor Study. Bone Marrow Transplant 2011, Epub ahead of print.

Prof. Dr. med André Tichelli
Hematology, University Hospital Basel
Petersgraben 4
CH–4031 Basel (Switzerland)
Tel. +44 61 265 42 77, E-Mail Tichelli@datacomm.ch

Häusermann P, Steiger J, Passweg J (eds): Transplantation Dermatology.
Curr Probl Dermatol. Basel, Karger, 2012, vol 43, pp 150–164

Drug Hypersensitivity Reactions during Hematopoietic Stem Cell Transplantation

Andreas J. Bircher · Kathrin Scherer Hofmeier

Allergy Unit, Department of Dermatology, University Hospital, Basel, Switzerland

Abstract

Drugs may elicit a considerable variety of clinical signs, often affecting the skin and the mucous membranes. The most common are maculopapular exanthema, urticaria and angioedema. More rarely pustular, vesiculobullous, vasculitic and lichenoid lesions may be observed. Apart from the morphology, also the chronology of the occurrence and the evolution of the single skin lesions and the exanthema are paramount in the clinical diagnosis. Often, the skin is the only affected organ; however, it may herald a systemic involvement of internal organs, such as in severe drug-induced hypersensitivity syndromes or anaphylaxis. Cutaneous manifestations, particularly maculopapular exanthemas have a high incidence among patients treated with hematopoietic stem cell transplantation. In many cases, a virus- or drug-induced origin or a combination of both is responsible. However, the transplantation itself may also induce similar skin changes. These exanthemas include most often graft-versus-host disease, and rarely engraftment syndrome or eruption of lymphocyte recovery. The elucidation of the underlying cause of the exanthemas occurring in immune compromised patients and the determination of the correct diagnosis remain challenging. An extensive differential diagnosis has to be put forward. This includes several groups of disorders with sometimes very similar cutaneous manifestations. Manifestations form the underlying disease, complications from therapy, infections and drug reactions are the most common differential diagnoses.

Hematopoietic stem cell transplantation (HSCT) is increasingly being used for the treatment of hematologic malignancies and occasionally for autoimmune disorders. The induction and preparation of HSCT causes severe immunosuppression; therefore, prophylactic and therapeutic administration of antimicrobials for opportunistic infections is necessary [1]. Sequential and parallel treatment with multiple drugs over prolonged periods in association with immune suppression and viral infections results in the frequent occurrence of cutaneous manifestations, particularly macular, papular and maculopapular exanthemas. They represent a considerable diagnostic challenge. The differential diagnoses include infectious and drug-induced exanthemas to a variety of different drugs and skin disorders caused by HSCT itself. The immunosuppressive therapy may additionally modify the appearance and manifestations of drug hypersensitivity reactions. Interestingly, immediate type reactions to drugs including urticaria, angioedema and anaphylaxis are apparently not more common than in other patient groups.

The two common toxic reactions associated with various cytostatic agents, mucositis [2] and the hand-foot syndrome also called palmoplantar erythrodysesthesia or chemotherapy-associated acral erythema [3], which are currently termed as toxic erythema of chemotherapy (TEC) [4] are not further reviewed. Rare reports of manifestations similar to TEC have been reported in patients with neoplasia or graft-versus-host disease (GVHD).

Differential Diagnosis

The differential diagnosis of cutaneous manifestations following HSCT should first be approached from a morphological and second from an etiological point of view [5]. That implies that first the diagnosis of a drug-related adverse event after exclusion of other cutaneous disorders should be made, followed by the identification of the potentially eliciting drug. Both steps represent a considerable challenge because adverse drug reactions and particularly exanthemas may mimic a vast variety of clinical conditions (fig. 1).

Infectious Exanthemas

Particularly infectious exanthemas of viral etiology, e.g. the human herpes viruses EBV, human herpesvirus 6 (HHV-6), CMV, as well as enterovirus, adenovirus, parvovirus B19 and HIV should be considered. The similarity of the confluent macular lesions typical for rubella and measles has resulted in the formerly used terms 'rubeoliform' and 'morbilliform' in the description of drug-induced exanthemas. The detailed analysis of the single lesions may allow to establish a certain likelihood of an infectious or drug-related etiology [6]. Disseminated herpes simplex infections or varicella zoster infections are usually not confounded with drug exanthemas due to their distinct manifestation. In the initial phase, however, they may have a macular appearance, and in immune-suppressed patients the skin lesions may appear atypical.

HHV-6B often reactivates in HSCT patients, and has been recognized as an important opportunistic pathogen for HSCT recipients. Apart from delayed platelet engraftment or myelosuppression, skin rash with or without GVHD and organ involvement (interstitial pneumonitis and encephalitis) has been observed [7]. Like all of the other herpesviruses HHV-6 has a tendency to establish latent infection in host cells after

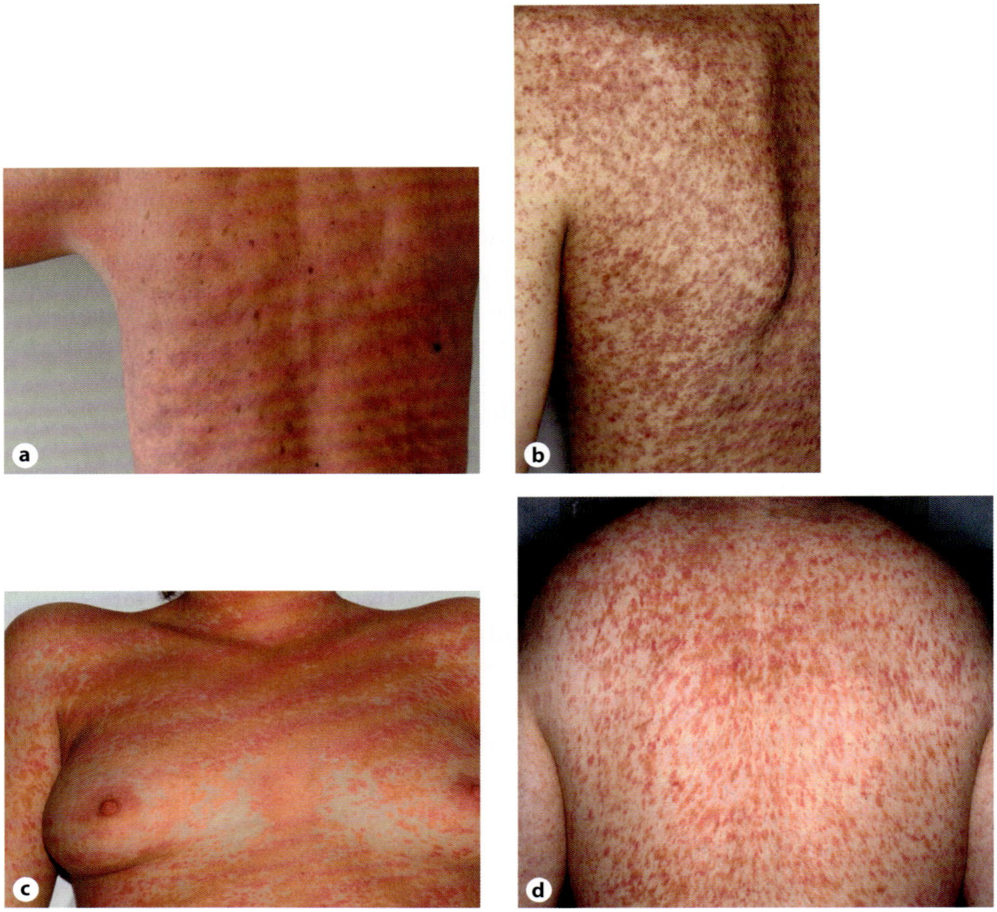

Fig. 1. **a** Maculopapular exanthema in DHS to amoxicillin. **b** Macular, partially hemorrhagic exanthema in acute GVHD. **c** Confluent macular and papular exanthema to aminopenicillin in acute EBV infection. **d** Macular exanthema from measles in an adult patient.

primary infection and may reactivate in immunocompromised situations, especially in the setting of HSCT. Skin eruptions occurring by day 30 after HSCT were found in 37.5%, half of the patients experienced it within 100 days after HSCT. [7]. Interestingly, human herpes viruses have also been implicated in the pathogenesis of the drug hypersensitivity syndrome (DHS; see below).

Exanthemas associated with bacterial or mycotic infections particularly with opportunistic microorganisms, manifest more likely with pustular or vasculitic lesions and may be associated with fever and systemic symptoms. Again, the skin lesions may be atypical in morphology, distribution and evolution in immunocompromised individuals.

Transplantation-Related Skin Disorders

An important differential diagnosis is hyperacute GVHD, and rarely exanthemas in the context of lymphocyte recovery (eruption of lymphocyte recovery ELR) or an engraftment syndrome are observed [1]. The earliest and most common manifestation is cutaneous GVHD. Typically, it manifests as maculopapular exanthema that often starts on palms and soles and later involves the whole body. Pruritus or tenderness in affected areas may be present. As the exanthema progresses, it may become confluent. In severe cases, blisters may occur. This may be confused with the severe bullous drug-induced disorders (see below). Patients receiving reduced intensity regimens, which do not result in marrow ablation, often have a later onset of GVHD. This is due both to the later engraftment and the damage from the preparative regimen, resulting in the production of cytokines that drive the immune responses resulting in clinical GVHD. Other organs involved in GVDH include gastrointestinal manifestations (diarrhea, nausea, vomiting), hepatic involvement and rarely noninfectious pulmonary involvement [8]. In ELR and engraftment syndrome, the skin manifestations are very similar to those observed in GVHD. Although ELR is confined to the skin, the other two systemic manifestations evolve as a result of profound cytokine release and neutrophil entrapment or the inhibition of autoreactive or alloreactive T cells. The considerable similarities of the clinical symptoms and pathogenetic mechanisms render the clinical differential diagnosis difficult. Finally, manifestations of immune reconstitution syndrome may be rarely involved in the pathogenesis of exanthemas and should be included in the differential diagnosis [9].

Specific Skin Diseases

More rarely, skin lesions typical for a distinct skin disorder, such as psoriasis, lichen planus, pityriasis rosea and eczemas may arise [6]. The personal history, the pattern of distribution of the lesions and histopathology may be helpful in differentiating these skin disorders from drug-induced or HSCT-related manifestations. Particularly psoriasis and lichen planus may present with the Koebner phenomenon, which means that slight trauma or inflammation may induce specific skin lesions in these patients, i.e. that an initial drug induced maculopapular exanthema may later turn into typical psoriatic lesions.

Clinical Manifestations of Drug Hypersensitivity

Drug hypersensitivity reactions affect most often the skin, which may also act as herald organ, e.g. in systemic hypersensitivity reactions such as anaphylaxis or the DHS. As opposed to the toxic-pharmacologic reactions such as hand-foot syndrome and mucositis, hypersensitivity reactions present with symptoms and signs, which are neither related to the dose nor the known pharmacological action of the drug in question. The skin may present a variety of different reaction patterns (table 1). For this reason, the term 'the great imitator' has been attributed to drug hypersensitivity reactions, because they can imitate a variety of other cutaneous diseases, as it has been previously attributed to syphilis. The correct identification and diagnosis of the skin lesions are paramount for the diagnosis of drug-induced hypersensitivity [10].

General Symptoms

Patients with mild reactions rarely have constitutional symptoms. In severe drug hypersensitivity reactions, general malaise, fatigue, headaches, elevated body temperature and gastrointestinal ailments (vomitus, diarrhea) may often mimic symptoms of other diseases such as viral or bacterial infections or direct consequences of the HSCT conditioning.

Drug Fever

Fever as an only manifestation of drug hypersensitivity is rare; many patients suffer from additional symptoms such as headache and myalgias or exanthemas. Physical factors, pyrogens and immune complexes are discussed. On the other hand, fever may precede or accompany particularly the more severe drug-induced exanthemas such as DHS or acute generalized exanthematous pustulosis.

Urticaria, Angioedema, and Anaphylaxis

A large number of factors can trigger mast cells and basophils such as drugs, foods, additives and infections, which renders the etiological differential diagnosis of those conditions difficult. Urticaria, angioedema and anaphylaxis can result from a type I (IgE antibody) or a type III (immune complex) reaction according to Coombs and Gell, but also from nonimmunological, so called pseudoallergic mechanisms as, for example, in NSAID intolerance [11].

Urticaria is characterized by disseminated rapidly emerging, migrating and itching wheals. It mainly affects the trunk and extremities, less often the face. The lesions appear typically within minutes and usually persist for less than 24 h at one location. Angioedema is characterized by a tense nonpitting edema, affecting mainly the face, lips, oral mucosa and male genitals. In severe cases, it affects the oropharynx and larynx. It is usually pale due to vasocompression and causes tingling and pressure sensations. Typical early symptoms of angioedema of the tongue and larynx that may

Table 1. Clinical manifestations, chronology and morphology of drug hypersensitivity reactions

Clinical manifestation	Chronology of elicitation (in previously sensitized patients)	Cutaneous findings and localization	Internal organ involvement	Systemic signs	Pertinent laboratory findings
Urticaria, Angioedema	Immediate Typically minutes to 1–2 h, angioedema up to 6 h Rapid change and resolution (wheals <24 h) Angioedema 24–72h	Urticarial wheals, pale swelling surrounded by erythematous border Pruritus No cutaneous sequelae Trunk, face, generalized, mucosae	In anaphylaxis respiratory tract Gastrointestinal tract Cardiovascular system	Mild fever	Mast cell tryptase (in anaphylaxis) Rarely specific IgE to few allergens (penicillins, latex, chlorhexidine)
Fixed drug exanthema	Delayed Typically 1–24 h Resolution 3–5 days	Erythematous or lilac macule or plaque, central bulla, erosion, permanent hyperpigmentation burning, pruritus Fixed (identical) acral localization, mucosa	None	None	None
Maculopapular exanthema	Delayed typically 6–24 h, peak at 48–72 h Resolution 5–7 days	Macules, papules confluence, desquamation Trunk, proximal extremities, dissemination, pruritus	None	Mild fever	Mild eosinophilia
SDRIFE (Baboon syndrome)	Delayed typically 6–24 h Peak at 48–72 h Resolution 5 – 7 days	Erythema Papules (rarely pustules) Flexural/ intertriginous areas, buttocks rarely dissemination	None	Mild fever	None
Pustular exanthema (AGEP)	Delayed typically 6–12 h up to 24–48 h Resolution 5–7 days	Confluent erythema, pinpoint nonfollicular pustules, pruritus, massive desquamation intertriginous areas, trunk, generalized dissemination	Possible but rare	High fever (>38°C)	Neutrophilia

Table 1. Continued

Clinical manifestation	Chronology of elicitation (in previously sensitized patients)	Cutaneous findings and localization	Internal organ involvement	Systemic signs	Pertinent laboratory findings
DHS Drug-related eosinophilia with systemic symptoms (DRESS)	Delayed Typically several days up to several weeks in newly sensitized patients Resolution weeks	Maculopapular exanthema Generalized erythroderma Centrofacial edema	Required Lymphadenopathy Hepatitis Pneumonitis Nephritis	Fever Malaise Fatigue	Eosinophilia, atypical lymphocytes Possibly cytopenias Pathological liver, renal function tests
Vesiculobullous exanthemas (SJS, TEN)	Delayed Typically several days up to several weeks in newly sensitized patients Resolution weeks	Macules, bullae, epidermolysis, Initially painful skin trunk, face dissemination Generalized mucositis (conjunctiva, oral, genital)	Internal mucosas Respiratory tract Gastrointestinal tract	Fever Malaise Fatigue	Lymphopenia

Modified from Bircher and Scherer [10].

develop into asphyxia and hypoxia are the urge to clear the throat, hoarseness, throat tightness, blurred speech and salivation [11].

In anaphylaxis, the spectrum includes several or all of these symptoms such as pruritus, urticaria, and angioedema (90%), dyspnea and bronchospasm (60%), dizziness and syncope (29%), flush (28%), abdominal colics and diarrhea (26%), swelling of the tongue, edema of the larynx, dysphonia, and dysphagia (24%), nausea and vomiting (20%), hypotension (20%), rhinitis (16%), conjunctivitis (12%) and headaches, and pruritus without skin changes (<5% each). Further unspecific early symptoms of impending anaphylaxis are agitation, excitation, feeling of impending doom, and mortal fear [12, 13].

Maculopapular Exanthemas

Macular and papular exanthemas are the most common delayed manifestations of drug hypersensitivity. Often, they are called 'rash' or 'eruption' which, from a dermatological point of view, only designates the sudden, concomitant appearance of disseminated lesions. For a distinct clinical diagnosis these terms are not sufficient.

They manifest initially with erythematous macules and/or infiltrated papules, affecting particularly trunk and proximal extremities.

The differential diagnosis as mentioned before includes infectious exanthemas and HSCT-related skin manifestations. In more severe reactions, elevated eosinophil counts can be observed in a number of patients, which helps to distinguish them from viral exanthemas. In stronger reactions, exanthemas are confluent, resulting in erythroderma. Typically, a more or less pronounced desquamation occurs after clearing of the inflammatory lesions within 7–10 days.

For a peculiar contact allergen- and drug-related exanthema appearing in a symmetrical distribution in intertriginous and flexural areas, the term baboon syndrome has been previously coined [14]. To delineate this particular drug hypersensitivity reaction from other skin disorders, the neutral acronym SDRIFE that stands for Symmetrical Drug-Related Intertriginous and Flexural Exanthema has been proposed [14].

A sharply delineated erythema of the perigenital and perianal area is associated with the affection of the large folds, such as the axilla, the elbows and the knees. Systemic symptoms are absent and in contrast to most other drug exanthemas, males are more often affected than females.

Most of these exanthemas result from a type IV (T cell-mediated) pathogenesis; in maculopapular exanthemas, cytotoxic CD4+ T cells seem to play the major role. While at least 5–7 days are required for expansion of drug-reactive cells and development of symptoms at the initial drug exposure, a sensitized individual develops symptoms typically 1–2 days after renewed drug exposure. First signs such as a discrete erythema may already appear after a few hours [10]. For common elicitors, see below.

Acute Generalized Exanthematic Pustulosis

In maculopapular exanthemas, few isolated pustules may be observed. In acute generalized exanthematic pustulosis (AGEP), however, on a diffuse widespread erythema, multiple small sterile pustules associated with pruritus or burning appear. The initial lesions often manifest in the face or intertriginous areas and then disseminate within hours. Fever and leukocytosis are mandatory diagnostic prerequisites. A diagnostic algorithm for this not uncommon drug hypersensitivity reaction has been proposed [15]. AGEP is most often elicited by antibiotics, particularly aminopenicillins and cephalosporins, sometimes exposure to mercury vapors, but has also been observed with a large number of other drugs [16].

Drug Hypersensitivity Syndrome

For the DHS, also the acronym DRESS (Drug Related Eosinophilia with Systemic Symptoms) has been proposed [17]. In this syndrome affecting multiple organs, a macular and/or papular, rarely hemorrhagic or bullous exanthema and an erythematous centrofacial swelling are typical. Fever and general malaise may be accompanied by one or several manifestations such as lymphadenopathy, hepatitis (in 50%), nephritis (in 10%) and more rarely pneumonitis. In the peripheral blood eosinophilia (in 90%), lymphocytosis, atypical lymphocytes, agranulocytosis and anemia may be observed [18]. Nephritis, pneumonitis, pancreatitis have also been documented and, dependent on the drug, other organs such as the myocardium, the thyroid gland and the gastrointestinal tract may be involved. Mortality reaches up to 10%, hepatitis is the most important cause for lethal outcome, and undiagnosed myocarditis has also resulted in fatal outcomes. As one pathogenic factor reactivation of HHV-6 has been implicated [19]. As demonstrated in GVHD, also other members of the herpes virus group have been shown to be reactivated in DRESS/DHS. This raises interesting questions on a common pathogenic pathway in both conditions, which to some extent also share clinical features [20]. In its initial phase, DRESS/DHS can be confused with acute viral infections such as primoinfection with EBV or HIV [21] or GVHD.

The period between the intake of the eliciting drug and the start of clinical manifestations lasts up to several days in previously sensitized patients. As opposed to the common maculopapular exanthemas from antibiotics, in newly sensitized individuals a delay of 3–4 weeks is often encountered, for some drugs even months. Graft failure in the context of a severe DHS/DRESS to phenytoin has been reported [22]. The drugs most often involved in DHS/DRESS are the aromatic antiepileptic drugs (carbamazepine, phenytoin, phenobarbital, lamotrigine), allopurinol, abacavir and minocycline.

Severe Vesiculobullous Exanthemas

The severe vesiculobullous exanthemas also called SCAR (severe cutaneous adverse reactions) are not one entity, but include a range of disorders of different severity and mortality. They include minor and major forms of erythema exsudativum multiforme (EEM), Stevens-Johnson syndrome (SJS) and toxic epidermal necrolysis (TEN or Lyell's disease) [23]. EEM and SJS are characterized by target lesions with often central bullae formation, which arise on the extremities and the trunk. TEN begins with a macular, often dusk red exanthema, the skin may be painful upon touch. Atypical target lesions may be present. Bullae rapidly arise on the trunk and become generalized later. Skin involvement is ≤10% in SJS, and >30% in TEN. The Nikolsky sign (movement of bullae upon tangential pressure) is positive. In SJS as well as TEN, at least one mucosa (stomatitis, conjunctivitis, genital mucosa) is involved. Mortality is about 10% in SJS, up to 30% in TEN. Sequelae on skin and mucosa are frequent. Acute GVHD may initially present with similar skin lesions as TEN and may be difficult to distinguish [24].

Particularly in children below the age of 6, staphylococcal scalded skin syndrome (SSSS) should be differentiated histologically from TEN. In both, the cleavage plane is situated in layers of the epidermis, in TEN the complete epidermal layer may become apoptotic. Skin and blister fluid are usually sterile in SSSS since the skin lesions are caused by exfoliative toxins excreted by *Staphylococcus aureus*. In TEN, the skin may be colonized by *S. aureus*, since secondary bacterial skin infections are found frequently [25].

Stomatitis

Mucosal involvement, in particular stomatitis or balanitis, could represent a localized drug reaction such as fixed drug eruption, but have to be taken seriously if more than one mucosal area is extensively affected and erosions and ulcerations occur. In SJS/TEN, severe mucositis of more than one mucosa usually appears early and is followed by epidermal blister formation and necrolysis. Conjunctival involvement, in particular, warrants early cooperation with ophthalmologists because persistent ocular complications are frequent.

Vasculitis

Nonblanchable erythematous lesions (purpura) represent vasculitis of cutaneous blood vessels or a deficiency in the coagulation cascade. Hemorrhagic or palpable lesions are a sign of perivascular inflammation after destruction of blood vessels and should prompt a search for systemic vasculitis with involvement of internal organs or thrombocytopenia. Bullous transformation and necrosis may follow, which can be extensive depending on the size of vessel affected. Drugs may rarely elicit cutaneous so-called allergic or systemic vasculitis, sometimes infections in immunocompromised hosts may mimic vasculitis. Affection of internal organs such as the kidneys, the gastrointestinal tract, the liver and the central nervous system has to be excluded [11].

Special Manifestations

Some special manifestations of drug exanthemas may mimic other skin disorders or represent complication of an infectious agent. An overview is presented in Bircher [5].

Psoriasiform and Pityriasiform Exanthemas

A number of drugs have been implicated in the elicitation or exacerbation of psoriasis [26]. The strongest evidence exists for lithium, beta-blockers and antimalarials. It may take several weeks to months until the psoriatic lesions appear. The paradoxal elicitation or exacerbation of psoriasis has been documented for TNF-α antagonists for psoriasis and sorafenib, a RAF and tyrosine kinase inhibitor. In patients with a psoriatic background, an initially macular or papular drug-induced exanthema may turn into psoriatic lesions (Koebner phenomenon).

Pityriasis rosea is a common, probably infectious skin disorder. An association with HHV-6 and -7, and recently also with HHV-8 has been suggested. Drug-induced pityriasis rosea has often an atypical clinical presentation; in histopathology, an interface dermatitis with eosinophils is found. Lichen planus-like changes may follow, leaving marked hyperpigmentation. Many drugs have been incriminated as possible triggers of pityriasis rosea-like eruptions, such as gold, captopril, tyrosine kinase inhibitors, and nonsteroidal anti-inflammatory agents among many others.

Lichenoid and Pseudolymphomatous Manifestations

Lichen planus or lichen planus-like reactions to drugs have also been reported. The oral mucosa may also be affected. In terms of location, morphology and histology, lichen planus and drug-induced lichenoid eruptions are identical. Most often gold, antimalarials, methyldopa, beta-blockers and lithium salts have been incriminated.

Initial macules may slowly proceed into very pruritic infiltrated nodules and plaques with the clinicohistological presentation of a pseudolymphoma. They have a slower and more protracted time course, often obscuring the relation to the eliciting drugs. Histology is mandatory to establish the diagnosis and to exclude malignant lymphoma [17].

Interstitial Granulomatous Drug Reaction

Interstitial granulomatous drug reaction is a rare drug-related reaction pattern [5]. It is characterized by erythematous and violaceous, nonpruritic, sometimes painful plaques and nodes in intertriginous areas [27]. It appears very late within a time range of weeks to months. Eliciting drugs include biologicals such as anakinra, adalimumab and TNF-α antagonists [28], gancyclovir, ACE inhibitors, furosemide, calcium antagonists, beta-blockers, sennosides, herbal medicines, antihistamines, anticonvulsants and antidepressants. The diagnosis has to be confirmed by histopathology.

Erythema Nodosum

Erythema nodosum-like drug reactions, histologically a septal panniculitis, have been observed to sulfonamides, oral contraceptives, salicylates and azathioprine. Clinically painful pretibial inflammatory nodules and plaques are present. From clinical and histopathological aspects, the etiology cannot be differentiated [5].

Acute Febrile Neutrophilic Dermatosis (Sweet's Syndrome)

Sweet's syndrome comprises a symptom complex including fever, neutrophilia, and tender erythematous papules, nodules, and plaques located on the face, neck, chest, and extremities. Three forms are distinguished: classical (idiopathic), malignancy-associated and drug-induced Sweet's syndrome. For the diagnosis of the drug-induced variant, five criteria are required: (a) abrupt onset of painful erythematous plaques or nodules, (b) a dense neutrophilic infiltrate without evidence of leukocytoclastic vasculitis, (c) fever >38°C, (d) temporal relationship between drug ingestion and manifestation, OR temporally related recurrence after reexposure, and (e) temporally related resolution of lesions after drug withdrawal or treatment with systemic corticosteroids. A large number of drugs have been implicated; however, best evidence exists for GM-CSF, all-trans-retinoic acid, vaccines and probably minocycline. Other reported drugs include bortezimib, azathioprine and sulfonamides [5].

Eliciting Drugs

The drugs most often involved in uncomplicated maculopapular exanthemas include the antimicrobial drugs (e.g. betalactam antibiotics, sulfonamide antibiotics), antimycotics, aromatic anticonvulsant drugs such as carbamazepine, phenytoine, lamotrigine, allopurinol, and antihypertensive drugs (e.g. calcium antagonists, nonaromatic sulfonamide diuretics). Rarely, also contrast media and even corticosteroids have been implicated. However, in an immune compromised patient with an exanthema, every given drug within a time period of up to 4 weeks before onset of symptoms and signs should be taken into consideration. Textbooks may help to identify more commonly eliciting drugs [29].

Diagnostic Procedures

The diagnostic steps depend on the clinical phase of the reaction. In an acutely ill patient suffering from a probable drug hypersensitivity reaction, the detailed history, complete analysis of all administered drugs and the exact clinical descriptions are the most important and often only diagnostic options. Skin biopsy is often recommended, which can be useful to exclude GVHD [30]. However, to reach high sensitivity in diagnosing drug hypersensitivity is difficult. Peripheral or tissue eosinophils are sometimes used as an indication for a hypersensitivity reaction. It requires, however a large number of eosinophils per high power field to be able to distinguish drug exanthemas from GVHD [31], and HSCT patients regularly receive large doses of corticosteroids decreasing eosinophil numbers. Cultures from biopsies, however, may help to identify infectious agents.

In the acute phase, often under extensive immune suppression, skin tests cannot be performed, and in vitro test using effector cell stimulation such as lymphocyte or basophil activation tests have generally a low sensitivity and should not be performed in lymphopenic patients.

The clinical diagnosis requires a detailed description of the morphology, particularly the cutaneous efflorescences and signs. The term 'rash' or eruption is not specific enough [10]. The clinical investigation comprises a complete examination of the skin and its appendages, including the mucous membranes of the mouth, eyes and genitals. The type and distribution of the lesions as well as their evolution (table 1) should be noted. Once the clinical diagnosis of a drug exanthema is likely, an attempt to identify eliciting drugs should be made.

The chronology of events is a useful clinical approach to narrow in on identifying eliciting drugs.

The time period between the first dose and the occurrence of first symptoms varies. A clear distinction between an immunologically naïve person and a previously sensitized individual should be made [10]. Sensitization to a drug or its metabolites takes at least 5–7 days of exposure for the expansion of drug-reactive lymphocytes, but for unknown reasons it may take up to several weeks as for example in DHS. It may, however, also occur through another similar molecule and elicit an allergic reaction upon first exposure to a molecule by cross-reactivity, although this may be overestimated [32]. Particularly intake of a drug with irregular frequency and changing intervals may facilitate sensitization, whereas continuous intake results more likely in tolerance. Sensitization may be influenced by cofactors such as dose, metabolism, dosing intervals, administration route, concomitant medications and particularly the immunologic reactivity of the patient. Once an individual is sensitized, the time between the eliciting dose and the first occurrence of symptoms varies depending on the pathomechanism and type of exanthema. In IgE-mediated reactions, the typical eliciting phase varies from a few minutes to some hours. In T cell-mediated reactions, the time delay ranges between a few hours to 2 days. Many factors, among them the route of administration (intravenous > intramuscular > subcutaneous > topical > oral), drug metabolism and other cofactors (food intake, drug interactions), play a modifying role [10].

Based on the information gathered by history, chronology and clinical examination, a pathogenetic hypothesis of the reaction can be formulated and may be later applied in an allergological workup, which is recommended to be performed in a time window of 4 weeks to 6 months after complete resolution, if possible.

References

1 Nellen RGL, Van Marion AMW, Frank J, Poblete-Gutiérrez P, Steijlen PM: Eruption of lymphocyte recovery or autologous graft-versus-host disease? Int J Dermatol 2008;47:32–34.
2 Degen A, Alter M, Schenck F, Satzger I, Völker B, Kapp A, Gutzmer R: The hand-foot-syndrome associated with medical tumor therapy – classification and management. J Dtsch Dermatol Ges 2010;8:652–661.
3 Worthington HV, Clarkson JE, Bryan G, Furness S, Glenny AM, Littlewood A, McCabe MG, Meyer S, Khalid T: Interventions for preventing oral mucositis for patients with cancer receiving treatment. Cochrane Database Syst Rev 2011;4:CD000978.
4 Bolognia JL, Cooper DL, Glusac EJ: Toxic erythema of chemotherapy: a useful clinical term. J Am Acad Dermatol 2008;59:524–529.
5 Bircher AJ: Uncomplicated drug-induced disseminated exanthemas; in French L (ed): Chemical Immunology. Basel, Karger, 2012, in press.
6 Drago F, Rampini P, Rampini E, Rebora A: Atypical exanthems: morphology and laboratory investigations may lead to an aetiological diagnosis in about 70% of cases. Br J Dermatol 2002;147:255–260.
7 Wang L-R, Dong L-J, Zhang M-J, Lu D-P: The impact of human herpesvirus 6B reactivation on early complications following allogeneic hematopoietic stem cell transplantation. Biol Blood Marrow Transplant 2006;12:1031–1037.
8 Jacobsohn DA, Vogelsang GB: Acute graft versus host disease. Orphanet J Rare Dis 2007;2:35.
9 Avigan D, Wu Z, Joyce R, Elias A, Richardson P, McDermott D, Levine J, Kennedy L, Giallombardo N, Hurley D, Gong J, Kufe D: Immune reconstitution following high-dose chemotherapy with stem cell rescue in patients with advanced breast cancer. Bone Marrow Transplant 2000;26:169–176.
10 Bircher AJ, Scherer K: Delayed cutaneous manifestations of drug hypersensitivity; in Pichler WJ (ed): Drug Hypersensitivity. Philadelphia, Saunders, 2010, vol 94, pp 711–725.
11 Scherer K, Bircher AJ: Danger signs in drug hypersensitivity; in Pichler WJ (ed): Drug Hypersensitivity. Philadelphia, Saunders, 2010, vol 94, pp 681–689.
12 Kemp SF, Lockey RF, Wolf BL, Lieberman P: Anaphylaxis: a review of 266 cases. Arch Intern Med 1995;155:1749–1754.
13 Webb L, Lieberman P: Anaphylaxis: a review of 601 cases. Ann Allergy Asthma Immunol 2006;97:39–43.
14 Hausermann P, Harr T, Bircher AJ: Baboon syndrome resulting from systemic drugs: is there strife between SDRIFE and allergic contact dermatitis syndrome? Contact Dermatitis 2004;51:297–310.
15 Sidoroff A, Halevy S, Bavinck JNB, Vaillant L, Roujeau J-C: Acute generalized exanthematous pustulosis (AGEP) – a clinical reaction pattern. J Cutan Pathol 2001;28:113–119.
16 Roujeau J-C, Bioulac-Sage P, Bourseau C, Guillaume J-C, Bernard P, Lok C, Plantin P, Claudy A, Delavierre C, Vaillant L, Wechsler J, Danan G, Benichou C, Beylot C: Acute generalized exanthematous pustulosis: analysis of 63 cases. Arch Dermatol 1991;127:1333–1338.
17 Bocquet H, Bagot M, Roujeau JC: Drug-induced pseudolymphoma and drug hypersensitivity syndrome (drug rash with eosinophilia and systemic symptoms: DRESS). Semin Cutan Med Surg 1996;15:250–257.
18 Prussick R, Knowles S, Shear NH: Cutaneous drug reactions. Curr Probl Dermatol 1994;6:83–122.
19 Seishima M, Yamanaka S, Fujisawa T, Tohyama M, Hashimoto K: Reactivation of human herpesvirus (HHV) family members other than HHV-6 in drug-induced hypersensitivity syndrome. Br J Dermatol 2006;155:344–349.
20 Shiohara T, Takahashi R, Kano Y: Drug-induced hypersensitivity syndrome and viral reactivation; in Pichler WJ (ed): Drug Hypersensitivity. Basel, Karger, 2007, pp 251–266.
21 Kano Y, Hiraharas K, Sakuma K, Shiohara T: Several herpesviruses can reactivate in a severe drug-induced multiorgan reaction in the same sequential order as in graft-versus-host disease. Br J Dermatol 2006;155:301–306.
22 Maecker B, Meissner B, Bettoni da Cunha-Riehm C, Sauer M, Welte K, Sykora KW: Severe graft failure presumably due to phenytoin-induced hypersensitivity syndrome in two patients after bone marrow transplantation. Bone Marrow Transplant 2008;41:833–835.
23 Wolf R, Orion E, Marcos B, Matz H: Life-threatening acute adverse cutaneous drug reactions. Clin Dermatol 2005;23:171–181.
24 Arvidson J, Kildal M, Linde T, Gedeborg R: Toxic epidermal necrolysis and hemolytic uremic syndrome after allogeneic stem-cell transplantation. Pediatr Transplant 2007;11:689–693.
25 Zakrzewski JL, Lentin G, Such U, Duerr A, Tran V, Guenzelmann S, Braunschweig T, Riede UN, Koldehoff M: Toxic epidermal necrolysis: differential diagnosis of an epidermolytic dermopathy in a hematopoietic stem cell transplant recipient. Bone Marrow Transplant 2002;30:331–333.
26 Rongioletti F, Fiorucci C, Parodi A: Psoriasis induced or aggravated by drugs. J Rheumatol 2009;83:59–61.

27 Ramdial PK, Naidoo DK: Drug-induced cutaneous pathology. J Clin Pathol 2009;62:493–504.
28 Regula CG, Hennessy J, Clarke LE, Adams DR, Ioffreda MD, Graber EM, Helm KF: Interstitial granulomatous drug reaction to anakinra. J Am Acad Dermatol 2008;59:S25–S27.
29 Litt JZ: Litt's D.E.R.M. – Drug Eruptions & Reactions Manual, ed 16. London, Informa Healthcare, 2010.
30 Hepburn NC, McLaren KM, Turner ML, Beveridge GW: The role of skin biopsies in bone marrow transplant recipients. QJM 1993;86:715–717.
31 Weaver J, Bergfeld WF: Quantitative analysis of eosinophils in acute graft-versus-host disease compared with drug hypersensitivity reactions. Am J Dermatopathol 2010;32:31–34.
32 McConnell SA, Penzak SR, Warmack TS, Anaissie EJ, Gubbins PO: Incidence of Imipenem hypersensitivity reactions in febrile neutropenic bone marrow transplant patients with a history of penicillin allergy. Clin Infect Dis 2000;31:1512–1514.

Andreas J. Bircher
Allergy Unit
Department of Dermatology
University Hospital Basel
Petersgraben 4
CH-4031 Basel (Switzerland)
Tel. +41 61 265 43 59, E-Mail andreas.bircher@unibas.ch

Häusermann P, Steiger J, Passweg J (eds): Transplantation Dermatology.
Curr Probl Dermatol. Basel, Karger, 2012, vol 43, pp 165–170

Future Trends in Hematopoietic Stem Cell Transplantation

Jörg Halter[a] · Jakob Passweg[a] · Peter Häusermann[b]

Departments of [a]Hematology and [b]Dermatology, University Hospital Basel, Basel, Switzerland

Abstract

The procedure of hematopoietic stem cell transplantation (HSCT) will keep expanding over the next decades. The list of indications for autologous or allogeneic HSCT of nonmalignant and malignant hematological disorders will grow. Other life-threatening diseases such as genetic, metabolic or autoimmune disorders including systemic sclerosis will undergo critical evaluation for that treatment. As a consequence of continuous research and clinical progress in that field, more and more patients will survive HSCT, and physicians will be confronted with organ-specific late and very late effects including chronic graft-versus-host disease (cGVHD). Changes of eligibility criteria for HSCT, quality assessment of the stem cell graft, graft manipulation, and new developments in donor selection might possibly impact patients' health status and epidemiology as well as presentations of posttransplant complications. Efforts to diminish GVHD while forcing graft-versus-tumor effects will persist to be one of the major goals, and advances in prophylaxis and treatment of cGVHD will remain high priority. Changes in stem cell sources and graft manipulation might have additional influence on immune reconstitution and posttransplant disorders of infectious and immunological type. The recent publications of the National Institutes of Health consensus development project on various aspects of chronic GVHD has rightly positioned cGVHD as a serious and difficult to treat pleiotropic systemic disease with tremendous impact on long-term outcome. In this chapter, we will point out some of the most important issues and trends related to HSCT.

Significance of Chronic Graft-versus-Host Disease

Chronic graft-versus-host disease (cGVHD) is a systemic multiorgan disorder after hematopoietic stem cell transplantation (HSCT) and the leading cause of late nonrelapse mortality. This disease was recognized and first classified more than 30 years ago, and although considerable progress has been made in the prevention of acute GVHD, major progress to understand, prevent or efficiently treat cGVHD has not been achieved yet [1, 2]. Faced with numerous unresolved issues and challenges of a disease that shares features of autoimmunity and immunodeficiency, the National Institutes of Health (NIH) established a consensus development project on cGVHD in order to better characterize and standardize clinical diagnosis and staging, pathology, define biomarkers and response criteria, propose ancillary therapy and supportive cares and design clinical trials [3–8]. In spite of the potential usefulness of the NIH criteria, Socie et al. [9] recently reviewed the ongoing unresolved issues that include: (1) difference (if any) in GVHD-specific survival between patients with late acute GVHD compared to those with classical cGVHD or with overlap syndrome, (2) predictive value of the old or new classification for survival and discontinuation of immunosuppressive therapy, (3) discriminating capacity of the different classifications for disease severity. There is not only a need for better understanding the pathogenesis of cGVHD, its disease definition and severity scoring. The few reports on efficacy of treatments in randomized clinical trials, the need for glucocorticoid-sparing regimens and the lack of validated end points for clinical trials are some of the major limitations and therewith the main challenges for the future [summarized in 9]. Improved understanding of the pathophysiology of cGVHD will be the basis for the development of more effective treatments of cGVHD and future approaches to enhance immune reconstitution and graft-versus-tumor effects, while diminishing the risk of infections will be of critical importance [9].

Influence of the NIH Consensus Project on Chronic Graft-versus-Host Disease on European Networks

The NIH consensus project on cGVHD had crucial influence on European centers performing HSCT. The renewed recognition of cGVHD as one of the most important systemic complications with negative impact on quality of life and patient survival and its limitations in diagnosis, staging and treatment have led representative groups from Germany, Austria and Switzerland to force the inner European network and equally standardize clinical practice of cGVHD. Consensus conferences were implemented and held on a yearly basis. In 2009, the meeting was organized in Regensburg, Germany. Shortly afterwards, the first recommendations were published so far addressing first- and second-line treatments of cGVHD and supportive therapy of chronic cutaneous and musculoskeletal GVHD [10–12]. In the near future, many more aspects on cGVHD will be published including standardized criteria and treatment for genital cGVHD and pathology.

The Chronic Graft-versus-Host Disease Consortium

The chronic GVHD Consortium was established as a consequence of the NIH consensus development project to test the new criteria of individual organ scoring and the algorithm for calculating global severity (mild, moderate, severe) of cGVHD. According to the first published longitudinal studies in patients with cGVHD, global severity scoring of cGVHD reliably differentiated prognosis, nonrelapse mortality and survival [13]. This study further underlined the important fact for dermatologists, that the skin was one of only three organs that determined the global severity score of cGVHD in the majority of cases. A second study of the consortium found that the presence of acute features (overlap syndrome) was a marker for adverse prognosis, greater functional impairment, and higher symptom burden [14]. These findings support the prognostic importance of the proposed designation of classic and overlap cGVHD, and argue for increased awareness and accurate classification in clinical practice as well as in research.

Summary on Chronic Graft-versus-Host Disease

Worldwide, cGVHD will be increasingly recognized as a systemic disease complicating allogeneic HSCT with tremendous implications for health care systems, health care workers and health care costs. Dermatologists, ophthalmologists, rheumatologists and many more physicians of other specialties will be confronted in their daily practice with patients suffering from various aspects of that disease. Physiotherapists, ergotherapists and professionals working in social and psychological areas will have their specific role in the treatment, support and guidance of these patients. The critical impact on sexuality and family planning of patients and related party will force further working groups to investigate time, clinical dedication and research in that particular medical field. To sustain and even optimize diagnostic and therapeutic accuracy on cGVHD, it will be critically important that interdisciplinary groups and international teams continue to study and investigate cGVHD. The need to effectively educate all involved primary health care workers will be equally important as will be the step-up of international networks to investigate, prevent and treat cGVHD.

New Developments

As usual, it is difficult to state where a particular field in medicine is moving to. Recent years have seen an increase in the use of this technology in Europe reaching 30,000 patients transplanted yearly with roughly 60% being autologous and 40% being allogeneic transplants. Using the EBMT activity survey registering transplants done in Europe since 1990, there were about 260,000 patients treated. Assuming long-term survival of 30–40%, it will be obvious to the reader that dermatologists will increasingly encounter long-term survivors of such a procedure.

Recent trends in allogeneic HSCT have been the use of cord blood as a stem cell source and increasing use of unrelated donors. Furthermore, haploidentical bone marrow transplantation may become more frequently performed during the next years since new transplant regimens no longer require highly demanding lab equipment for in vitro graft manipulation [15]. These developments are due to the fact that family size is not growing in Europe, and that donors other than HLA-matched siblings are required. This has led to a continued expansion of unrelated donor registries now reaching 19,000,000 donors registered worldwide (www.bmdw.org) with numbers still increasing. Unrelated donor cord blood banks have also evolved, and in Europe more than 700 cord blood transplants are reported annually. A similar number of transplants from mismatched family donors are done. The trend therefore goes to identifying donors other than HLA identical siblings for patients in need of a HSCT without such a donor. The consequences on GVHD presentation are manifold. Unrelated donors are known to be associated with increased GVHD risks, although at the present time it is not clear whether a young fully matched unrelated donor is not superior to an older sibling; this has increasingly become an issue as patient age is also increasing, and patients up to age 70 are now routinely undergoing allogeneic (and autologous) HSCT. On the other hand, cord blood transplants have lower GVHD risks, and GVHD presentation may be more atypical as the T lymphocyte content of cord blood products is lower and because T lymphocytes are more naive than in adult donors. Furthermore, immune reconstitution is delayed in cord blood or haploidentical bone marrow transplantation [16], leading to early and late posttransplant infections which are in part different from what is usually expected after 'standard' HSCT [17]. Some of these infections may also present lesions on the skin. Therefore, especially viral or fungal infectious disease should be considered early in differential diagnosis of skin lesions, bearing in mind that they may present in an atypical form, either because of an unusual time interval after transplantation or because of atypical lesions due to an intrinsic impaired immune response or concomitant immunosuppressive treatment. Finally, the increasing use of drugs for treatment or prophylaxis of infectious diseases will increase the number of cutaneous drug reactions seen by dermatologists which might be difficult to differentiate from cGVHD [18] or predispose to secondary skin malignancies.

Cellular Therapy

Approximately 20 years ago, the infusion of donor lymphocytes for patients relapsing after an allogeneic HSCT, thus exploiting the graft versus leukemia effect, has initiated the era of cellular therapy. This is the era where a lot of development is taking place. This may range from infusion of unselected lymphocytes of the donor, which may be given in a single large dose or fractionated [19] and titrated by repeated dosing, to selectively depleting T lymphocyte subsets to decrease GVHD risk [20], to positively selecting lymphocyte populations possibly associated with antitumor or anti-infectious agents such natural killer cells [21] which may be selected and infused or expanded and activated in vitro using cytokines, to selecting T lymphocytes with specific antiviral properties and expanding them in vitro for therapeutic use [22], which may reach sophisticated levels of gene-modified T cells with transduced T cell receptors to target antigens present in the tumor, as has been recently demonstrated with T cells targeting chronic lymphocytic leukemia cells [23], and to gene-modified hematopoietic stem cells which may correct defects such as the ones seen in primary immunodeficiency syndromes [24].

It is quite likely that such cellular therapies will play an increasing role in the future, and that dermatologists will be confronted with manifestations on the skin which may or may not be related to such cellular manipulations as the skin functions as a window through which the immune system sees the outside world, and as is true for all windows, the outside world may observe what is going on inside. Dermatology has a central role in GVHD diagnosis, classification and management and, as always, progress in medicine starts with the correct diagnosis.

References

1 Shulman HM, Sullivan KM, Weiden PL, et al: Chronic graft-versus-host syndrome in man. A long-term clinicopathologic study of 20 Seattle patients. Am J Med 1980;69:204–217.

2 Lee SJ, Vogelsang G, Flowers ME: Chronic graft-versus-host disease. Biol Blood Marrow Transplant 2003;9:215–233.

3 Filipovich AH, Weisdorf D, Pavletic S, et al: National Institutes of Health consensus development project on criteria for clinical trials in chronic graft-versus-host disease. I. Diagnosis and Staging Working Group Report. Biol Blood Marrow Transplant 2005;11:945–956.

4 Shulman HM, Kleiner D, Lee SJ, et al: Histopathologic diagnosis of chronic graft-versus-host disease: National Institutes of Health Consensus Development Project on Criteria for Clinical Trials in Chronic Graft-versus-Host Disease. II. Pathology Working Group Report. Biol Blood Marrow Transplant 2006;12:31–47.

5 Schultz KR, Miklos DB, Fowler D, et al: Toward biomarkers for chronic graft-versus-host disease: National Institutes of Health consensus development project on criteria for clinical trials in chronic graft-versus-host disease. III. Biomarker Working Group Report. Biol Blood Marrow Transplant 2006; 12:126–137.

6 Pavletic SZ, Martin P, Lee SJ, et al: Measuring therapeutic response in chronic graft-versus-host disease: National Institutes of Health Consensus Development Project on Criteria for Clinical Trials in Chronic Graft-versus-Host Disease. IV. Response Criteria Working Group Report. Biol Blood Marrow Transplant 2006;12:252–266.

7 Couriel D, Carpenter PA, Cutler C, et al: Ancillary therapy and supportive care of chronic graft-versus-host disease: National Institutes of health Consensus Development Project on Criteria for Clinical Trials in Chronic Graft-versus-Host Disease. V. Ancillary Therapy and Supportive Care Working Group Report. Biol Blood Marrow Transplant 2006;12: 375–396.

8 Martin PJ, Weisdorf D, Przepiorka D, et al: National Institutes of Health Consensus Development Project on Criteria for Clinical Trials in Chronic Graft-versus-Host Disease. VI. Design of Clinical Trials Working Group report. Biol Blood Marrow Transplant 2006;12:491–505.

9 Socie G, Ritz J, Martin PJ: Current challenges in chronic graft-versus-host disease. Biol Blood Marrow Transplant 2010;16:S146–S151.

10 Marks C, Stadler M, Hausermann P, et al: German-Austrian-Swiss Consensus Conference on clinical practice in chronic graft-versus-host disease (GVHD): guidance for supportive therapy of chronic cutaneous and musculoskeletal GVHD. Br J Dermatol 2011;165:18–29.

11 Wolff D, Gerbitz A, Ayuk F, et al: Consensus conference on clinical practice in chronic graft-versus-host disease (GVHD): first-line and topical treatment of chronic GVHD. Biol Blood Marrow Transplant 2010;16:1611–1628.

12 Wolff D, Schleuning M, von Harsdorf S, et al: Consensus Conference on Clinical Practice in Chronic GVHD: second-line treatment of chronic graft-versus-host disease. Biol Blood Marrow Transplant 2011;17:1–17.

13 Arai S, Jagasia M, Storer B, et al: Global and organ-specific chronic graft-versus-host disease severity according to the 2005 NIH Consensus Criteria. Blood 2011;118:4242–4249.

14 Pidala J, Vogelsang G, Martin P, et al: Overlap subtype of chronic graft vs. host disease is associated with adverse prognosis, functional impairment, and inferior patient reported outcomes: a chronic graft vs. host disease Consortium study. Haematologica 2011, Epub ahead of print.

15 Luznik L, O'Donnell PV, Symons HJ, Chen AR, et al: HLA-haploidentical bone marrow transplantation for hematologic malignancies using nonmyeloablative conditioning and high-dose, posttransplantation cyclophosphamide. Biol Blood Marrow Transplant 2008;14:641–650.

16 Jacobson CA, Turki AT, McDonough SM, Stevenson KE, Kim HT, Kao G, Herrera MI, Reynolds CG, Alyea EP, Ho VT, Koreth J, Armand P, Chen YB, Ballen K, Soiffer RJ, Antin JH, Cutler CS, Ritz J: Immune reconstitution after double umbilical cord blood stem cell transplantation: comparison with unrelated peripheral blood stem cell transplantation. Biol Blood Marrow Transplant 2011, Epub ahead of print.

17 Safdar A, Rodriguez GH, De Lima MJ, Petropoulos D, Chemaly RF, Worth LL, Shpall EJ, Rolston KV, Raad II, Chan KW, Champlin RE: Infections in 100 cord blood transplantations: spectrum of early and late posttransplant infections in adult and pediatric patients 1996–2005. Medicine (Baltimore) 2007;86: 324–333.

18 Patel AR, Turner ML, Baird K, Gea-Banacloche J, Mitchell S, Pavletic SZ, Wise B, Cowen EW: Voriconazole-induced phototoxicity masquerading as chronic graft-versus-host disease of the skin in allogeneic hematopoietic cell transplant recipients. Biol Blood Marrow Transplant 2009;15:370–376.

19 Chalandon Y, Passweg JR, Schmid C, Olavarria E, Dazzi F, Simula MP, Ljungman P, Schattenberg A, de Witte T, Lenhoff S, Jacobs P, Volin L, Iacobelli S, Finke J, Niederwieser D, Guglielmi C: Chronic Leukemia Working Party of European Group for Blood and Marrow Transplantation: Outcome of patients developing GVHD after DLI given to treat CML relapse: a study by the Chronic Leukemia Working Party of the EBMT. Bone Marrow Transplant 2010;45:558–564.

20 Orti G, Lowdell M, Fielding A, Samuel E, Pang K, Kottaridis P, Morris E, Thomson K, Peggs K, Mackinnon S, Chakraverty R: Phase I study of high-stringency CD8 depletion of donor leukocyte infusions after allogeneic hematopoietic stem cell transplantation. Transplantation 2009;88:1312–1318.

21 Brehm C, Huenecke S, Quaiser A, Esser R, Bremm M, Kloess S, Soerensen J, Kreyenberg H, Seidl C, Becker PS, Mühl H, Klingebiel T, Bader P, Passweg JR, Schwabe D, Koehl U: IL-2 stimulated but not unstimulated NK cells induce selective disappearance of peripheral blood cells: concomitant results to a phase I/II study. PLoS One 2011;6:e27351.

22 Feuchtinger T, Richard C, Joachim S, Scheible MH, Schumm M, Hamprecht K, Martin D, Jahn G, Handgretinger R, Lang P: Clinical grade generation of hexon-specific T cells for adoptive T-cell transfer as a treatment of adenovirus infection after allogeneic stem cell transplantation. J Immunother 2008; 31:199–206.

23 Porter DL, Levine BL, Kalos M, Bagg A, June CH: Chimeric antigen receptor-modified T cells in chronic lymphoid leukemia. N Engl J Med 2011;365: 725–733.

24 Boztug K, Schmidt M, Schwarzer A, Banerjee PP, Díez IA, Dewey RA, Böhm M, Nowrouzi A, Ball CR, Glimm H, Naundorf S, Kühlcke K, Blasczyk R, Kondratenko I, Maródi L, Orange JS, von Kalle C, Klein C: Stem-cell gene therapy for the Wiskott-Aldrich syndrome. N Engl J Med 2010;363:1918–1927.

PD Dr. Peter Häusermann
Department of Dermatology
University Hospital Basel
Petersgraben 4
CH–4031 Basel (Switzerland)
Tel. +41 61 328 67 87, E-Mail phaeusermann@uhbs.ch

Häusermann P, Steiger J, Passweg J (eds): Transplantation Dermatology.
Curr Probl Dermatol. Basel, Karger, 2012, vol 43, pp 171–196

Photoprotection in Transplant Recipients

Christian Surber[a] · Mark Pittelkow[c] · Stephan Lautenschlager[b]

[a]Department of Dermatology, University Hospital of Basel, Basel, [b]Outpatient Clinic of Dermatology, Triemli Hospital, Zurich, Switzerland; [c]Departments of Dermatology and Biochemistry and Molecular Biology, Mayo Clinic, Rochester, Minn., USA

Abstract

Skin cancers remain the most commonly diagnosed neoplasms among organ transplant recipients (OTRs), comprising nearly 40% of all posttransplant malignancies. The occurrence of skin tumors has a considerable impact on the quality of life and the overall survival of OTRs. Ultraviolet radiation (UVR) is the major environmental cause of nonmelanoma skin cancers, and it is therefore pivotal to protect the skin from UVR in order to prevent de novo and progression of preinvasive and invasive malignancies. The present chapter delivers background information on UVR, photoprotection and accompanying concerns regarding vitamin D, as well as educational and behavioral aspects of photoprotection in OTRs; some common misconceptions and mistakes regarding photoprotection are addressed as well.

Skin cancers remain the most commonly diagnosed neoplasms among organ transplant recipients (OTRs), comprising nearly 40% of all posttransplant malignancies [1]. The occurrence of skin tumors has a considerable impact on the quality of life and the overall survival of OTRs [2]. In addition to the increased incidence of these tumors in the OTR population, the tumors tend to behave more aggressively than those in nontransplants. Most of the cutaneous malignancies diagnosed in OTRs are nonmelanoma skin cancers (NMSC), with squamous cell carcinomas (SCC) and basal cell carcinomas (BCC) accounting for more than 90% of the total (table 1) [3].

The reported average time to develop NMSC is estimated to range from 3 to 10 years after organ transplantation [2, 8–12]. Male gender, older age at transplantation, and longer follow-up after transplantation are independently associated with the onset of NMSC [10]. Other predictors of NMSC after organ transplantation are skin phototypes I–III according to the Fitzpatrick scale, an excessive sun exposure history, 'aggressive' immunosuppressive medication and genetic factors [8, 13, 14].

Cumulative ultraviolet radiation (UVR) is the primary responsible carcinogen for the induction and promotion of NMSC, as suggested by the fact that

Table 1. Population-based standardized incidence ratios of skin cancers in OTRs [4–7].

Skin cancer	Increase in incidence (×)
SCC	>65–220
BCC	>10–16
Melanoma	>2.2–8
Kaposi sarcoma	>84

Table 2. Risk factors for the development of skin cancer after organ transplantation

Skin cancer
Exposure to UVR
Fitzpatrick skin types I–III
Increased age at transplantation
Duration, degree, and type of immunosuppression
Type of organ transplant
Previous organ transplant
Personal history of actinic keratosis
HPV infection

UVR is presumably the only factor that is to a certain degree 'avoidable'. Sun avoidance and sun protection measures, including sunscreen application, are usually the cornerstones of dermatological education programs designed for OTRs (see the section 'Educational and Behavioral Aspects in Skin Cancer Prevention').

the lesions almost exclusively appear on UV-exposed skin [15]. Hence, patients working in typical outdoor occupations or spending most of their leisure time outdoors and patients living in countries with high UV indices are at higher risk. The determinants of skin cancer development in OTRs are well defined (table 2).

The significance of UVR is further emphasized by the observation that after the first SCC, the rate of subsequent NMSC can be decreased if patients change their behavior and protect themselves from the sun [16]. Unfortunately, several studies highlighted the poor compliance among OTRs with advice of sun protection measures [17, 18]. In addition, a high number of OTRs are no longer integrated into a daily occupational routine after transplantation. Recreational sun exposure – either in their home environment or during prolonged vacations – gains predominant importance for OTRs. This is supported by previous findings that OTRs who participated in outdoor recreation were more likely to subsequently develop NMSC

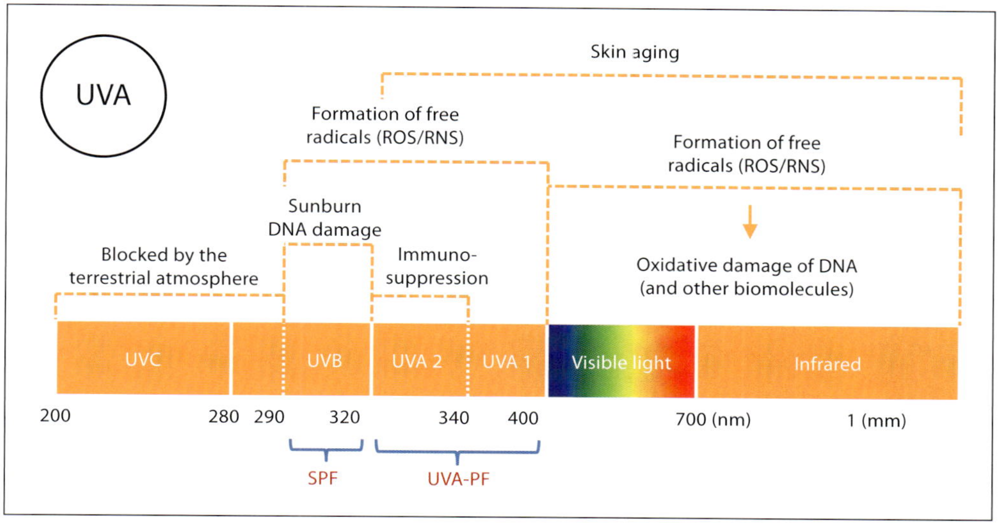

Fig. 1. UVR refers to solar radiation with wavelengths in the 200 to 400 nm range. Radiation in the 400 to 700 nm range is referred to as visible light. UVR is subdivided into UVC, UVB and UVA radiation. Penetration of UVR into skin is wavelength dependent and hence leads to different biological effects (e.g. sunburn, DNA damage, immune suppression, formation of free radicals, oxidative damage of DNA and other biomolecules). SPF is largely a measure of UVB protection. In Europe, a sufficient UVA protection of a sunscreen product is labeled with a dedicated UVA label as depicted above.

[17, 19]. UVR is presumably the only factor that is to a certain degree 'avoidable'. Sun avoidance and sun protection measures, including sunscreen application, are usually the cornerstones of dermatological education programs designed for OTRs.

In this chapter, background information on (A) UVR, (B) photoprotection and accompanying concerns regarding vitamin D, as well as educational and behavioral aspects of photoprotection in OTRs will be delivered – some common misconceptions and mistakes regarding photoprotection are addressed as well.

Ultraviolet Radiation

Physics of Ultraviolet Radiation

The electromagnetic spectrum covers a wavelength band of radiation ranging from 10^{-14} m (gamma radiation) to 10^4 m (radio waves). UVR refers to solar radiation with wavelengths in the 200 to 400 nm range. Radiation in the 400 to 700 nm range is referred to as visible light. UVR is subdivided into UVC, UVB and UVA radiation (fig. 1). Penetration of UVR into skin is wavelength dependent and hence leads to different biological effects [20–22]. The UVC band (200–290 nm) is known as the germicidal band and is primarily absorbed by the ozone layer (NB: industrial workers may experience UVC exposure, e.g. welding, UV drying of paint or finish). The UVB band (290–320 nm) – reaching the epidermis – is known as the erythemal band and is significantly attenuated by the atmosphere. UVA (320–400 nm) – reaching the basal layer of the epidermis and the upper dermis – is known as black light. It is further subdivided into UVA-1 (340–400 nm) and UVA-2 (320–340 nm). The shorter wavelengths of UVA-2 are more erythemogenic than UVA-1. Although UVA is more prevalent at the earth's surface, it is less effective than UVB in eliciting erythema in human skin [23].

Biological Effects of Ultraviolet Radiation

UVR exerts a number of important biological effects on the skin, influencing the immune system and vitamin D metabolism, as well as causing DNA damage, photoaging, skin cancer, and pigmentary changes through biologically complex mechanisms [24]. In addition, there are psychological effects, with many people reporting enhanced well-being after sun exposure, and social influences, with 20th and 21st century fashion dictating that in some cultures a suntan is attractive and a sign of increased socioeconomic status [25].

Since the 1890s, even before the discovery of DNA and the concept of genetic mutations, sunlight exposure was implicated in the etiology of skin cancer [26, 27]. Over time, significant scientific evidence has been collected and has linked UVR with skin cancer formation [28].

The exact mechanism of UVR-induced cutaneous carcinogenesis is multifactorial and has not been totally elucidated. It is a complex interplay between gene mutation, inflammation, and immunosuppression. Erythema is the clinically visible immediate effect on the skin from UVR. Evidence suggests that clinical erythema correlates with DNA damage. Wavelengths of UVR that are most efficient at producing erythema are also the most efficient at producing pyrimidine dimers [29, 30]. However, some of the deleterious effects of UVR occur before the erythema threshold is reached. Such suberythemal effects of UVR include inflammation, photoaging, diminished antigen responsiveness and depletion of epidermal Langerhans cells [31]. The tumor suppressor, p53 protein, is also induced, which is a strong indication that DNA damage is occurring during suberythematous ultraviolet (UV) exposures [32]. Although much of the literature documents the effects of UVB on skin, many studies in recent years have highlighted the role UVA radiation plays in inducing damage to the skin by causing immunosuppression, DNA mutations, lipid and protein oxidative damage, and photoaging [33].

All these effects and their strong association with cutaneous malignancies have led to the official recognition of UVR as an environmental carcinogen [34, 35]!

Ultraviolet Radiation and Immunosuppression

In general, exposure to UVR can cause suppression of specific immune responses. The pathways leading to the downregulation are complex, starting from the absorption of UV photons by chromophores in the skin and ending with local and systemic changes in immune mediators, the generation of T and B regulatory cells and inhibition of effector and memory T cell activation. The consequences for human health are thought to be both beneficial (e.g. T cell-mediated autoimmune diseases, asthma) and harmful (e.g. skin cancer, cutaneous lupus erythematosus, and infectious diseases) [36–38].

In immunosuppressed patients such as OTRs, the importance of the immune system in controlling the development of sun-induced cutaneous malignancies is readily apparent from the particularly high incidence of skin cancer arising almost entirely on sun-exposed areas of the body. The etiology of skin cancer in OTRs is multifactorial and includes host factors such as skin type, and environmental factors such as sun exposure and immunosuppression. The latter contributes to carcinogenesis through a number of mechanisms. Obviously, immunosuppressants prevent allograft rejection by suppressing host immune recognition of allograft antigens, but they also cause global dysfunction of cellular and humoral immunity, leading to reduced immune surveillance. This may result in uncontrolled proliferation, dysplasia and cancer. In addition, the immunocompromised host is vulnerable to a series of infections with virus-associated cancers, e.g. anogenital cancers (mucosal human papillomaviruses, HPV) or NMSC (genus β-HPV). Some older immunosuppressants (e.g. ciclosporin, azathioprine) have direct or indirect carcinogenic effects. Newer immunosuppressants (e.g. everolimus, sirolimus) seem to induce fewer NMSC, and some show antineoplastic properties [39].

Photoprotection

Environmental Photoprotection

Ozone, present in the stratosphere – 10–50 km above the surface of the earth – absorbs high quantities of shortwave UVB and UVC, but only a little UVA radiation. The ozone concentration varies naturally according to temperature, weather, latitude, and altitude. The atmosphere is thinner at higher altitudes, resulting in an increase in the intensity of UVR by 4% for every 300 m of elevation. The average increase in UVB intensity per degree of latitude is about 3% [40, 23]. The time of day also affects the intensity of UVR. At the solar zenith, the sun's rays pass through less of the atmosphere than they do at any other time point; thus, the atmosphere absorbs substantially less UVR. It is noteworthy that there are considerable deviations between true solar time and standard time [41], e.g. the shift between standard time and true solar

Table 3. Factors that influence UV protection of clothing

Factors that increase protection	Factors that offer lower levels of protection
Tightly woven textiles	Loosely woven textiles
Thicker fabrics	Thinner fabrics
Denim, wool, synthetic materials	Cotton, linen
Dry materials	Wet materials
Dark-color fabrics	Light-color fabrics

Hints for patients and consumers that certain textiles are less suitable for UVR protection are highly recommended [summarized in 46].

time adds up to about 2 h 40 min at the Spanish coast of the Atlantic Ocean, i.e. noon is not at 12:00 but rather at 2:40 p.m. (14:40 h CEST).

Photoprotective Clothing

It is generally recognized that textiles are a reliable means of photoprotection [42]. Nowadays, all sun protection programs urge the use of clothing in combination with hats and sunscreens for UVR protection. The protective quality is highly dependent on the property of the textiles (table 3) [43, 44]. Standardization of the protective properties has been advocated by various authorities [45].

Topical Photoprotection

Bewildering arrays of sunscreen products in various forms that make wide ranges of product claims – including non-sunscreen claims – are on the market. Like an umbrella shields people from the unwanted effects of rain, sunscreen products evenly spread over the skin should shield people from the unwanted effects of UVR ('photon rain'). All sunscreen products consist of UV absorbers and a carrier system (vehicle) into which they are incorporated [46, 47].

UV Absorber

UV absorber molecules are commonly used to reduce the penetration of solar UVR into the skin. They reduce the damaging radiation by absorption, scattering or reflection (directed scattering). UV absorbers have been available since 1928 and today play a predominant role in photoprotection and skin cancer prevention [48, 49]. They have become a quasi-exclusive mode of protection, even though seeking shade and wearing protective clothing provides more protection. Research and industry initially focused on improving the magnitude of photoprotection by increasing the sun protection factor (SPF) – defined as the minimal erythema dose (MED) of protected skin divided by the MED of unprotected skin. SPF is a measure for the reduction of the erythemal band (290–320 nm) of the UVR (≥UVB) that is responsible for the most obvious effect – sunburn. Hence, SPF is largely a measure of UVB protection. The importance of adequate UVA protection (320–400 nm) became apparent with improved understanding of UVA-induced damage to the skin causing immunosuppression, DNA mutations, lipid and protein oxidative damage, and photoaging via oxygen radical species as UVA energy interacts with endogenous photosensitizers. The recent understanding has led to the need for higher UVA protection and the development of new UV absorbers [50] and formulations. Regulatory bodies around the world have implemented guidelines and regulations on testing and labeling sunscreens for UVB and UVA protection [51–54].

About 55 UV absorbers are approved for use in sunscreen products globally. However, significant differences exist regarding regional and national approvals and the permitted maximal concentration of these absorbers in the formulations. There are less than 20 absorbers currently approved in the US, compared with approximately 30 in Australia and the EU. Only 10 UV absorbers are uniformly approved worldwide. This gap may arise from the different regulatory status of the absorbers and the products (OTC drugs vs. cosmetic products), necessitating a more or less rigorous and extensive approval process.

Typically, topical UV absorbers are classified into two categories: inorganic (formerly designated physical) agents and organic (formerly designated chemical). However, other categorizations exist (see text below).

Inorganic Agents

Inorganic agents act by scattering or reflecting (directed scattering) visible, UV, and infrared radiation over a broad spectrum (depending on the surface coating/quality, inorganic sunscreens may also absorb radiation). Today, the major inorganic agents are zinc oxide and titanium dioxide. Their protective qualities are slightly different. Zinc oxide offers better UVA protection, whereas titanium dioxide provides better UVB protection [55]. Because of aesthetic concerns, inorganic agents were unpopular until recently, when micronized forms were introduced. The micronized forms (10–50 nm) decrease visible light scattering and therefore improve cosmetic acceptability compared with their nonmicronized, whitish forms. Because of their lack of penetration [56] and their photostability, inorganic agents have been recommended for children and sunscreen-allergic individuals [57]. Inorganic, opaque sunscreens have also been recommended to protect against visible light-induced photosensitivity diseases [58]. Despite some recently raised concerns about safety, there is no evidence for absorption of physical sunscreens [59].

Organic Agents

Organic agents act by absorbing UV and thereby activating the agent's electrons from a passive to an excited state. When returning to the stable state condition, energy is emitted as insignificant quantities of heat and fluorescent radiation. The agents can be broadly divided into UVB, UVA, or broadband absorbers. Apart from being nontoxic and not causing irritation or contact allergy, the absorbers should be photochemically stable in sunlight. The exposure of UV-absorbing agents to sunlight may lead to photochemical reactions that can compromise both the physical attributes of the UV absorbers (color, appearance, etc.) and their chemical properties leading to undesirable reactions and by-products [60]. If a sensitive absorber is important for the performance of a product and cannot be replaced by a more stable filter, this can be overcome by adding a specific absorber to protect the sensitive one. UVB absorbers have been commonly used worldwide for many decades. Only in the past decade have UVA and broadband absorbers been developed and introduced. Since an absorber should protect against the entire UVR spectrum, different filters generally have to be combined in the same product. The increasing need for broadband agents and improved photostability has led to the introduction of a new generation of absorbers [61], including methylene bisbenzotriazolyl tetramethylbutylphenol (Tinosorb M) and bis-ethylhexyloxyphenol methoxyphenol triazine (Tinosorb S), both manufactured by BASF (Ludwigshafen, Germany), as well as terephthalylidene dicamphor sulfonic acid (Mexoryl SX) and drometrizol trisiloxane (Mexoryl XL), produced by L'Oréal (Clichy, France).

UV Absorber and Vehicle Type

While the labeled product UV efficacy (see below) is certainly important, perhaps more important is the true UV protection that people will achieve when they use the product in real life. Therefore, the ideal sunscreen is a product that people will use regularly and properly. Although this sounds trivial, in reality, achieving a uniform and adequate coating of the skin is quite a challenge, because the topography of the skin is very uneven. A first key principle for either formulating or choosing highly effective sunscreen products is providing a uniform film of sunscreen filters on the skin surface. The second – even more important – key principle is customer/patient compliance. Compliance encompasses (a) how regularly the product is used (frequency), (b) how much product is applied at each use (dose) and (c) how completely UV-exposed skin is covered with product (area covered). To achieve compliance, the product has to be formulated in a cosmetically elegant form to please the customer/patient. The following challenges have to be addressed [47].

Selecting UV Absorbers. Selecting UV absorbers to incorporate into a vehicle have a great impact on all major performance parameters of the final product – photoprotective quality (magnitude and wavelength range), applicability, spreadability and durability on the skin, compatibility with the skin and finally the sensory feel/aspect of the skin. The magnitude and breadth of UV attenuation vary widely between the different absorbers (see above). Higher concentrations of UV absorber generally increase the magnitude of UVR attenuation – total UV absorber concentration may range from 5 to more than 30%, correlating with the increase in the labeled SPF. Thus, to formulate a sunscreen product that provides both a high SPF and protection against a broad spectrum of UVR (UVA in addition to UVB) always requires the use of a combination of UV absorbers, in high concentrations, to achieve the necessary magnitude and breadth of UV attenuation. The UV absorbers can be categorized by their physicochemical characteristics into four groups – polar oils, oil-soluble crystalline solids, water-soluble salts and insoluble particulates. All possess significant handicaps regarding subsequent skin feel (greasy), skin appearance (opaque, whitish) and formulation characteristics (sticky). UVA filters tend to change the color (yellow) of light fabric treated with optical color brightener. In addition, UV absorbers are in general the most expensive materials in a sunscreen product, accounting for most of the total cost of the formula. The newer UV absorbers that are all well characterized and optimized in many respects are the most expensive ones. Hence low-priced sunscreen products rarely contain modern UV absorbers.

Selecting/Formulating the Vehicle. The vehicle of a product is always the sum of many different ingredients that – when mixed together and packed – result in a specific product form such as lotion, cream, gel, stick, spray or wipe. The physicochemical characteristics of the ingredients determine the practicable product form that can be created and the choice of UV filters that can be incorporated into it. The key concept of formulating is based on the material polarities. In its simplest sense, ingredients and UV absorbers can be grouped based on how polar they are, with very nonpolar or hydrophobic/lipophilic ingredients like mineral oil and silicones at one end of the scale and very polar or hydrophilic/lipophobic ingredients such as water, glycerin, and glycols at the other end of the scale. All of the ingredients used in sunscreen formulations can be placed on this scale, with ingredients with similar polarity generally being mutually soluble, and ingredients with very different polarity generally not being miscible with each other. The same concept applies to the UV absorbers – polar or hydrophilic absorbers will dissolve in polar or hydrophilic ingredients and nonpolar or lipophilic absorbers will dissolve in nonpolar or lipophilic ingredients. Materials with large differences in polarity will be immiscible. In addition, ingredients or specific combinations thereof determine the viscosity of the product. With this background, the broad range of sunscreen product forms can be described by the combination of their polarity and the viscosity. Thus, products can be categorized by whether they are (a) water based, (b) oil based, (c) ethanol/oil based, or (d) emulsions that contain both water and oil phases (fig. 2). Emulsion type vehicles include ingredients spanning a large range of polarity, and can therefore take up different UV absorbers with a similar range of polarity. This allows maximum flexibility to select the most efficient UV absorber combination, thus providing optimal photoprotection quality (magnitude and wavelength range), applicability, spreadability and durability on the skin, compatibility with the skin and skin feel. Thus, emulsion type sunscreen

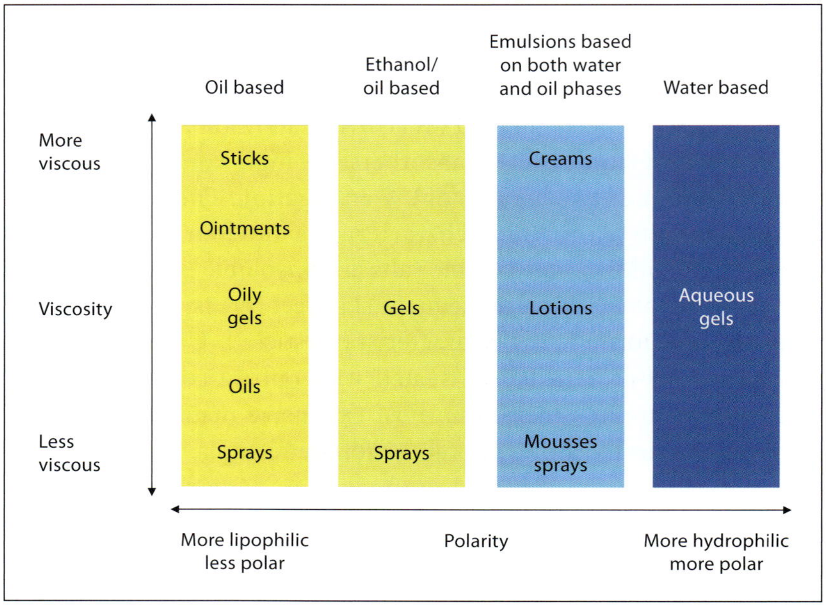

Fig. 2. Formulation types by overall formula polarity and product viscosity [47]. More polar formulas tend to offer weaker water resistance. For OTRs using sunscreens on a daily basis, the formulations should be more polar (hydrophilic = >'light' feeling) to increase a pleasant sensory feeling and hence to improve compliance. The nonpolar lipstick supplements the protection range for lips.

products (lotions, creams) have become the most common formulation forms on the market.

Product and Skin Feel. UV absorbers comprise a very large portion of a sunscreen product formulation. The largest single component of most marketed sunscreen products is a volatile carrier material – typically water. Thus, when a layer of a sunscreen product is applied to the skin, most of the product evaporates (metamorphosis of the vehicle) [62], leaving behind a layer of nonvolatile material consisting of UV absorber and vehicle components. As the product SPF is increased, the UV absorber concentration is also increased (up to 30%) leaving behind even more nonvolatile material. Even if significant work is done to try to mitigate the greasy, draggy, or sticky effects of specific UV absorbers, the skin will always be left with some 'coating' feeling.

Controversy and Everyday Error in Photoprotection

Controversy surrounding sunscreen efficacy and safety has stimulated a lively debate on their use and properties. Some misconceptions and mistakes regarding photoprotection are complicating the discussion.

Efficacy of Sunscreen Products

In terms of acute ultraviolet damage and squamous cell cancer, including actinic keratoses (AKs), studies have shown a direct protective effect of sunscreen use in human beings [63–67]. A systematic review by Dennis et al. [68] that examined 18 heterogeneous case-control studies failed to show any association between melanoma and sunscreen use. Different factors must be taken into account to explain the current lack of proof of preventive effects. First, the median SPF of commonly used sunscreens before the early 1990s was 4–10, and these sunscreens incorporated UV absorbers that were limited largely to the UVB waveband [48, 69]. Only by 1997 had the median SPF risen to about 15. Second, higher protection has been expected to induce longer sun exposure by delaying warning signs such as sunburn, or by providing a false impression of safety in the sun. In this regard, two randomized trials in students during their vacations have shown that application of a high SPF prompted them to increase the duration of their sun exposure [70, 71]. A prospective study by Thieden et al. [72] has shown that people use sunscreen when they know they are going to stay out for a long time and thus apply sunscreen as a tanning aid to avoid sunburn [73, 74]. Third, failure to apply sunscreen properly must be emphasized: sunscreens are frequently not applied before exposure [75] or soon after the onset of exposure [76]. Additionally, the SPF of a sunscreen is assessed after phototesting in vivo at an internationally agreed application amount of 2 mg/cm^2 [51, 53]. Several studies have shown that consumers apply much less than this, achieving only 20–50% of the protection expected from the product label [77, 78]. The uniformity of sunscreen application, failure to apply to all exposed skin, resistance to water immersion and the number of applications per day are known to influence protection [79]. Considering these factors, Diffey [80] concludes that it is not surprising that case-control studies have failed to find any association between the use of sunscreens and the risk of melanoma, especially given the limited effects of older sunscreens in modifying solar ultraviolet exposure (SPF >20, no UVA protection). Therefore, to expect that newer formulations of sunscreens will lead to a benefit as a protective agent against melanoma is reasonable [81], although such a benefit might not be seen for several decades [80]. However, their use in practice could be difficult, time consuming, and expensive, and they can, in general, be used only in addition to the more reliable measures of protective clothing and reduction of ultraviolet exposure during peak hours of solar radiation.

Safety of Sunscreen Products

Since OTRs are advised to protect themselves daily with sunscreens, questions regarding long-term safety have been raised.

Adverse Reactions to UVR Filters

Adverse reactions from UVR filters – including allergic and irritant contact dermatitis, phototoxic and photoallergic reactions and contact urticaria – have been reported [67, 82–84]. Most of these adverse reactions were due to irritant rather than allergic reactions to either the UVR filters, to the ingredients forming the formulations or to the combination thereof. The prevalence of these adverse reactions to UVR filters in the general population is not known [85, 86]. Despite the large increase in the use of UVR filters over the past decades, the development of photoconditional reactions remains rare. Furthermore, most of the common UVR filter photoallergens, including PABA, amyl dimethyl PABA, and benzophenone-10, are now rarely used in modern sunscreen products [85]. Benzophenone-3 (UVA filter) – still often used – is the most common contact photoallergen [82, 85]. Other UVA filters such as avobenzone (Parsol 1789) and sulisobenzone (benzo phenone-4) and the UVB filters such as methylbenzylidene camphor, octyl methoxycinnamate, and ensulizole, are known to induce contact allergic and photoallergic reactions only rarely. In the general population, there is no evidence that allergic reactions represent a common clinical problem. There is no documented information on adverse reactions to UVR filters in OTRs.

Vitamin D Deficiency and Photoprotection

Ninety percent of all requisite vitamin D is formed within the skin through the action of UVR [87]. Furthermore, several studies have suggested an association between vitamin D deficiency and several forms of cancer (e.g. colon, breast, prostate) including malignant melanoma [88–90]. Based on clinical experiments, the suppression of cutaneous vitamin D synthesis by sunscreens has been postulated [91, 92]. However, in larger clinical trials, the long-term use of sunscreens had little or no effect on vitamin D synthesis, and did not induce osteoporosis or secondary hyperparathyroidism [93, 94]. Conscientiously staying indoors and wearing protective clothing explicitly compromised the vitamin D synthesis [95].

The rigorous sun avoidance programs consisting of (a) seeking shade/staying indoors, (b) wearing protective clothes and (c) using sunscreens that are messaged to OTRs may cause a vitamin D deficiency [96, 97]. In addition, the skin of elderly people is less efficient in producing vitamin D in response to UVR [98]. It is therefore of importance to monitor the vitamin D status of OTRs and to supplement vitamin D if necessary. To estimate the vitamin D status, the serum 25(OH)-D_3 concentration is determined. The optimal concentration is >75 nM or >30 ng/ml. Values <30 nM or <12 ng/ml are considered as highly insufficient. Vitamin D supplementation is straightforward and cost-efficient. Despite the fact that the correct usage of sunscreens theoretically reduces vitamin D levels, in practice there is no evidence of this [99].

Absorption and Endocrine Effects of UVR Filters

Depending upon the physiochemical characteristics, any topically applied xenobiotic has the potential to be absorbed through the skin. Solubility, hydro-/lipophilicity, molecular weight of the xenobiotic and vehicle system carrying the xenobiotic determines the potential for absorption. Hence, it is obvious that UV filters may have the potential to be absorbed [100, 101]. However, these safety issues are addressed in national and international regulations. Once sufficient safety information is available, regulatory bodies approve the UV filters and their concentrations for concomitant use. More recently, a series of molecules have been designed with high molecular weights (over 500 Da) [102] to diminish their permeation through skin [50]. Nonetheless, there are concerns about the endocrine effect of UV filters, and the conclusion was reached that daily exposure to sunscreen formulations might have estrogenic effects in human beings [103, 104]. Questions have been raised about the methodological grounds used. In the animal experiments, topical exposure to UV filters was judged to be unrealistically high compared with potential human exposure scenarios. Wang et al. [101] indicate that the number of years of daily application required to obtain the equivalent levels of oxybenzone the experimental animals were exposed to are essentially unattainable, varying – depending on the scenario applied – between 35 and 277 years of daily application. The biological relevance of the estrogenic effect of UV filters has not yet been fully established, and additional long-term studies are required [105]. Clinically relevant disturbances of hormonal homeostasis have not been observed in humans.

Sun Protection Factor

SPF stands for sun protection factor. The SPF rating of sunscreens indicates the level of protection against UVR. The SPF rating is calculated by comparing the amount of time needed to produce sunburn on protected skin with the amount of time needed to cause sunburn on unprotected skin – the higher the SPF, the greater the sun protection. The SPF numbers on a product may range from as low as 2 to over 100. These numbers refer to the product's ability to attenuate the sun's 'burning rays' which basically derive from UVB radiation.

In this context, one often encounters two misconceptions.

The SPF of 2 absorbs 50%, SPF 15 93.3%, SPF 30 96.7% and SPF 50+ 98.3% of UVB radiation. Very many misunderstand this accurate statement, concluding that higher SPF numbers attenuate only a tiny percentage more and therefore do not offer substantial extra protection. As depicted in figure 3, relevant for the characterization of UVB protection is not the UV dose (%) filtered out by the sunscreen but rather the UV dose that reaches the skin and is part of the sunburn dose. Hence, the UV dose that is reaching the skin is halved between SPF 15 and 30 and again between SPF 30 and 50+. This means that the protection doubles between SPF 15 and 30 and between 30 and 50+. Nonetheless, the augmentation of the protection is limited. Products labeled with SPF higher than 50+ require large amounts of UV absorbers, often making spreadability more difficult, reducing the sensory attractiveness of the product, and tempting the consumer or patient to use less product. However, in real life situations one may conclude that in the SPF range 15–50+ the higher SPF delivers significant extra protection!

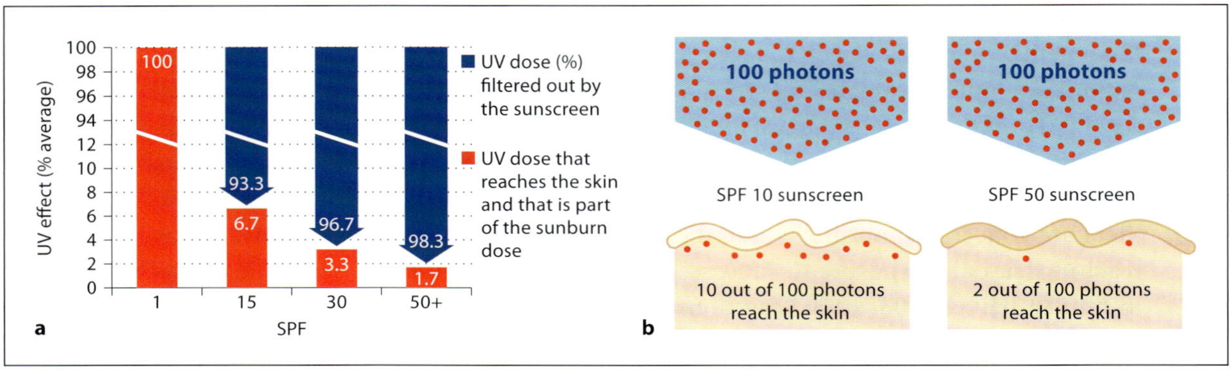

Fig. 3. a, b Relevant for the characterization of UVB protection is not the UV dose (%) filtered out by the sunscreen but the UV dose that penetrates the skin and is part of the sunburn dose. Hence, the UV dose that is reaching the skin is halved between SPF 15 and 30 and again between SPF 30 and 50+. This means that the protection doubles between SPF 15 and 30 and between 30 and 50+ (see also http://www.youtube.com/watch?v = 8cc8qRr7oMQ).

In theory, the SPF may serve as a factor to calculate the increased protection time by simply multiplying the SPF by the length of time it takes the consumer/patient to suffer a burn without sunscreen. This time is skin type dependent (e.g. skin type I approx. 10 min). A range of computer and smartphone applications offers the option to calculate the personal protection time. However, there are a number of caveats with this approach. The layperson is often unable to determine the own skin type, the 2 mg/cm^2 dose upon which the labeled SPF is based on is not applied by most consumers/patients, a significant amount of the applied sunscreen is lost during many recreational activities, and the labeled SPF refers to the midday sun. Hence, the calculation is studded by a number of uncertainties and is therefore unsuitable for everyday situations because it may impart a false sense of security among consumers and patients.

Water Resistance

According to regulatory agencies [106, 107], sunscreen products tested with two 20-min immersion periods (i.e. 40 min total) are allowed to include the 'water resistant' statement and sunscreen products tested with four 20-min immersion periods (i.e. 80 min total) are allowed to include the 'very water resistant' statement. In the US, the terms 'waterproof' or 'sweat proof' are no longer permitted on sunscreen labels, as the regulators see these claims as misleading. Despite the fact that the determination of the water resistance is highly standardized and the sunscreen industry has made some efforts to optimize for water resistance [108], its relevance may be debatable. In most real life situations, consumers or patients towel themselves after bathing or wipe sweat from their skin after perspiration. This will remove most of the sunscreen product from the skin and will necessitate reapplication. Prolonged protection with a water resistant or very water resistant sunscreen product during the stay in the water is likely; however, the time in the water remains shorter than the time outside the water – deviations may apply for isolated activities. Hence, the value of this quality remains limited. Unfortunately, the label is popular with consumer organizations comparing different products by their water resistance. The relevance is probably overvalued and may impart a false sense of security among consumers.

According to the new FDA sunscreen requirements, which come into effect in 2012, water resistance claims have to be accompanied by the recommendations to reapply after swimming or sweating, immediately after towel drying, and at least every 2 h.

Lifetime Ultraviolet Dose

Since 1986, it has been thought that people get 80% of their lifetime ultraviolet (UV) dose before they reach the age of 18 years. This is a misconception [109]. It is based on mathematical calculations, which assume that young adults receive a UV dose three times higher than older adults and that the incidence of skin cancer increases in relation to the square of the UV dose [110]. Based on these assumptions, the same authors calculated that using sunscreen of SPF 15 or higher during the first 18 years of life would give a 78% reduction in the incidence or development of NMSC. These findings were subsequently misconstrued and taken to mean that individuals would have been exposed to 80% of their lifetime UV dose by the time they reached 18 years. It was thus assumed that the incidence of NMSC correlates linearly with UV exposure. It is important to realize that this misconception spread around the world and can still be found today on various internet sites. A communication from Godar et al. [111] presented new calculations which show that the previous assumptions are wrong. The authors calculated the UV dose to which Americans are exposed throughout their lifetimes, based on the time spent in the open air. From these data, they calculated the cumulative, seasonal, annual and lifetime UV doses in the northern and southern US and found that Americans get only 23% of their lifetime UV dose before the age of 18. The UV exposure rises to 46% of the lifetime dose by the age of 40 and to about 74% by the age of 59. This means that the UV dose is roughly equal over the years with about 25% exposure in each of the following periods: the first 18 years of life, ages 19–40, ages 41–59, and finally ages 60–78. These findings are probably valid worldwide, as others have reported similar UV exposure patterns [112, 113]. The findings have significant consequences for sun protection measures. Until recently, the corresponding educational campaigns always emphasized that the use of sunscreen, sunglasses, UV-protective clothing, hats and parasols was particularly important for children and young people. As a result, adults may have concluded that sun protection measures were less important for them, as most of the UV damage to their skin had

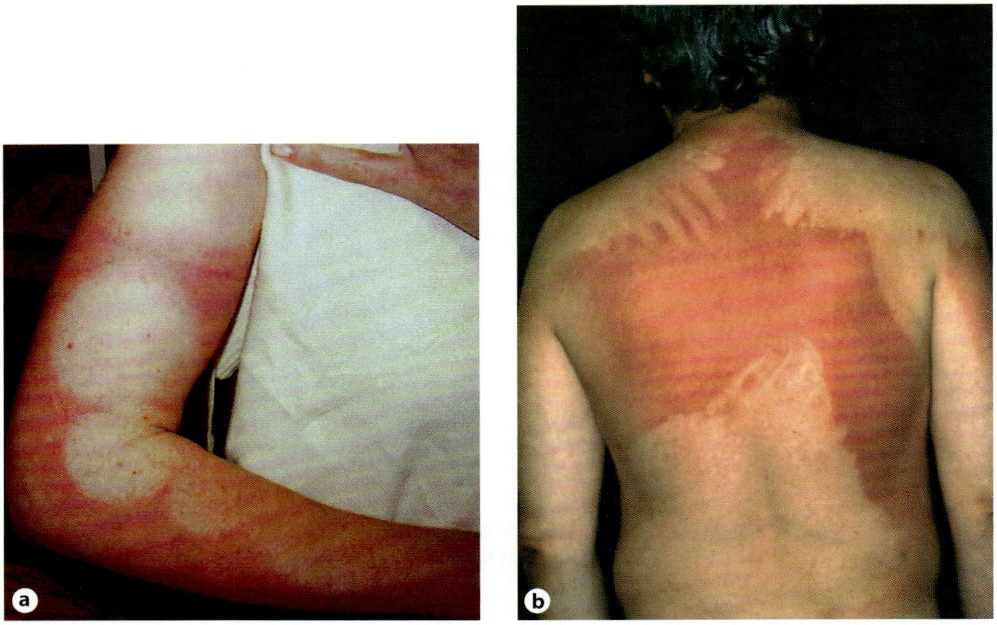

Fig. 4. Application of vehicle. **a** Sun-protected skin within the diameter of the spray's mist with surrounding sunburn. The popular light and sprayable formulations are often inadequately spread over the skin. **b** Self-application of sun protection product is often incomplete. Complete protection requires the help of a third party.

already been done by the time they were 19 years old. The calculations presented by Godar et al. [111], however, provide evidence that continued sun protection is essential. It is quite possible that inadequate sun protection in the middle-aged and elderly causes progression of UV-induced damage sustained in childhood and adolescence to more serious lesions. To reduce the risk of skin cancer more effectively, future campaigns must make the need for lifelong UV protection absolutely clear.

Summary

In summary, the efficacy of sunscreens in reducing the damaging effects of UVR is widely and thoroughly documented. UVA- and UVB-attenuating products protect against sunburn as well as more subtle suberythemal skin damage. While some concerns over the long-term safety of UV filters have been raised, the benefits of sunscreens clearly outweigh their potential risks. However, the principal barrier to attaining these benefits is patient/consumer compliance. Failure to prevent sun-related skin damage is usually due to the way sun-protective measures are observed and the way sunscreen products are applied rather than the technical inadequacy of the product (fig. 4). Taking advantage of improved technologies and product efficacy definitely requires patient education and public health measures encouraging sunscreen use.

Prevention of Skin Cancer in Organ Transplant Recipients

Possible preventive strategies include: (A) primary prevention of de novo preinvasive and invasive malignancies; (B) prevention of progression of premalignant lesions to invasive tumors, and (C) prevention of second primary tumors.

Primary Prevention of de novo Preinvasive and Invasive Malignancies

As outlined above, UVR is the principal carcinogen responsible for most skin cancers. Expert consensus guidelines all recommend strict UV photoprotection after transplant to reduce skin cancer risk [9, 114]. Advice usually includes avoidance of sunburn, intentional tanning and unnecessary UVR exposure. Sunscreens with broad-spectrum, high-factor UVB and UVA protection are recommended, together with the use of protective clothing including broad-brimmed hats and sunglasses. But does sunscreen use after transplantation translate into a reduction in skin (pre-) malignancy? In the general population, there is convincing evidence that sunscreens reduce AK and SCC [63, 64, 115]. New findings from a follow-up [81] of a community-based trial [116] of sunscreen use to prevent skin cancer provide reassurance in view of the widespread uncertainty about sunscreen's ability to prevent melanoma [117–119]. Recently, a randomized clinical trial of liposomal sunscreen use in OTR showed significant reduction in AK and SCC – but not BCC – after 24 months [120] (fig. 5).

Strict photoprotection measures would therefore appear justified in OTRs at high risk of developing SCC. Studies have shown that information regarding such photoprotective measures is best delivered in a specialist clinic setting [121] and compliance is improved by intensive educational reinforcement [122, 123] – see also the section 'Educational and Behavioral Aspects in Skin Cancer Prevention' below.

Prevention of Progression of Premalignant Lesions to Invasive Tumors

It is assumed that AK and Bowen's disease are precursors of SCC. The rate of progression from an individual AK to SCC is controversial, ranging from 0.25 to 20% per year/per lesion in the general population [124]. A recent prospective study showed that the risk of progression for a specific AK was relatively low, but that 65% of all primary SCC arose directly in AK [125]. The remaining SCC are presumed to arise from

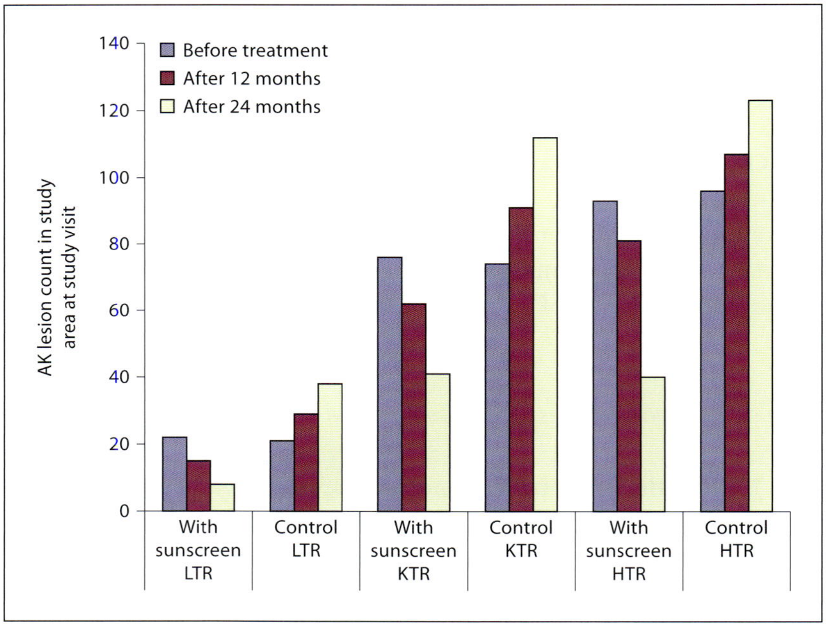

Fig. 5. Actinic keratosis (AK) lesion counts before, and 12 and 24 months after treatment. LTR = Liver transplant recipient; KTR = kidney transplant recipient; HTR = heart transplant recipient. In the sunscreen groups, the lesion counts decreased, whereas lesion counts increased in the control groups.

subclinical AK, providing a rationale for treating the whole 'field' and not just individual lesions. Cryotherapy and surgery are used as 'lesion-directed' treatments of individual AK/Bowen's lesions. Photodynamic therapy (PDT) using topical aminolevulinic or methyl aminolevulinic acid creams is an alternative nonsurgical option for treating individual AKs or larger fields of thin, nonhyperkeratotic AK. Only recently has an easily manageable aminolevulinic acid patch been launched to treat individual lesions using the PDT approach [126]. Larger areas of multiple and confluent (pre-) malignancies are more amenable to field-directed therapies such as 5-fluorouracil, imiquimod, and diclofenac semisolid formulations [127].

Prevention of Second Primary Tumors

Over 60% of OTRs will develop more than one skin malignancy and, after a first keratinocyte skin cancer, 75% will have a second within 5 years [6, 16]. The time interval between subsequent keratinocyte skin cancers shortens progressively. Current preventive strategies include alteration of immunosuppressive drug regimens [128] and systemic retinoids [129, 130].

Future Prospects for Prevention of Skin Cancer in Organ Transplant Recipients

Future prospects for prevention include a number of approaches [131]. Topical approaches include: (A) T4 endonuclease V, an enzyme involved in the repair of DNA damage after exposure to UVR [132, 133], (B) α-difluoromethylornithine, an irreversible inhibitor of ornithine decarboxylase [134, 135], (C) resiquimod, a more potent toll-like receptor 7/8 agonist than imiquimod [136], (D) ingenol mebutate, an extract from *Euphorbia peplus* [137, 138], and (E) betulinic acid, a pentacyclic triterpene from the outer bark of the birch [139]. Systemic approaches include: (A) capecitabine, a prodrug of 5-fluorouracil [140], and (B) afamelanotide, a chemical analogue of the α-melanocyte-stimulating hormone [141].

Educational and Behavioral Aspects in Skin Cancer Prevention

Because the most important element of skin cancer prevention in OTR is minimization of exposure to UVR, education regarding sun protection and avoidance is the cornerstone of any effective prevention program. However, numerous studies have shown both knowledge of the importance of photoprotection and compliance with photoprotective measures to be consistently inadequate among OTRs [17, 142–145]. Before the advent of multidisciplinary transplant clinics, Seukeran et al. [18] proposed that these deficiencies might be attributable, at least in part, to insufficient input by dermatologists in the process of preventive education. It is thus incumbent on the dermatologist to provide rigorous, repeated, and persuasive instruction to patients regarding the necessity of photoprotection and the most efficacious means thereof. Several studies have shown that the multidisciplinary approach is particularly well suited to the accomplishment of this goal. Ismail et al. [121] reported that, among patients attending their specialist OTR dermatology clinic, 98% recalled receiving photoprotection advice, and 95% reported regular sunscreen use, compared with 77 and 67%, respectively, of patients who did not attend. Clowers-Webb et al. [122] described significantly more compliant sun-protective behavior among OTRs in a multidisciplinary setting who received intensive versus standard preventive education. Ulrich et al. [120] found that, regardless of general photoprotection education, provision of free sunscreen and specific training regarding its correct application resulted in significantly more photoprotection compliance (measured as sunscreen use 5.6 days/week, compared with 0.3 days/week in the control group), with a concomitant decline in NMSC incidence. The dermatologist in the multidisciplinary setting should frequently and repeatedly encourage all OTRs to apply sunscreen (of sufficient SPF) every day, not just when sun exposure is expected, and advise avoidance of sun exposure between 10:00 a.m. and 4:00 p.m., abstention from exposure to artificial sources of UVR (tanning beds), and dressing in sun-protective clothes including long-sleeved shirts, long pants, and broad-brimmed hats (table 4).

Table 4. Recommended sun protection practices for OTRs.

Action
Use daily broad-spectrum (UVA and UVB protection) sunscreen with SPF >30
Apply sunscreen daily as part of the morning hygiene routine, and then reapply as needed throughout the day
Apply product 15–30 min before actual sun exposure
Apply '2 coats' to cover all exposed areas adequately (a total of approximately 30 ml of sunscreen is required to cover exposed areas of the body completely)
Include areas often overlooked such as back of neck, ears, and lips
In the periorbital area, use waxy stick sunscreen that will not melt or run when exposed to sweat
Reapply sunscreen every 2–3 h or after getting wet or excessive perspiration
Remember that after towel drying (water/sweat) sunscreen mechanically removed from the skin has to be reapplied
Use sunscreen even on cloudy days
Wear a wide-brimmed hat
Wear UV-blocking sunglasses
Wear protective clothing that has tight weave
Minimize activity at peak sun exposure between 10 a.m. and 4 p.m. and seek shade
Avoid any exposure to artificial sources of UVR (tanning beds)

Conclusions

It is indisputable that UVR exposure is both directly and indirectly linked to skin cancer. NMSC is the most frequent cancer diagnosis in fair-skinned populations, and the incidence is increasing worldwide. OTRs experience high rates of NMSC due to their immunosuppressive treatment, and the relative risk is dramatically higher than in the immunocompetent population. UVR is the major environmental cause of NMSC, and it is pivotal to protect the skin from UVR in order to prevent the development of NMSC.

Bewildering arrays of sunscreen products in various forms that make wide ranges of product claims are on the market. Like umbrellas shield people from the unwanted effects of rain, sunscreen products evenly spread over the skin shield people from the unwanted effects of UVR (photon rain). The efficacy of sunscreens in reducing the damaging effects of UVR is thoroughly documented. UVA- and UVB-attenuating products protect against sunburn as well as more subtle suberythemal skin damage. While some concerns over the long-term safety of UV filters have been raised, the benefits of sunscreens clearly outweigh their potential risks.

The principal obstacle to attaining these benefits is patient compliance. Failure to prevent sun-related skin damage is usually due to the way sun protective measures are observed and the way sunscreen products are applied rather than technical inadequacy of the products. In numerous studies, it has been shown that both knowledge of the importance of photoprotection and compliance with photoprotective measures are consistently inadequate among OTRs. In real life, it has been shown that frequent and repeated education and encouragement of OTRs to apply sunscreen every day, to avoid direct UVR exposure and to dress in sun-protective clothes is a successful means to prevent de novo and progression of preinvasive and invasive malignancies. Multidisciplinary settings are most likely to offer environments that facilitate medical care, supervision, frequent and repeated education, and encouragement of OTRs to comply with the all sun protection measures.

References

1 Penn I: Post-transplant malignancy: the role of immunosuppression. Drug Saf 2000;23:101–113.

2 Euvrard S, Kanitakis J, Claudy A: Skin cancers after organ transplantation. Engl J Med 2003;348:1681–1691

3 Tessari G, Naldi L, Boschiero L, Nacchia F, Fior F, Forni A, Rugiu C, Faggian G, Sassi F, Gotti E, Fiocchi R, Talamini G, Girolomon G: Incidence and clinical predictors of a subsequent non-melanoma skin cancer in solid organ transplant recipients with a first non-melanoma skin cancer: a multicenter cohort study. Arch Dermatol 2010;146:294–299

4 Jensen P, Hansen S, Møller B, Leivestad T, Pfeffer P, Geiran O, Fauchald P, Simonsen S: Skin cancer in kidney and heart transplant recipients and different long-term immunosuppressive therapy regimens. J Am Acad Dermatol 1999;40:177–186.

5 Hartevelt MM, Bavinck JN, Kootte AM, Vermeer BJ, Vandenbroucke JP: Incidence of skin cancer after renal transplantation in The Netherlands. Transplant 1990;49:506–509.

6 Wisgerhof HC, Edelbroek JR, de Fijter JW, Haasnoot GW, Claas FH, Willemze R, Bavinck JN: Subsequent squamous- and basal-cell carcinomas in kidney-transplant recipients after the first skin cancer: cumulative incidence and risk factors. Transplantation 2010 27;89:1231–1238.

7 Brewer JD, Colegio OR, Phillips PK, Roenigk RK, Jacobs MA, Van de Beek D, Dierkhising RA, Kremers WK, McGregor CG, Otley CC: Incidence of and risk factors for skin cancer after heart transplant. Arch Dermatol 2009;145:1391–1396.

8 Bouwes Bavinck JN, Euvrard S, Naldi L, Ingo Nindl I, Proby CM, Neale R, Abeni D, Tessari GP, Feltkamp MCW, Claudy A, Stockfleth E, Harwood CA: Keratotic skin lesions and other risk factors are associated with skin cancer in organ-transplant recipients: a case-control study in the Netherlands, United Kingdom, Germany, France, and Italy. J Invest Dermatol 2007;27:1647–1656

9 Ulrich C, Kanitakis J, Stockfleth E, Euvrard S: Skin cancer in organ transplant recipients: where do we stand today? Am J Transplant 2008;8:2192–2198.

10 Naldi L, Fortina AB, Lovati S, Barba A, Gotti E, Tessari G, Schena D, Diociaiuti A, Nanni G, La Parola IL, Masini C, Piaserico S, Peserico A, Cainelli T, Remuzzi G: Risk of nonmelanoma skin cancer in Italian organ transplant recipients. A registry-based study. Transplantation 2000;70:1479–1484.

11 Bouwes Bavinck JN, Hardie DR, Green A, Cutmore S, MacNaught A, O'Sullivan B, Siskind V, Van Der Woude FJ, Hardie IR: The risk of skin cancer in renal transplant recipients in Queensland, Australia. A follow-up study. Transplantation 1996;61:715–721.

12 Wong G, Chapman JR: Cancers after renal transplantation. Transplant Rev (Orlando) 2008;22:141–149.

13 Villeneuve PJ, Schaubel DE, Fenton SS, Shepherd FA, Jiang Y, Mao Y: Cancer incidence among Canadian kidney transplant recipients. Am J Transplant 2007;7:941–948.

14 Fortina AB, Caforio AL, Piaserico S, Alaibac M, Tona F, Feltrin G, Livi U, Peserico A: Skin cancer in heart transplant recipients: frequency and risk factor analysis. J Heart Lung Transplant 2000;19:249–255.

15 Armstrong BK, Kricker A: The epidemiology of UV induced skin cancer. J Photochem Photobiol 2001; 63:8–18.

16 Euvrard S, Kanitakis J, Decullier E, Butnaru AC, Lefrancois N, Boissonnat P, Sebbag L, Garnier JL, Pouteil-Noble C, Cahen R, Morelon E, Touraine JL, Claudy A, Chapuis F: Subsequent skin cancers in kidney and heart transplant recipients after the first squamous cell carcinoma. Transplantation 2006;81: 1093–1100.

17 Moloney FJ, Almarzouqi E, O'Kelly P, Conlon P, Murphy GM: Sunscreen use before and after transplantation and assessment of risk factors associated with skin cancer development in renal transplant recipients. Arch Dermatol 2005;141:978–984.
18 Seukeran DC, Newstead CG, Cunliffe WJ: The compliance of renal transplant recipients with advice about sun protection measures. Brit J Dermatol 1998;138:301–303.
19 Urwin HR, Jones PW, Harden PN, Ramsay HM, Hawley CM, Nicol DL, Fryer AA: Predicting risk of nonmelanoma skin cancer and premalignant skin lesions in renal transplant recipients. Transplantation 2009;87:1667–1671.
20 Everett MA, Yeargers E, Sayre RM, Olson RL: Penetration of epidermis by ultraviolet rays. Photochem Photobiol 1966;5:533–542.
21 Bruls, WAG, Slaper H, van der Leun JC, Berrens L: Transmission of human epidermis and stratum corneum as a function of thickness in the ultraviolet and visible wavelengths. Photochem Photobiol 1984;40:485–494.
22 Meinhardt M, Krebs R, Anders A, Heinrich U, Tronnier H: Absorption spectra of human skin in vivo in the ultraviolet wavelength range measured by optoacoustics. Photochem and Photobiol 2009; 85:70–77.
23 Matts PJ: Solar ultraviolet radiation: definitions and terminology. Dermatol Clin 2006;24:1–8.
24 Seité S, Fourtanier A, Moyal D, Young AR: Photodamage to human skin by suberythemal exposure to solar ultraviolet radiation can be attenuated by sunscreens: a review. Br J Dermatol 2010; 163:903–914.
25 Matts PJ, Fink B: Chronic sun damage and the perception of age, health and attractiveness. Photochem Photobiol Sci. 2010;9:421–431.
26 Urbach F: The historical aspects of photocarcinogenesis. Front Biosci 2002;7:e85–e90.
27 Jackson R, Finkelstein H: Historical aspects of nonmelanoma skin cancer. Clin Dermatol 1995;13: 517–525.
28 Narayanan DL, Saladi RN, Fox JL: Ultraviolet radiation and skin cancer. Int J Dermatol 2010;49:978–986.
29 Hacham H, Freeman SE, Gange RW: Do pyrimidine dimer yields correlate with erythema induction in human skin irradiated in situ with ultraviolet light (275–365 nm)? Photochem Photobiol 1991;53: 559–563.
30 Pfeifer GP, Besaratinia A: UV wavelength-dependent DNA damage and human non-melanoma and melanoma skin cancer. Photochem Photobiol Sci 2011;11:90–97.
31 Cooper K, Oberhelman L, Hamilton T: UV exposure reduces immunization rates and promotes tolerance to epicutaneous antigens in humans: relationship to dose, CD1a-DR+ epidermal macrophages induction, and Langerhans cell depletion. Proc Natl Acad Sci USA 1992;89:8497–8501.
32 Healy E, Reynolds NJ, Smith MD: Dissociation of erythema and p53 protein and mRNA following application of skin irritants. J Invest Dermatol 1994;103:493–499.
33 Marrot L, Meunier JR: Skin DNA photodamage and its biological consequences. J Am Acad Dermatol 2008;58(5 Suppl 2):S139–S148.
34 http://monographs.iarc.fr/ENG/Classification/index.php
35 El Ghissassi F, Baan R, Straif K, Grosse Y, Secretan B, Bouvard V, Benbrahim-Tallaa L, Guha N, Freeman C, Galichet L, Cogliano V: WHO International Agency for Research on Cancer Monograph Working Group: A review of human carcinogens – part D: radiation. Lancet Oncol 2009; 10:751–752.
36 Schwarz T, Schwarz A: Molecular mechanisms of ultraviolet radiation-induced immunosuppression. Eur J Cell Biol 2011;90:560–564.
37 Norval M, Halliday GM: The consequences of UV-induced immunosuppression for human health. Photochem Photobiol 2011;87:965–977.
38 Lucas RM, McMichael AJ, Armstrong BK, Smith WT: Estimating the global disease burden due to ultraviolet radiation exposure. Int J Epidemiol 2008; 37:654–667.
39 Gallagher MP, Kelly PJ, Jardine M, Perkovic V, Cass A, Craig JC, Eris J, Webster AC: Long-term cancer risk of immunosuppressive regimens after kidney transplantation. J Am Soc Nephrol 2010;21:852–858.
40 Rigel DS, Rigel EG, Riegel AC: Effects of altitude and latitude on ambient UVB radiation. J Am Acad Dermatol 1999;40:114–116.
41 Stick C: Solar time – the importance of standard time for the UV-exposure of the skin. JDDG 2007;5: 788–792.
42 Hatch KL, Osterwalder U: Garments as ultraviolet radiation screening materials. Dermatol Clin 2006; 24:85–100.
43 Ghazi S, Couteau C, Coiffard LJ: What level of protection can be obtained using sun protective clothing? Determination effectiveness suing an in vitro method. Int J Pharm 2010;397:144–146.
44 Gambichler T, Hatch KL, Avermaete A, Bader A, Herde M, Altmeyer P, Hoffmann K: Ultraviolet protection factor of fabrics: comparison of laboratory and field-based measurements. Photodermatol Photoimmunol Photomed 2002;18:135–140.

45 Gambichler T, Laperre J, Hoffmann K: The European standard for sun-protective clothing: EN 13758. J Eur Acad Dermatol Venereol 2006;20: 125–130.

46 Lautenschlager S, Wulf HC, Pittelkow MR: Photoprotection. Lancet 2007;370:528–537.

47 Tanner PR: Sunscreen product formulation. Dermatol Clin 2006:24:53–62.

48 Couteau C, Coiffard L: History of sun protection. Rev Hist Pharm (Paris) 2010;58:151–162.

49 Urbach F: The historical aspects of sunscreens. J Photochem Photobiol B 2001;64:99–104

50 Herzog B, Hueglin D, Osterwalder U: New sunscreen actives; in Saath NA, editor: Suncreens: Regulations and Commercial Development, ed 3, New York, NY, Taylor&Francis, 2005, 291–320.

51 ISO 24444:2010 Cosmetics – Sun protection test methods – In vivo determination of the sun protection factor (SPF).

52 European Commission: Recommendation on the efficacy of sunscreen products and the claims made relating thereto. Official Journal of the European Union 2007;2006/647/EC.

53 COLIPA, CTFA SA, JCIA, CTFA: International sun protection factor (SPF) test method. The European Cosmetic, Toiletry and Perfumery Association, 2006.

54 DIN 67502 February 2005. Berlin, Beuth, 2005.

55 Pinnell SR, Fairhurst D, Gillies R, Mitchnick, MA, Kollias N: Microfine zinc oxide is a superior sunscreen ingredient to microfine titanium dioxide. Dermatol Surg 2000;26:309–314.

56 Song Z, Kelf TA, Sanchez WH, Roberts, Rička J, Frenz M, Zvyagin AV: Characterization of optical properties of ZnO nanoparticles for quantitative imaging of transdermal transport. Biomed Opt Epress 2011;3:3321–3333.

57 Palm MD, O'Donoghue MN: Update on photoprotection. Dermatol Ther 2007:20;360–376.

58 Moseley H, Cameron H, MacLeod T, Clark C, Dawe R, Ferguson J: New sunscreens confer improved protection for photosensitive patients in the blue light region. Br J Dermatol 2001;145:789–794.

59 Osmond MJ, McCall MJ: Zinc oxide nanoparticles in modern sunscreens: an analysis of potential exposure and hazard. Nanotoxicology 2010;4: 15–41.

60 Shaath NA: Ultraviolet filters. Photochem Photobiol Sci 2010;9:464–469.

61 Tuchinda C, Lim HW, Osterwalder U, Rougier A: Novel emerging sunscreen technologies. Dermatol Clin 2006;24:105–117.

62 Surber C, Smith EW: The mystical effects of dermatological vehicles. Dermatology 2005;210:157–168

63 Thompson SC, Jolley D, Marks R: Reduction of solar keratosis by regular sunscreen use. N Engl J Med 1993;329:1147–1151.

64 Green A, Neale R, Battistutta D: Daily sunscreen application and betacarotene supplementation in prevention of basal-cell and squamous-cell carcinomas of the skin: a randomized controlled trial. Lancet 1999;354:2955–2529.

65 Young AR, Sheehan JM, Chadwick CA, Potten CS: Protection by ultraviolet A and B sunscreens against in situ dipyrimidine photolesions in human epidermis is comparable to protection against sunburn. J Invest Dermatol 2000;115:37–41.

66 Roberts LK, Beasley DG, Learn DB, Gidden LD, Beard J, Stanfield JW: Ultraviolet spectral energy differences affect the ability of sunscreen lotions to prevent ultra-violet induced immunosuppression. Photochem Photobiol 1996;63:874–884.

67 Naylor MF, Farmer KC: The case for sunscreens: a review of their use in preventing actinic damage and neoplasia. Arch Dermatol 1997;133:1146–1154.

68 Dennis LK, Beane Freeman LE, Van Beck MJ: Sunscreen use and the risk for melanoma: a quantitative review. Ann Intern Med 2003;139:966–978.

69 Rebut D: The sunscreen industry in Europe: Past, present and future. In Lowe N. Saath NA, eds. Sunscreens: Development, evaluation and regulatory aspects. New York: Marcel Dekker, 1990, pp 161–171.

70 Autier P, Dore JF, Negrier S: Sunscreen use and duration of sun exposure: a double-blind, randomized trial. J Natl Cancer Inst 1999;91:1304–1309.

71 Autier C: Sunscreen use and intentional exposure to ultraviolet A and B radiation: a double blind randomized trial using personal dosimeters. Br J Cancer 2000;83:1243–1248.

72 Thieden E, Philipsen PA, Sandby-Moller J, Wulf HC: Sunscreen use related to UV exposure, age, sex, and occupation based on personal dosimeter readings and sun-exposure behavior diaries. Arch Dermatol 2005;141:967–973.

73 Robinson JK: Sun exposure, sun protection, and vitamin D. JAMA 2005;294:1541–1543.

74 Dupuy A, Dunnant A, Grob JJ: Randomized controlled trial testing the impact of high-protection sunscreens on sun-exposure behavior. Arch Dermatol 2005;141:950–956.

75 Robinson JK, Rademaler AW: Sun protection by families at the beach. Arch Pediatr Adolesc Med 1998;152:466–470.

76 Diffey BL: When should sunscreen be reapplied? J Am Acad Dermatol 2001;45:882–885.

77 Wulf HC, Stender IM, Lock-Anderson J: Sunscreens used at the beach do not protect against erythema: a new definition of SPF is proposed. Photodermatol Photoimmunol Photomed 1997;13:129–132.

78 Bech-Thomsen N, Wulf HC: Sunbather's application of sunscreen is probably inadequate to obtain the sun protection factor assigned to the preparation. Photodermatol Photoimmunol Photomed 1992–1993;9:242–244.

79 Diffey BL: Sunscreens: use and misuse. In: Giacomoni PU, ed. Sun Protection in Man. Amsterdam: Elsevier, 2001, pp 521–534.

80 Diffey BL: Sunscreens and melanoma: the future looks bright. Br J Dermatol 2005;153:378–381.

81 Green AC, Williams GM, Logan V, Strutton GM: Reduced melanoma after regular sunscreen use: randomized trial follow-up. J Clin Oncol 2011;29:257–263.

82 Schauder S, Ippen H: Contact and photo contact sensitivity to sunscreens. Review of a 15 year experience and the literature. Contact Dermatitis 1997;37:221–232.

83 Lange-Asschenfeldt B, Huegel R, Brasch J: Anaphylactic reaction caused by the UVA absorber disodium phenyl dibenzimidazole tetrasulfonate. Acta Derm Venerol 2005;85:280–281.

84 Foley P, Nixon R, Marks R, Frowen K, Thompson S: The frequency of reactions to sunscreens: Results of a longitudinal population-based study on the regular use of sunscreens in Australia. Br J Dermatol 1993;128:512–518.

85 Darvay A, White IR, Rycroft RJ. Jones AB, Hawk JL, McFadden JP: Photallergic contact dermatitis is uncommon. Br J Dermatol 2001;145:597–601.

86 Wong T, Orton D: Sunscreen allergy and its investigation. Clin Dermatol 2011;29:306–310.

87 Holick MF: Vitamin D: A millennium perspective. J Cell Biochem 2003;88:187–194.

88 Grant WB, Garland CF: Evidence supporting the role of vitamin D in reducing the risk of cancer. J Intern Med 2002;252:178–179.

89 Mohr SB, Gorham ED, Alcaraz JE, Kane CJ, Macera CA, Parsons JK, Wingard DL, Garland CF: Serum 25-hydroxyvitamin D and prevention of breast cancer: pooled analysis. Anticancer Res. 2011;31: 2939–2948.

90 Loke TW, Sevfi D, Khadra M: Prostate cancer incidence in Australia correlates inversely with solar radiation. BJU Int 2011;108(Suppl 2):66–70.

91 Matsuoka LY, Wortsman J, Hanifan N, Holick MF: Chronic sunscreen use decreases circulating concentrations of 25-hydroxyvitamin D: a preliminary study. Arch Dermatol 1988;124:1802–1804.

92 Norval M, Wulf HC: Does chronic sunscreen use reduce vitamin D production to insufficient levels? Br J Dermatol 2009;161:732–736.

93 Farrerons J, Barnadas M, López-Navidad A, Renau A, Rodríguez J, Yoldi B, Alomar A: Sunscreen and risk of osteoporosis in the elderly: a two-year follow-up. Dermatology 2001;202:27–30.

94 Farrerons J, Barnadas M, Rodriguez J: Clinically prescribed sunscreen (sun protection factor 15) does not decrease serum vitamin D concentrations sufficiently either to induce changes on parathyroid function or on metabolic markers. Br J Dermatol 1998;139:422–427.

95 Cusack C, Danby C, Fallon JC, Ho WL, Murray B, Brady J, O'Kelly P, Ambrose N, Kearns G, Murphy GM: Photo protective behavior and sunscreen use: impact on vitamin D levels in cutaneous lupus erythematosus. Photodermatol Photoimmunol Photomed 2008;24:260–267.

96 Saha HH, Salmela KT, Ahonen PJ, Pietilä KO, Mörsky PJ, Mustonen JT, Lalla ML, Pasternack AI: Sequential changes in vitamin D and calcium metabolism after successful renal transplantation. Scand J Urol Nephrol 1994;28:21–27.

97 Palmer SC, McGregor DO, Strippoli GF: Interventions for preventing bone disease in kidney transplant recipients. Cochrane Database Syst Rev 2007;CD005015.

98 Holick MF, MatsuokaLy, Wortsman J: Age, vitamin D, and solar ultraviolet. Lancet 1989;ii:1104–1105.

99 Burnett ME, Wang SQ: Current sunscreen controversies: a critical review. Photodermatol Photoimmunol Photomed 2011;27:58–67.

100 Chatelain E, Gabard B, Surber C: Skin penetration and sun protection factor of five UV filters: Effect of the vehicle. Skin Pharmacol Appl Skin Physiol 2003;16:28–35.

101 Wang SQ, Burnett ME, Li HW: Safety of oxybenzone: putting numbers into perspective. Arch Dermatol 2011;147:865.

102 Bos JD, Meinardii MM: The Dalton rule for skin penetration of chemical compounds and drugs. Exp Dermatol 2000;9:165–169

103 Heneweer M, Muusse M, Berg M, Sanderson JT: Additive estrogenic effects of mixtures of frequently used UV filters on pS2-gene transcription in MCF-7 cells. Toxicol Appl Pharmacol 2005;208:170–177.

104 Schlumpf M, Cotton B, Conscience M, Haller V, Steinmann, Lichtensteiger W: In vitro and in vivo estrogenicity of UV screens. Environ Health Perspect 2001;109:239–244.

105 Witorsch RJ, Thomas JA: Personal care products and endocrine disruption: a critical review of the literature. Crit Rev Toxicol 2010;40 Suppl 3:1–30.

106 COLIPA. Guideline for evaluating sun product water resistance. The European Cosmetic, Toiletry and Perfumery Association, 2005.

107 http://www.fda.gov/ForConsumers/ConsumerUpdates/ucm258416.htm.

108 Poh Agin P: Water resistance and extended wear sunscreens. Dermatol Clin 2006;24:75–79.
109 Krutmann J: Sonnenschutz: Die Korrektur eines Irrtums. Hautarzt 2003;54:674.
110 Stern RS, Weinstein MC, Baker SG: Risk reduction for nonmelanoma skin cancer with childhood sunscreeen use. Arch Dermatol 1986;122:537–545.
111 Godar DE, Urbach F, Gasparro FP, van der Leun JC: UV doses of young adults. Photochem and Photobiol 2003;77:453–457
112 Thieden E, Philipsen PA, Sandby-Møller J, Heydenreich J, Wulf HC: Proportion of lifetime UV dose received by children, teenagers and adults based on time-stamped personal dosimetry. J Invest Dermatol 2004;123:1147–1150.
113 Diffey BL: The impact of topical photoprotectants intended for daily use on lifetime ultraviolet exposure. J Cosmet Dermatol 2011;10:245–250.
114 KDIGO clinical practice guideline for the care of kidney transplant recipients. Kidney Disease: Improving Global Outcomes. Cancer of the skin and lip. Am J Transplant 2009;9(suppl 3):S84–S85.
115 Gordon LG, Scuffham PA, van der Pols JC, McBride P, Williams GM, Green AC: Regular sunscreen use is a cost-effective approach to skin cancer prevention in subtropical settings. J Invest Dermatol 2009;129:2766–2771.
116 Green A, Williams G, Neale R, Hart V, Leslie D, Parsons P, Marks GC, Philip Gaffney P, Battistutta D, Frost C, Lang C, Russell A: Daily sunscreen application and beta carotene supplementation in prevention of basal-cell and squamous-cell carcinomas of the skin: a randomised controlled trial. Lancet 1999;354:723–729.
117 Gallagher RP: Sunscreens in melanoma and skin cancer prevention. CMAJ 2005;173:244–245.
118 Berwick M: Counterpoint: Sunscreen use is a safe and effective approach to skin cancer prevention. Cancer Epidemiol Biomarkers Prev 2007;16:1923–1924.
119 Lazovich D, Vogel RI, Berwick M, Weinstock MA, Warshaw EM, Anderson KE: Melanoma risk in relation to sue of sunscreen or other sun protection methods. Cancer Epidemiol Biomarkers Prev 2011; 20:2583–2593
120 Ulrich C, Jürgensen JS, Degen A, Hackethal M, Ulrich M, Patel MJ, J. Eberle J, Terhorst D, Sterry W, Stockfleth E: Prevention of non-melanoma skin cancer in organ transplant patients by regular use of a sunscreen: a 24 months, prospective, case-control study. Br J Derm 2009;161(Suppl. 3):78–84.
121 Ismail F, Mitchel L, Casabonne D, Gulati A, Newton R, Proby CM, Harwood CA: Specialist dermatology clinics for organ transplantrecipients significantly improve compliance with photoprotection and levels of skin cancer awareness. Br J Dermatol 2006;155: 916–925.
122 Clowers-Webb HE, Christenson LJ, Phillips PK, Roenigk RK, Nguyen TH, Weaver AL, Otley CC: Educational outcomes regarding skin cancer in organ transplant recipients: randomized intervention of intensive vs. standard education. Arch Dermatol 2006;142:712–718.
123 Tavadia S, Dawn G, Payne C: Skin cancer awareness in Scottish cardiac transplant recipients. Clin Exp Dermatol 2006;31:354–357.
124 Quaedvlieg PJ, Tirsi E, Thissen MR, Krekels GA: Actinic keratosis: how to differentiate the good from the bad? Eur J Dermatol 2006;4:335–339.
125 Criscione VD, Weinstock MA, Naylor MF: Actinic keratosis: natural history and risk of malignant transformation in the Veterans Affairs Topical Tretinoin Chemoprevention Trial. Cancer 2009;115: 2523–2530.
126 Hauschild A, Stockfleth E, Popp G, Borrosch F, Brüning H, Dominicus R, Mensing H, Reinhold U, Reich K, Moor AC, Stocker M, Ortland C, Brunnert M, Szeimies RM: Optimization of photodynamic therapy with a novel self-adhesive 5-aminolaevulinic acid patch: results of two randomized controlled phase III studies. Br J Dermatol 2009;160: 1066–1074.
127 Stockfleth E: Topical management of actinic keratosis and field cancerisation. G Ital Dermatol Venereol 2009;144:459–462.
128 Salgo R, Gossmann J, Schöfer H: Switch to a sirolimus-based immunosuppression in long-term renal transplant recipients: reduced rate of (pre-)malignancies and nonmelanoma skin cancer in a prospective, randomized clinical trial. Transplant 2010; 10:1385–1393.
129 Bouwes Bavnick JN, Tieben LM, van der Woude, FJ: Prevention of skin cancer and reduction of keratotic skin lesions during acitretin therapy in renal transplant recipients: a double-blind, placebo-controlled study. J Clin Oncol 1995;13:1933–1938.
130 Athar M, Walsh SB, Kopelovich L, Elmets CA: Pathogenesis of nonmelanoma skin cancers in organ transplant recipients. Arch Biochem Biophys. 2011; 508:159–163.
131 Amini S, Viera MH, Valins W, Berman B: Nonsurgical innovations in the treatment of nonmelanoma skin cancer. J Clin Aesthet Dermatol 2010;3:20–34.
132 www.clinicaltrials.gov; NCT00089180.

133 Yarosh D: Effect of topically applied T4 endonuclease V in liposomes on skin cancer in xeroderma pigemtosum: a radomized study. Lancet 2001;357: 926–929.

134 Camp WL, Turnham JW, Athar M, Elmets CA: New agents for prevention of ultraviolet-induced nonmelanoma skin cancer. Semin Cutan Med Surg 2011;30:6–13.

135 Bailey HH, Kim K, Verma AK, Sielaff K, Larson PO, Snow S, Lenaghan T, Viner JL, Douglas J, Dreckschmidt NE, Hamielec M, Pomplun M, Sharata HH, Puchalsky D, Berg ER, Havighurst TC, Carbone PP: A randomized, double-blind, placebo-controlled phase 3 skin cancer prevention study of alpha-difluoromethylornithine in subjects with previous history of skin cancer. Cancer Prev Res (Phila) 2010;3:35–47.

136 Szeimies RM, Bichel J, Ortonne JP, Stockfleth E, Lee J, Meng TC: A phase II dose-ranging study of topical resiquimod to treat actinic keratosis. Br J Dermatol 2008;159:205–210.

137 Siller G, Rosen R, Freeman M, Welburn P, Katsamas J, Ogbourne SM: PEP005 (ingenol mebutate) gel for the topical treatment of superficial basal cell carcinoma: results of a randomized phase IIa trial. Australas J Dermatol 2010;51:99–105.

138 Rosen RH, Gupta AK, Tyring SK: Dual mechanism of action of ingenol mebutate gel for topical treatment of actinic keratoses: rapid lesion necrosis followed by lesion-specific immune response. J Am Acad Dermatol 2011, Epub ahead of print.

139 Galgon T, Wohlrab W, Dräger B: Betulinic acid induces apoptosis in skin cancer cells and differentiation in normal human keratinocytes. Exp Dermatol 2005;14:736–743.

140 Jirakulaporn T, Endrizzi B, Lindgren B, Mathew J, Lee PK, Dudek AZ: Capecitabine for skin cancer prevention in solid organ transplant recipients. Clin Transplant 2011;25:541–548.

141 Langan EA, Nie Z, Rhodes LE: Melanotropic peptides: more than just 'Barbie drugs' and 'sun-tan jabs'? Br J Dermatol 2010;163:451–455.

142 Cowen EW, Billingsley EM: Awareness of skin cancer by kidney transplant patients. J Am Acad Dermatol 1999;40:697–701.

143 Robinson JK, Rigel DS: Sun protection attitudes and behaviors of solid-organ transplant recipients. Dermatol Surg 2004;30:610–615.

144 Donovan JCH, Rosen CF, Shaw JC: Evaluation of sun-protective practices of organ transplant recipients. Am J Transplantation 2004;4:1852–1858.

145 Mahé E, Morelon E, Fermanian J, Lechaton S, Pruvost C, Ducasse MF, Mamzer-Bruneel MF, Kreis H, Bodemer C, de Prost Y: Renal-transplant recipients and sun protection. Transplantation 2004;78: 741–744.

Prof. Dr. phil. Christian Surber
Dermatologische Universitätsklinik Basel
Universitätsspital Basel
Petersgraben 4
CH–4031 Basel (Switzerland)
Tel. +41 79 366 5050, E-Mail christian.surber@unibas.ch

Author Index

Subject Index